Assessing Well-Being

Social Indicators Research Series

Volume 39

This new series aims to provide a public forum for single treatises and collections of papers on social indicators research that are too long to be published in our journal Social Indicators Research. Like the journal, the book series deals with statistical assessments of the quality of life from a broad perspective. It welcomes the research on a wide variety of substantive areas, including health, crime, housing, education, family life, leisure activities, transportation, mobility, economics, work, religion and environmental issues. These areas of research will focus on the impact of key issues such as health on the overall quality of life and vice versa. An international review board, consisting of Ruut Veenhoven, Joachim Vogel, Ed Diener, Torbjorn Moum, Mirjam A.G. Sprangers and Wolfgang Glatzer, will ensure the high quality of the series as a whole.

For futher volumes:
http://www.springer.com/series/6548

Ed Diener
Editor

Assessing Well-Being

The Collected Works of Ed Diener

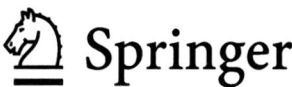 Springer

Editor
Prof. Ed Diener
University of Illinois
Dept. Psychology
603 E. Daniel St.
Champaign IL 61820
USA
ediener@uiuc.edu

ISSN 1387-6570
ISBN 978-90-481-2353-7   e-ISBN 978-90-481-2354-4
DOI 10.1007/978-90-481-2354-4
Springer Dordrecht Heidelberg London New York

Library of Congress Control Number: 2009926878

Cover design: Boekhorst Design BV

Printed on acid-free paper

Springer is part of Springer Science+Business Media (www.springer.com)

Contents

Contributors

Raksha Arora The Gallup Organization, Washington, DC 20004, USA, Raksha-Arora@gallup.com

Robert Biswas-Diener Center for Applied Positive Psychology, robert@cappeu.org

Dong-won Choi Department of Psychology, California State University, East Bay, Hayward, CA 94542, USA, dong-won.choi@csueastbay.edu

Ed Diener Department of Psychology, University of Illinois, Urbana-Champaign, Champaign, IL 61820, USA, ediener@uiuc.edu

James Harter The Gallup Organization, Washington, DC 20004, USA, Jim_Harter@gallup.com

Daniel Kahneman Princeton University, Princeton, NJ 08544-1013, USA, kahneman@princeton.edu

Chu Kim-Prieto Department of Psychology, College of New Jersey, Ewing, NJ 08628, USA, kim@tcnj.edu

Randy J. Larsen Department of Psychology, Washington University, St. Louis, Missouri 63130, USA, rlarsen@artsci.wustl.edu

Richard E. Lucas Department of Psychology, Michigan State University, East Lansing, MI 48824, USA, lucasri@msu.edu

Shigehiro Oishi Department of Psychology, University of Virginia, Charlottesville, VA 22904, soishi@virginia.edu

William Pavot Department of Psychology, Southwest Minnesota State University, Marshall, NM 56258, USA, pavot@southwestmsu.edu

Ed Sandvik

Ulrich Schimmack University of Toronto, Mississauga, Ontario, L5L 1C6, Canada, uli.schimmack@utoronto.ca

Christie Napa Scollon School of Social Sciences, Singapore Management University, Singapore 178903, cscollon@smu.edu.sg

Larry Seidlitz

William Tov Singapore Management University, Singapore 178903,
williamtov@smu.edu.sg

Derrick Wirtz East Carolina University, Greenville, NC 27858, USA,
WirtzD@ecu.edu

Endorsements

Over the past several decades Professor Diener has contributed more than any other psychologist to the rigorous research of subjective well-being. The collection of this work in this series is going to be of invaluable help to anyone interested in the study of happiness, life-satisfaction, and the emerging discipline of positive psychology

Mihaly Csikszentmihalyi, Professor of Psychology and Management, Claremont Graduate University

---

Ed Diener, the Jedi Master of the world's happiness researchers, has inspired and informed all of us who have studied and written about happiness. His life's work epitomizes a humanly significant psychological science. How wonderful to have his pioneering writings collected and preserved for future students of human well-being, and for practitioners and social policy makers who are working to promote human flourishing.

David G. Myers, Hope College, and author, *The Pursuit of Happiness*

Ed Diener's work on life satisfaction – theory and research – has been ground-breaking. Having his collected works available will be a great boon to psychologists and policy-makers alike.

Christopher Peterson, Professor of Psychology, University of Michigan

---

By looking at happiness and well-being in many different cultures and societies, from East to West, from New York City to Calcutta slums, and beyond, Ed Diener has forever transformed the field of culture in psychology. Filled with bold theoretical insights and rigorous and, yet, imaginative empirical studies, this volume will be absolutely indispensable for all social and behavioral scientists interested in transformative power of culture on human psychology.

Shinobu Kitayama, Professor and Director of the Culture and Cognition Program, University of Michigan

---

Ed Diener is one of the most productive psychologists in the world working in the field of perceived quality of life or, as he prefers, subjective well-being. He has served the profession as a researcher, writer, teacher, officer in professional organizations, editor of leading journals, a member of the editorial board of still more journals as well as a member of the board of the Social Indicators Research Book Series. As an admirer of his work and a good friend, I have learned a lot from him, from his students, his relatives and collaborators. The idea of producing a collection of his works came to me as a result of spending a great deal of time trying to keep up with his work. What a wonderful public and professional service it would be, I thought, as well as a time-saver for me, if we could get a substantial number of his works assembled in one collection. In these three volumes we have not only a fine selection of past works but a good number of new ones as well. So, it is with considerable delight that I write these lines to thank Ed and to lend my support to this important publication.

Alex C. Michalos, Ph.D., F.R.S.C., Chancellor, Director, Institute for Social Research and Evaluation; Professor Emeritus, Political Science, University of Northern British Columbia

Editor's note concerning source publications

Diener & Larsen: Temporal Stability and Cross- Situational Consistency of affective, behavioral, and cognitive responses, *Journal of Personality and Social Psychology*, 47/4 (1984), American Psychological Association

Diener: Assessing Subjective Well-Being: Progress and Opportunities, *Social Indicators Research*, 31/2 (1994), Springer SBM

Diener, Scollon, & Lucas: Evolving conceptions of subjective well-being: The multifaceted nature of happiness, (P. Costa, I.C. Siegler) *Advances in Cell Aging and Gerontology: Recent Advances in Psychology and Aging, 15*, 2004, Elsevier

Pavot & Diener: Review of the Satisfaction With Life Scale, *Psychological Assessment*, 5/2 (1993), American Psychological Association

Sandvik, Diener, & Seidlitz: Subjective well-being: the convergence and stability of self-report and non-self-report measures, *Journal of Personality*, 61/3 (1993), Wiley-Blackwell Publishing

Lucas, Diener, & Larsen: Measuring Positive Emotions, (S.J. Lopez, C.R. Snyder) *Positive Psychological Assessment: A Handbook of Models and Measures*, 2003, American Psychological Association

Scollon, Kim Prieto, & Diener: Experience Sampling: Promises and Pitfalls, Strengths and Weaknesses, *Journal of Happiness Studies*, 4/1 (2003), Springer SBM

Schimmack, Diener, & Oishi: Life-satisfaction is a momentary judgment and a stable personality characteristic: The use of chronically accessible and stable sources, *Journal of Personality*, 70/3 (2002), Wiley-Blackwell Publishing

Diener, Sandvik, & Pavot: Happiness is the frequency, not intensity, of positive versus negative affect, (F. Strack, M. Argyle, N. Schwarz) *Subjective Well-Being: An interdisciplinary perspective*, 1991, Elsevier

Introduction – Measuring Well-Being: Collected Theory and Review Works

Ed Diener

Progress on Assessing Well-Being

Measurement is the most important activity in behavioral science, and perhaps the activity that is undervalued the most. It can be argued that scientific understanding and measurement go hand in hand. Indeed, this is the insight offered by Cronbach and Meehl (1955) when they argued that the development of a measure and the understanding of the underlying phenomena go hand-in-hand. Many people, even researchers themselves, think of measurement as a technical affair to be performed by the slower and less creative scientists, while the geniuses are busy formulating grand theories. In fact, Greenwald (2001, 2002) found that the majority of Nobel prizes in the sciences go to work on measurement rather than theory. And as argued above, theory and measurement usually advance together. To be able to measure something well means that we must have a good theory about that phenomenon. In addition, what sets science apart from other approaches to knowledge, such as philosophy or theology, is the heavy grounding it has in the empirical method. Thus, observing, recording, and measuring are core aspects of science, and their importance cannot be underestimated.

Several core issues occur in the measurement of subjective well-being. One is the definition and inclusion of some phenomena and the exclusion of others. What is subjective well-being, and what are its components? When people respond to well-being self-report measures, what are the psychological processes involved? For example, how much do they call on memory versus their general self-concept? How do they weight various areas of their lives? How do various methods, such as self-report, experience sampling, and informant reports, converge with one another? Finally, how large is the problem of measurement artifacts?

E. Diener (✉)
Department of Psychology, University of Illinois, Urbana-Champaign, Champaign, IL 61820, USA; The Gallup Organization
e-mail: ediener@uiuc.edu

E. Diener (ed.), *Assessing Well-Being: The Collected Works of Ed Diener*, Social Indicators Research Series 39, DOI 10.1007/978-90-481-2354-4_1, © Springer Science+Business Media B.V. 2009

Overview of this Volume

The papers in this book begin to answer the questions above, and in some cases provide substantial answers. The chapters cover the validity and other psychometric properties of the existing scales, but they also delve deeper in order to analyze the psychological properties that influence the measures. Thus, the chapters offer initial analyses of the psychological processes that influence scores, for example processes that affect respondents' answers to surveys.

The Diener and Larsen (1984) paper established that studying people's long-term well-being is worthy of study because there is some consistency across situations and over time in people's feelings of well-being. Without such stability, it would be no use studying the well-being of persons because the major variability would be due to situational factors and error. We found that there is much stability in people's reports of life satisfaction, although some change as well, and a moderate amount of stability in people's moods and emotions. This means that the study of "happy" versus "unhappy" individuals will capture the meaningful variation in feelings of well-being, but not all of it, because some of the variation will be due to situations and the interaction of situations and persons. The Diener and Larsen paper establishes a bedrock of study in this area because it provides support for the notion that people do differ from one another in a somewhat consistent way in terms of feelings and judgments of well-being.

The review of subjective well-being measurement that I wrote for *Social Indicators Research* in 1994 became a citation classic for that journal because it described the validity of the scales and what was known about the problems of measurement artifacts. In general, the news was encouraging because the validity evidence for the scales was generally positive and because the effects of artifacts, although present, were often relatively small. At the same time, the review pointed to areas where understanding was only beginning, such as in the influence of memory on the reporting of well-being, and where much more research was needed. I also described in this article a number of non-self-report measures of well-being.

In the following chapter by Diener, Scollon, and Lucas (2004), we present an updated review of measures of well-being and our theoretical understanding of the measures. We outline what is known about the structure of well-being and its discriminant validity from other concepts. We also present a theoretical model of well-being measures in terms of a time-sequence of responses to life events, varying from immediate reactions to summary judgments of life.

The Pavot and Diener (1993) article reviewed the Satisfaction with Life Scale that we created in the 1980s and the data on the scale at the time. The Diener, Emmons, Larsen, and Griffin (1985) paper in which the SWLS was first presented has become a citation classic within psychology, with over 1,600 citations, and the Pavot and Diener paper in this volume is the most comprehensive review of the scale. In 2008, Pavot and I published another review of the scale, which includes more material on the cognitive processes involved when people respond to the items, plus a review of more recent studies using the measure. However, the 1993 article is still the most thorough in terms of reviewing findings using this widely-used measure of life satisfaction.

The Sandvik, Diener, and Seidlitz (1993) paper is another that has received widespread attention because it documented the fact that self-report well-being scales correlate with a number of other methods of measuring the same concepts, such as with reports by knowledgeable "informants" (family and friends), experience sampling measurement, and the memory for good versus bad life events. A single factor was found to underlie measures using different methods, and a number of different well-being self-report measures were found to correlate with the non-self-report measures. Thus, although the self-report measures of well-being are imperfect, and can be influenced by response artifacts, they have substantial validity as shown by their correlations with measurements based on alternative methods.

Whereas the Pavot and Diener article reviewed the Satisfaction with Life Scale, the Lucas, Diener, and Larsen (2003) paper reviews various approaches to assessing positive emotions. As we wrote in the chapter in this volume in which we present new measures, we do not consider any of the existing measures of positive affect to be entirely acceptable for measuring subjective well-being in the affect area, and that is why we have created and validated a new measure.

A major method of measuring well-being besides the typical survey method is the Experience Sampling Method (ESM), also sometimes referred to as EMA (Ecological Momentary Assessment). In the Scollon et al. (2003) article, we review how this method is performed and the benefits and shortcomings of the approach. In this method, the participants are signaled through the day, usually at random moments, and asked to record what they are doing and feeling at the moment. In most modern studies a handheld computer is used to deliver the questions and record the responses. The approach is time-consuming for participants and researchers alike, but is likely to yield a more accurate assessment of people's emotional lives. Furthermore, the discrepancies between longer-term reports of emotions and those obtained from ESM can be revealing in terms of how people's memories differ from actual experience. There are alternative methods for recording naturally-occurring moods and emotions, for example the Daily Reconstruction Method (DRM; Kahneman, Krueger, Schkade, Schwarz, & Stone 2004).

The next chapters in this volume are concerned with the theoretical underpinnings of the measures. For example, Schimmack et al. (2002) discuss the types of information that people use when they make life satisfaction judgments, and the fact that when this information changes in their lives, the judgments also move. People make life satisfaction judgments based on information that is salient and relevant to them. Because of this, certain passing influences can affect the judgments. However, certain types of information can be chronically salient, such as a person's marriage quality, and are therefore used whenever life satisfaction is computed by that individual. To the degree that these sources of information are stable for people, and they often are, life satisfaction judgments are also fairly stable. Furthermore, we found that the effects of personality on life satisfaction were mediated by the influence of personality on a person's moods and emotions.

In the article by Diener, Sandvik, and Pavot (1991), we argue that overall well-being depends more on frequently feeling positive moods than on experiencing them intensely. This prediction derived from several ideas. First, we thought that frequency and duration of moods and emotions can be measured more accurately across people than intensity, which is harder to calibrate. Second, we argued that intense positive moods could have certain downsides, which was later supported in a study by Diener, Colvin, Pavot, and Allman (1991). For example, people who feel very intense positive moods might also have a propensity when they do feel negative, to feel intensely so. In the Diener, Sandvik, and Pavot article we found that broad measures of happiness, such as the Fordyce (1988) scale, were better predicted by the frequency of positive versus negative feelings than by their intensity. Furthermore, non-self-report measures of people's happiness, such as informant reports, are much better predicted by the frequency of a person's positive moods than by the intensity of their positive moods. This indicates that frequency/duration and intensity ought to be separately assessed in measuring subjective well-being. Although our findings require more extensive exploration and confirmation by other researchers, the findings offer possible insights into the true nature of "happiness." Thus, measurement does more than simply help us scale some phenomenon; it helps us understand the meaning of the phenomenon. Over time, understanding and measurement sophistication advance together.

The Diener, Kahneman et al. article is about income and well-being. It is presented in this volume rather than in Volume 37 with other articles about the effects of money because it so strongly makes the point that various measures of well-being reflect different phenomena and are associated with different predictors. In this case, we show that Cantril's Ladder, which is a broad judgment a respondent makes of his or her life in reference to the best and worst possible life that can be imagined, is compared to measures of affect—how a person felt yesterday. We show that the judgment is highly correlated with income, but that affect is much less associated with money. In contrast, feelings of autonomy or self-direction in everyday life are much more associated with positive emotions than with the global judgment of life. The results are interesting in themselves, but also make clear that we must include different types of measures when we assess subjective well-being.

Finally, in the Diener et al. article, we present a new set of measures for the first time. In this chapter, we offer several new scales of well-being and give psychometric evidence to support the reliability and validity of them. We present a new measure for assessing positive and negative feelings, a scale for calibrating psychological well-being, and also a measure of positive thinking. We also include our older Satisfaction with Life Scale and show how the new scales correlate with each other and with earlier scales designed to assess similar characteristics. Our hope is that these new scales will prove valuable to researchers.

For ages people have debated the true nature of happiness. Some maintain that it is virtue, others that it is meaning, and yet others that it is pleasure. However, these descriptions are philosophical and prescriptive whereas scientists focus on describing and understanding phenomena, not proclaiming which one is "truly" happiness. What scientists hope to do is determine how various forms of well-being relate to one another, and what their courses and consequences are. Although lay verbal definitions are often a starting point for exploration, measurement and other scientific explanations eventually help redefine phenomena and their interrelationships. In the realm of well-being, we are coming to that point where we no longer need to debate the nature of "true happiness," but instead can define types of well-being by their measurement, courses, and outcomes.

In conclusion, the articles in this volume represent our advance in understanding the components of well-being and their interrelationships, as well as the validation of the measures that has occurred in the last 25 years. We now have a much clearer idea of the types of artifacts that can influence the measures, although more work on this topic is needed. We have a much clearer idea of how various types of measures of well-being differ from one another and the psychological processes that influence the different measures. Importantly, we have alternatives to the self-report measures when these are called for. In the concluding chapter in this volume, I outline the research on well-being measures that is needed now.

References

Cronbach, L. J., & Meehl., P. E. (1955). Construct validity in psychological tests. *Psychological Bulletin, 52*, 281–302.

Diener, E. (1994). Assessing subjective well-being: Progress and opportunities. *Social Indicators Research, 31*, 103–157.

Diener, E., Colvin, C. R., Pavot, W. G., & Allman, A. (1991). The psychic costs of intense positive affect. *Journal of Personality & Social Psychology, 61*, 492–503.

Diener, E., Emmons, R. A., Larsen, R. J., & Griffin, S. (1985). The satisfaction with life scale. *Journal of Personality Assessment, 49*, 71–75.

Diener, E., & Larsen, R. J. (1984). Temporal stability and cross-situational consistency of affective, behavioral, and cognitive responses. *Journal of Personality and Social Psychology, 47*, 871–883.

Diener, E., Sandvik, E., & Pavot, W. (1991). Happiness is the frequency, not the intensity, of positive versus negative affect. In F. Strack, M. Argyle, & N. Schwarz (Eds.), *Subjective well-being: An interdisciplinary perspective*. New York: Pergamon.

Diener, E., Scollon, C. N., & Lucas, R. E. (2004). The evolving concept of subjective well-being: The multifaceted nature of happiness. In P. T. Costa & I. C. Siegler (Eds.), *Advances in cell aging and gerontology*, Vol. 15. Amsterdam: Elsevier.

Fordyce, M. (1988). A review of research on happiness measures: A sixty second index of happiness and mental health. *Social Indicators Research, 20*, 355–381.

Greenwald, A. G. (2001, October). *Nothing so practical as a good method*. Invited address at meeting of the Person Memory Interest Group, Coeur d'Alene, ID.

Greenwald, A. G. (2002, April). *Illusory competition between theories*. Paper presented at annual meeting of the Society of Experimental Psychologists, Berkeley, CA.

Kahneman, D., Krueger, A. B., Schkade, D. A., Schwarz, N., & Stone, A. (2004). A survey method for characterizing daily life experience: The day reconstruction method. *Science, 306*, 1776–1780.

Lucas, R. E., Diener, E., & Larsen, R. J. (2003). Measuring positive emotions. In S. J. Lopez & C. R. Snyder (Eds.), *Positive psychological assessment: A handbook of models and measures*. Washington, DC: American Psychological Association.

Pavot, W., & Diener, E. (1993). Review of the Satisfaction with Life Scale. *Psychological Assessment, 5*, 164–172.

Sandvik, E., Diener, E., & Seidlitz, L. (1993). Subjective well-being: The convergence and stability of self-report and non-self-report measures. *Journal of Personality, 61*, 317–342.

Schimmack, U., Diener, E., & Oishi, S. (2002). Life-satisfaction is a momentary judgment and a
    stable personality characteristic: The use of chronically accessible and stable sources. *Journal
    of Personality, 70,* 345–384.
Scollon, C. N., Kim-Prieto, C., & Diener, E. (2003). Experience sampling: Promises and pitfalls,
    strengths and weaknesses. *Journal of Happiness Studies: An Interdisciplinary Periodical on
    Subjective Well-Being, 4,* 5–34.

Temporal Stability and Cross-Situational Consistency of Affective, Behavioral, and Cognitive Responses

Ed Diener and Randy J. Larsen

Abstract Consistency and stability of feelings were examined in reports that were completed on 3,512 occasions randomly sampled from the lives of 42 subjects. The stability and consistency of responses depended on the situations, individuals, and responses involved. High degrees of consistency were unusual for single responses, although mean levels of responding tended to be both highly stable and consistent. The consistency and stability of variables covaried, suggesting a connection between the two. Persons who were more consistent across one pair of situations tended to be more consistent across other situational pairs. The results indicate that the question of whether personality consistency exists does not have a simple answer, and requires knowledge of the persons, situations, responses, and level of analysis involved.

When Mischel (1968) raised the issue of whether behavior is cross-situationally consistent and stable for persons over time, a controversy that has continued for over a decade was initiated within the field of personality. As Underwood and Moore wrote in 1981, "The issue of consistency is one of the most controversial and most fundamental issues for the future of personality psychology...." (p. 784). One major response to Mischel's critique has been the idea that personality theories do not require cross-situational consistency of behavior (e.g. Alker, 1972). Some personologists maintain that it is enough if behavior shows intrapsychic consistency. In other words, "Personality characteristics may be revealed in a variety of situations by different behaviors exemplifying the same trait" (Alker, 1972, p. 8). Another response to Mischel's thesis is that only some people are consistent on a particular trait (e.g., Bem & Allen, 1974). Yet a third response to Mischel, one that can be quite compatible with his social learning approach, is that personality should be studied idiographically. The idiographic approach suggests that each person may show a stable pattern of behavior across situations, but that he or she cannot be compared with others because the responses that covary will be unique to each individual. Finally, conceptualization of personality in terms of person by situation interactions

E. Diener (✉)
Department of Psychology, University of Illinois, Champaign, IL 61820, USA
e-mail: ediener@uiuc.edu

E. Diener (ed.), *Assessing Well-Being: The Collected Works of Ed Diener*,
Social Indicators Research Series 39, DOI 10.1007/978-90-481-2354-4_2,
© Springer Science+Business Media B.V. 2009

7

(Ekehammar, 1974) is yet another response to Mischel. Interactional approaches, like situational ones, rest on the assumptions of a person's inconsistency of responses across situations (Endler & Magnusson, 1976). However, they are compatible with some theories of personality, such as Murray's (1938), that stress the interplay between personal and situational forces. Note that each of these defenses against Mischel's critique of personality rests on the admission that a person's responses are not cross-situationally consistent. It is our contention that knowledge about response consistency across a variety of samples, responses, and natural settings is necessary before this debate can be resolved in an intelligent manner. Not all approaches to personality require the degree of consistency that a strong trait view might imply. However, we believe that consistency data ought to be gathered across a variety of responses and situations before a firm commitment to one of the approaches is made.

Why are the questions of consistency and stability of responding so important? The bedrock of the traditional idea of personality is that although individuals differ from one another, they show coherence in their behavior across time or place. Without such coherence there would be little point in a field that focuses on individuals. Instead, personologists would be better off studying momentary decisional processes, situational effects, and so forth, without reference to any ongoing stability in persons. However, even if one takes a coherence, interactional, or idiographic approach to personality, some patterned stability of individuals must be defended. In personological formulations, the person should at least be stable over time and across situations that are very similar.

One reason that the empirical base is not sufficient to completely answer questions about response consistency is that the answer is not likely to be simple. First, consistency and stability probably differ for different response domains. Even Mischel (1968) admitted that consistency probably occurs in the area of cognitive abilities and styles. Also, consistency can be conceptualized and measured in different ways. As already suggested, person consistency can occur either across situations ("consistency") or over time ("stability"). These two are related in that there is always some time difference when people are tested across situations and there is always some difference in the situations when people are tested over time.

Both consistency and stability can be considered either as correlations between single occasions or as the relation of responses between two situations or two periods of time based on the average of a number of occasions in each situation or time period. Responses on single occasions may not be particularly consistent because of a myriad of factors that may influence them. However, personal consistency may appear when responses are aggregated over several observations in a situation, and highly stable patterns may thus emerge. Jaccard (1974) showed that much higher predictability is gained when one is interested in such aggregates. Similarly, Epstein (1979) demonstrated across a number of response domains that reliability climbs as one aggregates more occasions over time. When one aggregates an individual's responses over occasions, there is a tacit admission that single responses are likely to be inconsistent. One is able to better predict a person's average responses over a number of occasions because the effect of moods, situations, and other factors is lessened or removed from what is being predicted.

In other words, when data are aggregated for individuals, other factors that influence single responses will tend to be controlled because they will be averaged out over occasions.

Stability of responding over both short and long time periods has been found in a number of studies (e.g., Block, 1971; Block, Buss, Block, & Gjerde, 1981; Costa, McCrae, & Arenberg, 1980; Olweus, 1979; Schaie & Parham 1976; Schuerger, Tait, & Tavernelli, 1982). Mischel (1979) recently wrote that there appears to be substantial temporal stability in behavior, but a small amount of cross-situational consistency. Indeed, he writes that the belief in personality traits comes about because of the perception of the stability in behavior (Mischel & Peake, 1982). However, there has been insufficient research on cross-situational consistency, especially in natural settings. For example, Koretzky, Kohn, and Jeger, 1978, using independent raters, found moderate cross-situational consistencies in delinquents for apathetic ($r = 0.42$) and angry/defiant ($r = 0.52$) behaviors. On the other hand, Dudycha (1936) found only small amounts of consistency for punctuality measured across a variety of settings. The low consistency found by Dudycha was based, however, not on ratings but on measurement of single responses. Note that findings of higher cross-situational consistencies such as those based on peer ratings are usually based on data that are implicitly averaged across occasions. One reason that rater judgments may show relatively high cross-situational consistency (e.g., Koretzky et al. 1978) is that raters base their judgments on a number of occasions.

The purpose of the present study was to examine the temporal stability and cross-situational consistency of positive and negative affect, as well as several other cognitive and behavioral responses. We studied whether aggregated responses were consistent across situations and stable over time, and we also estimated the consistency and stability that would have been obtained if single responses had been used. We also compared the stability and consistency of affect to (a) more cognitive judgmental feelings (e.g., life satisfaction), (b) feelings that denote behavioral predispositions or motivational propensities (e.g., sociability), and (c) broad behavioral responses (e.g., physical activity). We also examined consistency across differing types of situations. Another purpose of the present study was to compare different individuals in terms of consistency. If some individuals are highly consistent and others are highly inconsistent, then a totally nomothetic, individual-differences approach to affect is called into question.

It is our belief that science progresses by explaining regularities that are found in the world. We need to discover what responses are recurrent under what conditions in order to resolve the person/situation debate and move to more sophisticated theories of personality that are based on firm data. We are not advocating the kind of blind empiricism that has sometimes occurred in this area. However, we do advocate building a data base for a variety of response domains in order to determine and delimit the types of person consistency that may exist. We did not ask subjects to imagine how they might feel in a variety of situations. Rather, we assessed how they reported they felt on a number of occasions when in natural situations.

There is reason to believe that response consistency may be greater in the affective domain than in overt behavioral responses. Behavior is more subject to reinforcement contingencies, which may be highly idiosyncratic for specific situations.

On the other hand, the everyday stereotype of moods is that they may also be quite variable. However, Epstein (1982) presented evidence that suggested that feelings show more temporal stability than either behavior or impulses. We examined not only positive and negative affect over time in our respondents' everyday lives, but also the consistency of affect across specific situations.

A question relevant to the topic of response consistency is also a question that has plagued interactionists: namely, how to define situations. Debates have raged over whether situations should be defined subjectively or objectively, and also about how molar or molecular the situations should be (Moos & Insel, 1974). We have selected for study situations that differ in a number of ways. Our first situational dimension was degree of interaction with other people, varying from social interaction to being alone. This dimension can be objectively defined and seems to be one of the most fundamental and important ways in which situations can be categorized. The second situational contrast we used was work versus recreation. Although this issue is somewhat more subjective, there is fairly widespread agreement in our culture about what is work and what is play. In addition, this too seems to be an important situational subdivision in that there are very different expectancies and rewards in our culture for these two situations. Last, we used the situational typology of novel versus typical as subjectively judged by the person. We thought that this more abstract dimension might be relevant to the question of consistency because a person may develop a habitual way of responding to typical but not to novel situations. As can be seen, our situations depended more on culturally shared meanings and activity and less on the physical environment per se.

In summary, the present study was aimed at collecting ecologically valid data on the feelings of individuals across time and across situations. We hoped to determine the degree of stability and consistency for (a) various feelings and responses, (b) single versus aggregated responses, (c) different types of situations, and (d) the whole sample versus certain individuals who were particularly consistent or inconsistent.

Method

Participants

The subjects were 42 University of Illinois undergraduate students, equally divided between men and women. The participants were enrolled in an independent study course on life satisfaction in which they received a grade of satisfactory or unsatisfactory. The subjects were quite heterogeneous in terms of motivation for enrolling in the course, in personality, and in their seriousness as students. There were virtually no constraints on what university students could enroll in if they were interested.

Procedures

Participants completed mood forms at two random times every day for a six-week period. Each student wore a watch with an alarm that had been preset to go off at random times during the individuals' waking hours. The random times, which were based on sampling without replacement, were generated so that every 10-min period during the waking day was covered over the six weeks. Times were also selected so that the first one in a day would come in the morning or early afternoon, with the second one occurring in the later afternoon or evening. The subject would set his or her alarm according to this list for the next alarm time on each occasion that the alarm had just sounded. Several precautions were taken so that the alarm would not be expected, thus making the measurements nonreactive. For example, the next time the alarm was to go off was several hours to many hours later, and so the subject would have forgotten about it by that time. It was the experience of most subjects that they would think about the alarm for the first day or two, but thereafter the alarm would catch them unexpectedly.

When the alarm sounded, the subject was to focus on the feelings of that instant and then complete the mood questionnaire immediately. If it was impossible to do so (e.g., during a test), the student could postpone completing the form up until one hour later. If it was still impossible to complete the form, an extra random time later in the day was to replace the missed time. Under no circumstances were the mood forms to be completed several hours or a day later because memory distortion was thought to be a potential problem. In order to ensure compliance, students had to turn in the forms every day.

Mood Form

The mood form consisted of 41 self-report scales about feelings. Twenty-three of the scales were monopolar and answered on a scale ranging from 0 (*I felt it not at all*) to 6 (*extremely much*). Mood adjectives covered both positive affect (e.g., happy, joyful, and pleased) and negative affect (e.g., unhappy, frustrated, and de pressed). Positive and negative affect are treated separately throughout this report because we and others have found that the two vary independently across persons (Bradburn, 1969; Diener & Emmons, 1985; Zevon & Tellegen, 1982). When the re sults were analyzed, four adjectives were averaged to provide positive affect (happy, joyful, pleased, and enjoyment) and five negative adjectives were averaged for negative affect (depressed, unhappy, frustrated, angry, and worried/anxious). These items were selected based on factor analytic work in other studies we have conducted. Additional scales included adjective self-ratings such as "Productive" and "Satisfied with my life." There were also a series of bipolar adjective pairs (rated on a 9-point scale) such as: "crabby–cheerful," "physically active–inactive," "feeling ill–feeling well," "unaroused–aroused," "tired/lethargic–energetic," "see world as beautiful/good–ugly/bad," "low self-esteem–high self-esteem," and "sociable–want to be alone." Subjects responded to each bipolar pair on a 9-point scale; the midpoint (5) was labeled *Does not apply* and the two extremes (1 and 9) were anchored with *Very much* Subjects were to indicate how much they were feeling one or the other of the adjectives contained in each bipolar pair when their beeper went off.

For this report, in addition to the more purely affective adjectives, self-reports were also chosen to reflect several other response domains: cognitive judgmental (e.g., life satisfaction), motivational (e.g., sociability), and behavioral (e.g., physical activity). Thus comparisons across domains could be made and the relative degree of stability and consistency could be more readily judged.

Situations

Also reported on the mood form was the current activity in which the person was engaged. Subjects indicated whether they were working, recreating, or maintaining (e.g., eating, walking to class). We focused on the work and recreation situations for this report because they were seen as most dissimilar. Although subjects might indicate that they were in more than one situation at once (e.g., eating while studying), these times were excluded from the data analyses because they led to non-independence among situations. The second situation concerned sociality (degree of interaction with others). The most social situation was being involved in verbal conversation; next were the categories semisocial and social presence; last was being alone, not in the presence of others. In our analyses we again have focused on the two most dissimilar situations, social interaction versus being alone. The third situational dimension was more subjective: the degree of novelty in the situation. Subjects rated the situation as typical or novel on a 9-point bipolar scale. For purposes of data analysis, we excluded times that were marked at the midpoint of 5, and dichotomized the scale into two categories.

Artifact Checks

In addition to the Crowne–Marlowe scale (Crowne & Marlowe, 1964) measuring social desirability, we included two measures to indicate how each subject used the number system of the scales. A response style of using high or low numbers to report one's affect could potentially inflate consistency and stability estimates. The artifact measures indicated how intense of an emotional response each subject meant when he or she responded with a 2, a 4, and so on. On one measure, subjects described in detail how they felt when they marked, say, either a 2 or a 4 on positive and on negative affect separately. These four descriptions were then rated on a -100 to 100 scale by two independent raters who showed high interrater agreement for both the positive and negative descriptions ($rs = 0.90$ and 0.92). These ratings indicated the degree to which subjects used the number scale in a conservative or liberal direction in describing their feelings. After they were averaged across the two raters, the responses (2 and 4) for positive affect were summed, as was also done for negative affect. A high score on the positive sum and negative sum indicated responding in a conservative fashion on the scale, so that the scale numbers meant more extreme affect for the subject. In another effort to detect artifactual responding, we had subjects indicate where each of their scale numbers from 0 through 6 would be on a line. The line was marked continuously with positive affect words that had been prescaled for intensity and were placed at the appropriate position on the line. This provided subjects another opportunity to indicate the intensity of feeling they meant by their number responses. Thus we could check on the possibilitythat stability and consistency might be due to response style rather than affect per se.

Results

The first analyses considered the degree to which self-report artifacts may have biased the findings. Specifically, did social desirability or idiosyncratic use of the number scales inflate the consistency found? The first answer is that the degree of consistency varied so greatly among variables, with some being quite inconsistent, that it seems unlikely that artifacts had a strong effect. The artifact measures showed substantial correlations with each other (average $r = 0.63$) and low correlations with the Crowne–Marlowe (average $r = 0.18$), suggesting that some subjects did report using the number scales in characteristic ways. The ratings between these potential artifacts and subjects' response ratings were also quite modest. The artifact checks correlated an average of $r = 0.17$ with positive affect and an average of $r = 0.04$ with negative affect. The Crowne–Marlowe correlated -0.01 with positive affect and -0.34 with negative affect.

The Crowne–Marlowe score and the three scale usage scores were partialed out of key consistency and stability correlations. The three-week stability coefficients changed from 0.79 to 0.76 for positive affect and from 0.81 to 0.77 for negative affect. The consistency correlations also changed very little. These analyses indicated that response artifacts had very little substantive influence on the results or conclusions of this article and they are not considered further. Because response bias appeared to have so little impact on the findings, we thought it inadvisable to correct the data for response style variance. In addition, it is problematical whether such "artifacts" are totally spurious or whether they represent substantive differences between individuals. We did, however, correct the findings for another potential problem, measurement unreliability.

One difficulty in estimating true consistency and stability is that the measures may contain some degree of unreliability or error. For example, subjects may make numerical errors when reporting their behavior. Consistency and stability estimates can be corrected for such unreliability. In order to estimate the reliability of our measures, we have correlated (both over all occasions and also within situations) the average of individuals' responses from odd and even days over the six-week period and these are shown in Table 1. The average number of occasions in each situation are also shown. Other things being equal, scores based on larger aggregates show higher reliabilities. These odd/even-day correlations are good estimates of the reliability of the measures because they are based on a large number of observations within the same settings during the same time period. Internal consistency

Table 1 Odd–even reliabilities for responses within situations

	Situation pairs						
Response	All	Social	Alone	Novel	Typical	Work	Recreation
Affect							
Positive	0.83	0.88	0.74	0.85	0.94	0.91	0.91
Negative	0.87	0.87	0.86	0.82	0.97	0.94	0.90
Bodily feelings							
Aroused	0.86	0.86	0.76	0.63	0.83	0.88	0.86
Energetic	0.92	0.76	0.69	0.58	0.68	0.70	0.73
Feeling well	0.80	0.86	0.82	0.77	0.95	0.89	0.82
Behavior							
Physically active	0.88	0.90	0.64	0.82	0.72	0.86	0.88
Productive	0.92	0.82	0.64	0.76	0.82	0.84	0.89
Behavioral predispositions							
Sociable	0.96	0.74	0.75	0.66	0.88	0.82	0.80
Cheerful	0.95	0.76	0.76	0.82	0.90	0.81	0.77
Cognitive/judgmental							
World beautiful	0.95	0.94	0.84	0.92	0.97	0.93	0.89
Self-esteem	0.84	0.82	0.71	0.86	0.94	0.82	0.74
Satisfied with life	0.88	0.97	0.97	0.95	0.99	0.98	0.99

Note. Average number of occasions in each situation was as follows: Social = 25, alone = 19, novel = 24, typical = 57, work = 28, recreation = 28.

reliabilities (coefficient alpha) were also computed for the affect measures because they were composed of several items (Cronbach, 1951). The coefficients were 0.89 and 0.84, based on the full sample of moments for positive and negative affect, respectively. One can see that both types of reliability are acceptably high. In this report we present results that are both uncorrected and corrected for unreliability (based on the odd–even reliability estimates). One may desire to correct for measurement unreliability in order to estimate the true-score correlation between two measures (Ghiselli, Campbell, & Zedeck, 1981). However, such corrections may cloud substantive issues. For example, when the focus of concern is on the consistency and stability of responding, the reliability of that responding is the substantive issue that is being explored. Because it is impossible to totally separate unreliability that is due to one's measures from the lack of stability in the phenomenon, we have presented both the corrected and uncorrected correlations.

Table 2 shows the correlations for individuals' responses across pairs of situations. The correlations corrected for unreliability (Lord & Novick, 1968) are also shown. One can see that some variables show much greater cross-situational consistency than others, regardless of whether corrected or uncorrected correlations are examined. For example, life satisfaction shows very high consistency across all situation pairs, whereas the feeling of sociability is invariably inconsistent. For some variables such as activity, productivity, and cheerfulness, the degree of consistency depends very much on which situational pairs are being considered. Thus these results suggest clearly that the issue of consistency should not be treated in a global manner.

Table 2 Aggregated cross-situational consistency correlations

	Uncorrected			Corrected for unreliability		
Response	Social–alone	Novel–typical	Work–recreational	Social–alone	Novel–typical	Work–recreational
Affect						
Positive	0.58	0.67	0.70	0.72	0.75	0.77
Negative	0.70	0.80	0.74	0.81	0.90	0.81
Bodily feelings						
Aroused	0.50	0.56	0.60	0.62	0.77	0.69
Energetic	0.24	0.43	0.34	0.33	0.69	0.47
Feeling well	0.57	0.60	0.77	0.68	0.70	0.90
Behavior						
Physically active	0.11	0.58	0.47	0.15	0.76	0.54
Productive	0.29	0.56	0.16	0.40	0.71	0.19
Behavioral predispositions						
Sociable	0.10	0.15	0.01	0.13	0.20	0.01
Cheerful	0.13	0.47	0.37	0.17	0.55	0.47
Cognitive/judgmental						
World beautiful	0.80	0.84	0.78	0.90	0.89	0.86
Self-esteem	0.41	0.62	0.58	0.54	0.69	0.74
Satisfied with life	0.92	0.96	0.97	0.94	0.99	0.98

Situations were selected in order to increase their dissimilarity. If a variance components analysis were applied to these data, then using the extremes of the situational distributions would attenuate the person effects. This is not a problem in the present correltional analyses. However, to the extent that there is a linear person-situation interaction, selection of situational extremes will lead to an underestimation of consistency. If the interaction is nonlinear, the impact of selecting situational extremes would depend on the nature of the nonlinear function.

In Table 3 we present the consistency correlations disaggregated to single occasions. We have disaggregated the correlations based on the average number of occasions the subjects were in each situation, using a formula presented by Ghiselli (1981). These figures enable one to estimate the average value one would expect to obtain if two individual random moments were selected for each individual and then correlated. The most striking thing, of course, is the low value of most of these correlations. Only life satisfaction shows consistency correlations across single occasions that most would consider substantial. All other variables show very low cross-situational consistency correlations when single occasions are considered.

In Table 4 we present the temporal stability correlations computed across all situations. The first column represents the correlations for each variable when subjects' average scores for the first three weeks of the study are correlated with their average scores for the second three weeks. One can see that the temporal stability of different responses also varies greatly. A number of variables show high stability, but the stability of feel well/ill and feelings of sociability are quite modest. The middle column contains the three-week stability coefficients that have been corrected for the total odd–even unreliability estimates. The last column presents the values from

Table 3 Corrected cross-situational consistencies disaggregated to single occasions

	Situational pairs		
Response	Social–alone	Novel–typical	Work–recreation
Affect			
Positive	0.10	0.08	0.11
Negative	0.16	0.19	0.13
Bodily feelings			
Aroused	0.07	0.08	0.07
Energetic	0.02	0.06	0.03
Feeling well	0.09	0.06	0.25
Behavior			
Physically active	0.01	0.08	0.04
Productive	0.03	0.06	0.01
Behavioral predispositions			
Sociable	0.01	0.01	0.00
Cheerful	0.01	0.03	0.03
Cognitive/judgmental			
World beautiful	0.30	0.18	0.18
Self-esteem	0.05	0.06	0.09
Satisfied with life	0.44	0.70	0.67

the middle column that have been disaggregated down to single-occasion estimates of stability by a reverse application of the Spearman–Brown formula (Allen and Yen, 1979). When one considers the disaggregated figures, it is apparent that many variables are also not very stable when only single occasions are considered. Nevertheless, one can see that with the exception of life satisfaction, there is only modest stability for single responses on the other variables.

Table 4 Temporal stabilities across all situations

Response	Three-week aggregated uncorrected	Three-week aggregated corrected	Three-week disaggregated corrected
Affect			
Positive	0.79	0.95	0.48
Negative	0.81	0.93	0.39
Bodily feelings			
Aroused	0.81	0.95	0.45
Energetic	0.65	0.70	0.10
Feeling well	0.44	0.55	0.05
Behavior			
Physically active	0.58	0.66	0.08
Productive	0.65	0.71	0.10
Behavioral predispositions			
Sociable	0.34	0.35	0.03
Cheerful	0.76	0.80	0.16
Cognitive/judgmental			
World beautiful	0.89	0.93	0.40
Self esteem	0.70	0.84	0.20
Satisfied with life	0.87	0.99	0.87

Table 5 Corrected three-week stabilities within situations

	Situations					
Response	Social	Alone	Novel	Typical	Work	Recreation
Affect						
Positive	0.79	0.75	0.61	0.85	0.58	0.83
Negative	0.72	0.88	0.48	0.86	0.69	0.72
Bodily feelings						
Aroused	0.68	0.55	0.68	0.94	0.57	0.86
Energetic	0.32	0.94	0.71	0.86	0.73	0.65
Feeling well	0.05	0.50	0.41	0.49	0.19	0.65
Behavior						
Physically active	0.51	0.60	0.46	0.82	0.56	0.54
Productive	0.73	0.84	0.36	0.72	0.75	0.69
Behavioral predispositions						
Sociable	0.49	0.71	0.29	0.62	0.29	0.64
Cheerful	0.70	0.70	0.38	0.93	0.27	0.90
Cognitive/judgmental						
World beautiful	0.85	0.57	0.71	0.91	0.83	0.89
Self-esteem	0.51	0.70	0.39	0.81	0.61	0.62
Satisfied with life	0.93	0.91	0.90	0.93	0.91	0.93

One can see the result of considering stability within particular situations by referring to the values in Table 5. Life satisfaction is stable within every situation. Affect tends to be quite stable over time in typical situations, but only moderately stable in novel and work situations. Although one may notice greater stabilities for all variables in typical situations than in novel ones, one must remember that the number of observations is much smaller for novel situations.

When one compares the situational stabilities in Table 5 with the cross-situational consistencies presented in Table 2, it is difficult to draw general conclusions about whether there is more consistency or stability in aggregated behavior. However, one can also compare the disaggregated consistencies shown in Table 3 with the disaggregated stabilities shown in Table 4, thus correcting for differences in the number of observations. This comparison suggests that affect, arousal, and the cognitive variables show greater stability than they do consistency. Nonetheless, the stability of many variables between single occasions is very small (e.g., feeling well/ill and physical activity). The correlations for feeling well/ill were undoubtedly attenuated by ceiling effects because most subjects felt well most of the time.

The covariation between stability and consistency can also be examined. Are those responses that are most stable the same onesas those that are most consistent? After we created the positive and negative sums, there were 32 self-rating variables. The stability and consistency correlations for each were converted to Z scores and these were correlated across variables. The remarkably high correlation of 0.81 ($p < 0.001$) indicates that there was a strong tendency for variables that were inconsistent to also be those that were unstable. Is this simply due to the reliability of the measures? One can note from Table 1 that the overall reliability of the measures was similar and high. Thus differences in scale reliability cannot explain why the measures that are inconsistent also tend to be those that are unstable. Clearly, the variables that show coherence within individuals across time also tend to show it across situations.

Were some individuals more consistent across situations? Absolute value difference scores were taken between each pair of situations for each variable. For example, we computed the absolute value of average positive affect in social situations minus average positive affect in "alone" situations. This was done for each variable for each of the three pairs of situations. Such scores represent how much each individual changed from situation to situation. These change scores were then correlated between situational dimensions for each variable separately, and these correlations are shown in Table 6. A caveat is worth mentioning: Change scores are often highly unreliable even when the measures themselves are quite reliable. Thus correlations based on change scores can be highly attenuated (McNemar, 1969). Therefore, we computed the reliability of the change scores based on the formula suggested by Allen and Yen (1979). These reliability estimates for the change scores, although somewhat lower than the reliabilities for the component scores, were still substantial, averaging 0.61 across all variables. Nevertheless, the figures in Table 6 should be used to give a rough idea of whether some individuals are more consistent than others, without giving a precise estimate of the strength of this effect. It appears that there is a tendency for all variables for the more consistent people to be more consistent across all three situational dimensions. One should note that for variables such as life satisfaction, which are highly reliable, virtually all individuals must be consistent relative to one another. Therefore, some individuals must be virtually unchanging on such a variable, with others changing slightly for person consistency

Table 6 Correlations of absolute difference scores

Response	Difference score pairs		
	Novel–typical & social–alone	Social–alone & work–recreation	Novel–typical & work–recreation
Affect			
Positive	0.25	0.50	0.41
Negative	0.40	0.51	0.22
Bodily feelings			
Aroused	0.19	0.54	0.35
Energetic	0.00	0.16	0.42
Feeling well	0.21	0.24	0.54
Behavior			
Physically active	0.41	0.33	0.33
Productive	0.46	0.23	0.12
Behavioral predispositions			
Sociable	0.14	0.68	0.40
Cheerful	0.40	0.36	0.53
Cognitive/judgmental			
World beautiful	0.43	0.34	0.43
Self-esteem	0.21	0.14	0.15
Satisfied with life	0.18	0.36	0.46

differences to emerge. Although the correlations in Table 6 should not be taken as precise values, it should be noted that the correlations were all positive and definitely are not distributed around zero. This indicates that there is a tendency for some individuals to be more consistent than others across various situational pairs. This appeared to be true for all variables. Thus some individuals appear to be more consistent and others less so.

Discussion

In our study we sampled affect in subjects' everyday lives. Each subject completed approximately 84 mood reports that were scattered over a six-week period. In all we have a total of 3,512 occasions on which moods and other responses were reported. Because the reports were completed at random times, they represent an ecological sample of affect and a representative sample of the situations in which participants spent their time. In summary, our major findings were as follows:

1. The degree of consistency not only differed for different responses and sets of situations, but specific responses were more or less consistent in different sets of situations. This finding suggests that general statements about consistency may be overly simple. Similarly, arranging situations on a single similarity dimension may be too simple because different aspects of situations may influence different responses. Within-situation stability was also diverse, depending on the response and situation involved.
2. Despite the diversity in consistency just referred to, several general trends can be noted. Life satisfaction was invariably stable and consistent, whereas feelings of sociability were not so. Affect and arousal showed moderately strong stability. Nevertheless, even after aggregation some responses were very consistent and others were not. Thus person effects can be weak in some cases even if long-term trends are examined. In other cases, person effects for long-term means can be quite strong.
3. Aggregating data across occasions resulted in much higher stability and consistency estimates than those based on disaggregated estimates. Such aggregation is analogous to randomization and experimental control in laboratory research because aggregation helps reduce the influence of uncontrolled factors. There were striking differences between the correlations for aggregated data and those disaggregated to single occasions. This indicates that there are consistent and stable long-term trends in mean levels of responding for individuals, but in general single responses will show very low levels of consistency and stability. Recall that our responses were randomly sampled from the everyday lives of our respondents. The low estimated single occasion correlations suggest short-term fluctuations or variability in the responses of our subjects, even though there is a long-term trend in the mean level of their responses.
4. It appeared that most variables tended to show somewhat greater stability that consistency. This difference was most pronounced for affect, arousal, and the

cognitive variables. However, each of these also showed strong consistency when aggregated data were analyzed. Only one variable, feeling well/ill, showed somewhat more consistency than stability.

5. There has recently been interest in whether some individuals are more consistent than others (e.g., Campus, 1974; Chaplin & Goldberg, 1984; Kenrick & Braver 1982; Rushton, Jackson, & Paunonen, 1981). In our data it appeared that some individuals were more consistent across all types of situations than were others. Because every single correlation between change in one situational pair and another situational pair was positive, this is a strong indication that some individuals are consistently more consistent than others.

6. Stability and consistency strongly covaried across responses, indicating that a sharp demarcation cannot be drawn between the two. Although stability and consistency imply lack of change along the dimensions of time and situations, each always includes the other to some degree. Cross-situational consistency always occurs over time and temporal stability occurs over situations because no two situations can ever be truly identical. Those responses that were most stable over time were the same ones that were most consistent across situations. We cannot account for this finding by differences in the reliability of the measures. Mischel (1979) has stressed that stability exists in behavior because of the temporal stability of reinforcement contingencies, but that inconsistency across situations exists because persons recognize fine differences in the reinforcement systems of differing situations. The high correlations between stability and consistency indicate that certain additional factors must work to keep some responses relatively unchanging. Other responses appear to be more free to vary both across time and situation. Placing the locus of stability entirely in the environment fails to account for the high correlation found between the stability and consistency of variables. It is probable that some variables are more internally stable, whereas others are more reactive to environmental change.

There are several important implications of the aggregation data. On the prediction side, one can expect much stronger results when aggregated data are being used because situational and other effects tend to cancel out. Of course, aggregation across time or across persons has been used for decades in other areas of psychology in order to average out factors in which the scientist was not interested. However, there are potential problems with aggregation that should be noted. First, it is easy to lose sight of the fact that in focusing on a particular variable, one will be ignoring and averaging out other variables that also influence the behavior being studied. This can be a curse or a blessing depending on the purpose of the study and the phenomenon in which one is interested. Second, when aggregation is used it becomes more difficult to compare effect sizes. Because aggregation over greater numbers of incidents will almost inevitably lead to larger correlations, the size of the relations found will depend both on the number of occasions aggregated and on the underlying effect size per se. In other words, a correlation may be large simply because it is based on a larger aggregate, not because the underlying connection is larger. This makes effect size comparisons between variables and between studies difficult because the aggregated number of occasions usually differ. This problem is especially serious for personality correlations based on ratings made by knowledgeable informants because their ratings depend on different numbers of observations. One approach to solving the problem related to varying numbers of observations is to disaggregate to single responses as we have done and as discussed by Golding (1975).

On the conceptual side, the high degree of stability and consistency obtained when occasions are aggregated reaffirms the fact that behavior (as well as other responses such as affect) tends to be complexly determined. In predicting a single occasion, many factors, including uncontrolled ones, will influence a response. In most cases, nomothetic person effects are not so strong in determining single responses that they outweigh other factors. There are exceptions. Some cognitive judgments, at least once initially formed, tend to be very stable and consistent even for single occasions. Although for most types of responses persons are usually only mildly consistent across situations, the person consistency that does exist may be very interesting in terms of psychological theory. As Diener (1983) has pointed out, a recurrent phenomenon such as person consistency may be theoretically important regardless of effect size. The statistical strength of a relation is only one factor among many when its theoretical importance is judged. Even correlations of only .05 could be important in some cases. The fact that some level of nomothetic consistency exists for virtually all variables is a phenomenon requiring explanation. The present data reveal that small correlations across individual occasions can translate into large correlations if one is interested in long-term trends in behavior. Nevertheless, it should always be recalled that certain other important influences on single responses are averaged out if one aggregates the behavior of individuals. It is one thing to note that personality correlations for responses on single occasions are low, but quite another to maintain that they are zero. Virtually all studies and all the consistency correlations we presented are positive. They are not distributed around zero. Thus the likelihood that consistency is actually zero as proposed by Bem (1972) is extremely small.

If one is interested in long-term average levels of behavior, strong person effects can be found for many variables. This approach to personality has been advocated by Jaccard (1974), Epstein (1979, 1982) and more recently by Buss and Craik (1983). What is suggested is that there are stable and consistent mean differences in the behavior of individuals, but also variability around these mean levels so that individual responses are not strongly predicted by person differences. If one is interested in the single responses of individuals within specific situations, as is Mischel (Mischel & Peake, 1982), then nomothetic personality may not be very potent for most responses, although variables such as life satisfaction are an exception. The high correlations obtained in this study and by Epstein (1979, 1982) for aggregates do not mean that personality is any stronger in its ability to explain individual responses. However, if one is interested in long-term mean levels of behavior, there may be person effects that are strong, although some variables may show person effects that are small even at this level (e.g., feeling sociable). Which level of analysis a scientist chooses to study willdepend on the phenomena he or she is attempting to explain. The understanding of long-term person effects is a justifiable undertaking. When investigators aggregate data for persons, they will amplify person effects by averaging out short-term situational effects, as well as random errors of measurement (Diener & Larsen 1984). The explanation of specific behaviors in specific situations may also be justifiable but will undoubtedly require many variables. If one is interested in understanding momentary moods or emotion, the personality of the respondent would only be one small influence among many. However, the investigator might wish to understand long-term differences in happiness, in which case personality might play a larger role. Ultimately the goal must be to develop well-grounded theories to explain phenomena, and not simply debate the question of the "strength" of personality.

Because few behavioral responses show high consistency across single occasions, there is a temptation to use idiographic and interactional approaches. Whether these will be more successful in predicting single occasion behavior or whether these effects will also be overlaid by a large number of other factors has yet to be seen. Certainly in the domain of overt behavior in which response consistency is low, other approaches should be tried, but they do not necessarily have a better a priori probability of success.

One major conclusion that one can draw from the present study is that person consistency varies greatly, depending on the response domain, the situations being considered, and the particular persons involved. Given this complexity, it seems advisable to quit debating whether person consistency exists, and to begin exploring the factors that control consistency (e.g., Monson, Hesley, & Chernick, 1982; Snyder, 1982). At the level of theory, the degree of consistency that does exist suggests a place for nomothetic person variables, but also indicates that more refined theories must be developed. We need to determine why and when consistency and inconsistency occur (Diener, 1983). In this regard, we need to carefully consider why some variables, some situational dimensions, and some individuals tend to show larger amounts of consistency. However, we should not expect an overly simple answer to the question of when consistency will occur.

Acknowledgments We wish to express our appreciation to Robert Emmons, Laura Spera, and Sharon Griffin for their help in the data collection and analyses. This research was supported in part by National Institute of Mental Health Grant No. MH-15140 for research training in personality and social ecology.

References

Alker, H. A. (1972). Is personality situationally specific or intrapsychically consistent? *Journal of Personality, 40,* 1–16.

Allen, M. J., & Yen, W. M. (1979). *Introduction to measurement theory.* Monterey, CA: Brooks/Cole.

Bem, D. J. (1972). Constructing cross-situational consistencies in behavior: Some thoughts on Alker's critique of Mischel. *Journal of Personality, 40,* 17–26.

Bem, D. J., & Allen, A. (1974). On predicting some of the people some of the time: The search for cross-situational consistencies in behavior. *Psychological Review, 81,* 506–520.

Block, J. (1971). *Lives through time.* Berkeley, CA: Bancroft Books.

Block, J., Buss, D. M., Block, J. H., & Gjerde, P. F. (1981). The cognitive style of breadth of categorization: Longitudinal consistency of personality correlates. *Journal of Personality and Social Psychology, 40,* 770–779.

Bradburn, N. (1969). *The structure of psychological well being.* Chicago: Aldine.

Buss, D. M., & Craik, K. H. (1983). The act frequency approach to personality. *Psychological Review, 90,* 105–126.

Campus, N. (1974). Transituational consistency as a dimension of personality. *Journal of Personality and Social Psychology, 29,* 593–600.

Chaplin, W. F., & Goldberg, L. R. (1984). A failure to replicate the Bem and Allen study on individual differences in cross-situational consistencies. *Journal of Personality and Social Psychology, 47,* 1074–1090.

Costa, P. T., & McCrae, R. R., & Arenberg, D. (1980). Enduring dispositions in adult males. *Journal of Personality and Social Psychology, 38,* 793–800.

Cronbach, L. J. (1951). Coefficient alpha and the internal structure of tests. *Psychometrika, 16,* 297–334.

Crowne, D. P., & Marlowe, D. (1964). *The approval motive Studies in evaluative independence.* New York: Wiley.

Diener, E. (1983). *The phenomenon of person consistency.* Unpublished manuscript, University of Illinois.

Diener, E., & Emmons, R. A. (1985). The independence of positive and negative affect. *Journal of Personality and Social Psychology, 47,* 1105–1117.

Diener, E., & Larsen, R. J. (1984). *Limitations of aggregation.* Unpublished manuscript, University of Illinois.

Dudycha, G. J. (1936). An objective study of punctuality in relation to personality and achievement. *Archives of Psychology, 204,* 1–39.

Ekehammar, B. (1974). Interactionism in personality from a historical perspective. *Psychological Bulletin, 81,* 1026–1048.

Endler, N. S., & Magnusson, D. (1976). Toward an interactional psychology of personality. *Psychological Bulletin, 83,* 956–974.

Epstein, S. (1979). The stability of behavior: I. On predicting most of the people much of the time. *Journal of Personality and Social Psychology, 37,* 1097–1126.

Epstein, S. (1982). A research paradigm for the study of personality and emotions. In M. M. Page (Ed.), *Nebraska symposium on motivation 1981* (pp. 91–154). Lincoln: University of Nebraska Press.

Ghiselli, E. E., Campbell, J. P., & Zedeck, S. (1981). *Measurement theory for the behavioral sciences.* San Francisco: Freeman.

Golding, S. L. (1975). Flies in the ointment: Methodological problems in the analysis of the percentage of variance due to persons and situations. *Psychological Bulletin, 82,* 278–288.

Jaccard, J. J. (1974). Predicting social behavior from personality traits. *Journal of Research in Personality, 7,* 358–367.

Kenrick, D. T., & Braver, S. L. (1982). Personality: Idiographic and nomothetic! A rejoinder. *Psychological Review, 89,* 182–186.

Koretzky, M. B., Kohn, M., & Jeger, A. M. (1978). Cross-situational consistency among problem adolescents: An application of the two-factor model. *Journal of Personality and Social Psychology, 36,* 1054–1059.

Lord, F. M., & Novick, M. R. (1968). *Statistical theories of mental test scores.* Reading, MA: Addison-Wesley.

McNemar, Q. (1969). *Psychological statistics.* New York: Wiley.

Mischel, W. (1968). *Personality and assessment.* New York: Wiley.

Mischel, W. (1979). On the interface of cognition and personality: Beyond the person–situation debate. *American Psychologist, 34,* 740–754.

Mischel, W., & Peake, P. K. (1982). Beyond Déjà Vu in the search for cross-situational consistency. *Psychological Review, 89,* 730–755.

Monson, T. C., Hesley, J. W., & Chernick, L. (1982). Specifying when personality traits can and cannot predict behavior: An alternative to abandoning the attempt to predict single-act criteria. *Journal of Personality and Social Psychology, 43,* 385–399.

Moos, R. H., & Insel, P. M. (1974). *Issues in social ecology.* Palo Alto, CA: National Press Books.

Murray, H. A. (1938). *Explorations in personality.* New York: Oxford University Press.

Olweus, D. (1979). Stability of aggressive reaction patterns in males: A review. *Psychological Bulletin, 86,* 852–875.

Rushton, J. P., Jackson, D. N., & Paunonen, S. V. (1981). Personality: Nomothetic or idiographic? A response to Kenrick and Stringfield. *Psychological Review, 88,* 582–589.

Schaie, K. W., & Parham, I. A. (1976). Stability of adult personality: Fact or fable? *Journal of Personality and Social Psychology, 34,* 146–158.

Schuerger, J. M., Tait, E., & Tavernelli, M. (1982). Temporal stability of personality by question-naire. *Journal of Personality and Social Psychology, 43,* 176–182.

Snyder, M. (1982). *Understanding individuals and their social worlds.* Paper presented at the Annual Convention of the American Psychological Association, Washington, DC.

Underwood, B., & Moore, B. S. (1981). Sources of behavioral consistency. *Journal of Personality and Social Psychology, 40,* 780–785.

Zevon, M. A., & Tellegen, A. (1982). The structure of mood change: An idiographic/nomothetic analysis. *Journal of Personality and Social Psychology, 43,* 111–122.

Assessing Subjective Well-Being: Progress and Opportunities

Ed Diener

Abstract Subjective well-being (SWB) comprises people's longer-term levels of pleasant affect, lack of unpleasant affect, and life satisfaction. It displays moderately high levels of cross-situational consistency and temporal stability. Self-report measures of SWB show adequate validity, reliability, factor invariance, and sensitivity to change. Despite the success of the measures to date, more sophisticated approaches to defining and measuring SWB are now possible. Affect includes facial, physiological, motivational, behavioral, and cognitive components. Self-reports assess primarily the cognitive component of affect, and thus are unlikely to yield a complete picture of respondents' emotional lives. For example, denial may influence self-reports of SWB more than other components. Additionally, emotions are responses which vary on a number of dimensions such as intensity, suggesting that mean levels of affect as captured by existing measures do not give a complete account of SWB. Advances in cognitive psychology indicate that differences in memory retrieval, mood as information, and scaling processes can influence self-reports of SWB. Finally, theories of communication alert us to the types of information that are likely to be given in self-reports of SWB. These advances from psychology suggest that a multimethod approach to assessing SWB will create a more comprehensive depiction of the phenomenon. Not only will a multifaceted test battery yield more credible data, but inconsistencies between various measurement methods and between the various components of well-being. Knowledge of cognition, personality, and emotion will also aid in the development of sophisticated theoretical definitions of subjective well-being. For example, life satisfaction is theorized to be a judgment that respondents construct based on currently salient information. Finally, it is concluded that measuring negative reactions such as depression or anxiety give an incomplete picture of people's well-being, and that it is imperative to measure life satisfaction and positive emotions as well.

E. Diener (✉)
Department of Psychology, University of Illinois, Urbana-champaign, Champaign,
IL 61820, USA
e-mail: ediener@uiuc.edu

E. Diener (ed.), *Assessing Well-Being: The Collected Works of Ed Diener*,
Social Indicators Research Series 39, DOI 10.1007/978-90-481-2354-4_3,
© Springer Science+Business Media B.V. 2009

25

Assessing Subjective Well-Being: Progress and Opportunities

Since the Golden Age of Greek philosophy, western thinkers have been concerned with understanding "happiness." Aristotle laid down this agenda when he defined happiness as the summum bonum, the supreme good. He maintained that happiness is the only value which is final and sufficient: final in that all else is merely a means to this end, and sufficient in that once happiness is attained, nothing else is desired. It is little wonder, then, that scholars have been seeking this holy grail ever since. It is also unsurprising, given the difficulties that thinkers have in defining this concept, that folk wisdom maintains that happiness is highly desirable, but elusive. Nonetheless, researchers have created a number of self-report scales to measure "happiness." In recent decades behavioral scientists focused a spotlight on happiness, although relabeling the concept under new rubrics such as subjective well-being (SWB), morale, positive affect, and life satisfaction.

The overwhelming majority of work on subjective well-being has been based on self-report assessment. One widespread SWB measure is Bradburn's (1969) Affect Balance Scale which separately measures "positive" and "negative" affect. The respondent is asked whether, in the past few weeks, he or she experienced a series of 10 feelings such as "Depressed or very unhappy" and "On top of the world." Larsen, Diener, and Emmons (1985) report that this scale performs more poorly than several others, perhaps there are too few questions, in light of the narrowness of most items (e.g., "Upset because someone criticized you"). Nonetheless, the scale was the first to separately assess long-term levels of negative and positive affect.

A short, one-item scale to measure global well-being was developed by Andrews and Withey (1976) and has been used extensively in large-scale survey work. The question asks respondents "How do you feel about your life as a whole?" and instructs them to frame their answer in terms of what has happened in the last year and what they expect in the near future. The seven response options vary from "delighted" to "terrible" and the scale is therefore often called the D-T Scale. In the work of Andrews and Withey, this item is averaged across two administrations given about 20 minutes apart during the interview. The scale was designed to reflect both affective and cognitive components of well-being, and in a cluster analysis falls near the center of well-being items. A LISREL analysis showed the scale to have a surprisingly high validity coefficient (0.77) for two administrations of a single item (Andrews & Robinson, 1991). A similar scale was created by Fordyce (1988). His major question specifically mentions "happiness," and the response options list emotions varying from "elation" to "utter despair." Additional questions ask about the percent of time the respondent feels happy and unhappy. Thus, this scale is likely to reflect emotional well-being to a great extent and a life satisfaction judgment to a lesser extent than the D-T scale. Fordyce (1988) advertises the scale as one which shows "good reliability, exceptional stability, and a record of convergent, construct, and discriminative validity unparalleled in the field" (p. 355).

In contrast to the above scales, the Affectometer 2 (Kammann & Flett, 1983) and the Satisfaction with Life Scale (Diener & Emmons et al., 1985; Pavot & Diener,

1993b) are multi-item scales which are purposefully designed to more narrowly measure affective well-being and life satisfaction, respectively. The Affectometer 2 measures the balance of pleasant and unpleasant feelings in recent experience with items such as "I smile and laugh a lot" and "Nothing seems very much fun anymore." The Satisfaction with Life Scale (SWLS) was explicitly designed to measure cognitive judgments of life satisfaction rather than affect perse. Sample items, answered on a scale varying from "Strongly agree" to "Strongly disagree," are "If I could live my life over, I would change almost nothing," and, "My life is close to my ideal."

A number of reviews of well-being measurement are available and these focus primarily on the psychometric evaluation of existing scales (Andrews & Robinson, 1991; Diener, 1984; George & Bearon, 1980; Larsen et al., 1985; McKennell, 1974; Nydegger, 1977; Veenhoven, 1984). There are also a number of reviews of the historical definitions of happiness (Jones, 1953; Tatarkiewicz, 1976; Veenhoven, 1984). Finally, there are existing reviews of the correlates of subjective well-being (Andrews and Withey, 1976; Diener, 1984; Diener & Larsen, 1993; Veenhoven, 1984).

In the current review, I examine evidence showing that long-term well-being is a meaningful construct. There are cross-situational consistencies and temporal stabilities in subjective well-being. Further, I briefly review the evidence which demonstrates that self-report measures of SWB display adequate levels of validity and reliability. Despite the past success of SWB measures, information is accumulating in psychology which suggests that current measures and definitions of subjective well-being can be advanced. A major purpose of the present paper is to review advances in psychology as they relate to the assessment of well-being. Progress in basic areas of psychology now make possible more sophisticated understanding and measurement of subjective well-being. In the final section, recommendations are made for improving the definition and measurement of SWB.

Progress to Date: The Current Status of SWB Measurement

Defining Subjective Well-Being

Definitions of subjective well-being are often not made explicit in the literature, but are only implied by the measures which are used. Nonetheless, a current composite definition of SWB can be gleaned from the major works in the field. Diener (1984) suggests that there are three hallmarks to the area of SWB: First, it is subjective—it resides within the experience of the individual. Second, it is not just the absence of negative factors, but also includes positive measures. Third, it includes a global assessment rather than only a narrow assessment of one life domain. Although these hallmarks serve to delimit the area of study, they are not complete definitions of subjective well-being.

Veenhoven (1984) defines subjective well-being as the degree to which an individual judges the overall quality of her or his life as a whole in a favorable way. In other words, subjective well-being is how well the person likes the life he or she leads (p. 22). Andrews and Withey (1976) define subjective well-being as "both a cognitive evaluation and some degree of positive or negative feelings, i.e., affect" (p. 18). Veenhoven (1984) follows their lead in asserting that individuals use two components in evaluating their lives: their affects and their thoughts (p. 25). The affective component is hedonic level, the pleasantness experienced in feelings, emotions, and moods. Campbell, Converse, and Rodgers (1976) define satisfaction, the cognitive component, as "the perceived discrepancy between aspiration and achievement, ranging from the perception of fulfillment to that of deprivation. Satisfaction implies a judgmental or cognitive experience while happiness suggests an experience of feeling or affect" (p. 8).

Of course the most useful definition of subjective well-being will be based on a compelling theory. The implicit theory of SWB in the above definitions is the following. Humans are not only capable of appraising events, life circumstances, and themselves, but they make such appraisals continually. Appraisals of things in terms of goodness-badness is a human universal. Following the theory of Lazarus (1991), such appraisals are seen as leading to emotional reactions, which can be either pleasant or unpleasant. Other things being equal, pleasant experiences are perceived as desirable and valuable. Thus, a person who has pleasant emotional experiences is more likely to perceive his or her life as being desirable and positive.

People with high subjective well-being are those who make a preponderance of positive appraisals of their life events and circumstances. People who are "unhappy" are those who appraise a majority of factors in their life as harmful or as blocking their goals. Life satisfaction is a global judgment that people make when they consider their life as a whole, whereas the hedonic component of subjective well-being is the presence of ongoing pleasant affect (due to positive appraisals of ongoing events) much of the time and infrequent unpleasant affect (resulting from few on-line negative appraisals).

Life satisfaction and hedonic level are likely to correlate because both are influenced by appraisals of one's life events, activities, and circumstances. At the same time, life satisfaction and hedonic level are likely to diverge to some degree because life satisfaction is a global summary of one's life as a whole, whereas hedonic level consists of ongoing reactions to events (and may also be influenced by unconscious goals and biological factors which may influence mood). In support of this reasoning, Campbell, Converse, and Rodgers (1976) found that there is a strong general SWB factor, but that there are also components of SWB which may behave differently under some circumstances. Research shows that affect and cognitive satisfaction judgments can diverge (Andrews and Withey, 1976; Horley & Little, 1985; Judge, 1990; Lawton, 1983; Liang, 1985; Stock, Okun, & Benin, 1986), although many measures include both components (Chamberlain, 1988). Affective well-being and satisfaction sometimes move in different directions over time and have different correlates (Beiser, 1974; Campbell et al., 1976; DeHaes, Pennink, & Welvaart, 1987; Kushman & Lane, 1980). However, life satisfaction and affective well-being tend to fall together on a common well-being factor when a second order factor analysis is performed (Liang, 1985; McNeil, Stones, & Kozma, 1986), although this second order structure may not be longitudinally invariant (McCulloch, 1991). Thus, SWB is composed of partially separable affective and cognitive components, which nevertheless correlates at levels sufficient to say that they are parts of a higher order construct.

In the literature, the term "happiness" is sometimes used synonymously with subjective well-being. Most authors, however, avoid the use of the term "happiness" because of its varied popular meanings. For example, happiness may refer to the global experience of well-being, to the current feeling of joy, or to the experience of much positive affect over time. In contrast, the terms used in this field now possess more specific meanings. Subjective well-being refers to the global experience of positive reactions to one's life, and includes all of the lower-order components such as life satisfaction and hedonic level. Life satisfaction refers to a conscious global judgment of one's life. Hedonic level or balance refers to the pleasantness minus unpleasantness of one's emotional life.

Subjective well-being is likely to have both stable and changeable components. One's appraisals of ongoing life events can change, and therefore one's hedonic level can change. But at the same time, one's emotions are likely to return to an average baseline which is set by one's temperament and one's general life circumstances. Thus, although immediate emotions may change constantly, one's long-term subjective well-being is likely to have considerable stability. Similarly, one's life satisfaction might change if one's life circumstances change dramatically. There are likely to be many life circumstances, however, which are consistent over time and this leads to a degree of stability in life satisfaction.

One can decompose subjective well-being into finer and finer units. For example, life satisfaction can be broken down into satisfaction with various domains: work, love, and so forth. These domains in turn can be broken down more finely. Similarly, emotion can be divided into finer and finer categories. Unpleasant affect can be broken into discrete emotions such as anger, which can in turn be decomposed into anger over various types of events. The more global categories of hedonic level, life satisfaction, and subjective well-being serve a useful scientific role, however, because people show coherencies between their well-being in different domains (e.g., Campbell et al., 1976) and because specific positive or negative emotions tend to covary to some extent (e.g., McConville & Cooper, 1992). In other words, the reasons to study more molar as well as more molecular categories is that the smaller categories cohere in larger units. Thus, broader categories of well-being are useful scientifically because they point to more global psychological phenomena. At the same time, there are many circumstances in which narrow aspects of subjective well-being are scientifically useful.

Although useful as a starting point, the above definitions and theory must be refined as advances occur in the field. One message of this paper is that advances in other areas of psychology, including cognition and emotion, now allow us to proceed beyond the theory above. If we examine contributions in other areas of psychology, we can offer more refined definitions of subjective well-being and prescribe more sophisticated measurement approaches.

Existence of Long-Term Well-Being

Although well-being researchers recognize the influence of momentary factors in influencing life satisfaction and affective well-being, they are most interested in longer-term subjective well-being. Rather than study emotions which fluctuate from moment-to-moment, SWB researchers are primarily interested in factors which lead to specific levels of well-being over periods of weeks, months, or years. Thus, it is imperative to first demonstrate that there is some stability in moods and life satisfaction which transcends the moment-to-moment fluctuations which exist. Although verbal definitions of SWB have been advanced as described above, these definitions will be important only insofar as the phenomena they describe actually possess long term coherence at the empirical level.

SWB shows some temporal stability. For example, Headey and Wearing (1989) found stabilities in the 0.5–0.6 range over a six year period and Chamberlain and Zika (1992) found that the average six-month reliability across well-being measure was 0.69. Wessman and Ricks (1966) report a two-year stability of 0.67 for hedonic level. Others also report strong temporal reliabilities (e.g., Bradburn, 1969; Campbell et al., 1976; Kammann & Flett, 1983). Costa and McCrae (1988) report an impressive 0.57 correlation between spouse-ratings and self-ratings of positive affect separated by six years and a correlation of 0.49 for negative affect. Given these stabilities, one cannot conceive of well-being as simply a momentary phenomenon without enduring aspects. Because several of the studies relied on both self reports and informant reports, a methodological explanation of the temporal stabilities of SWB in terms of self-report artifacts seems untenable. Thus, long-term levels of life satisfaction and hedonic level do exist.

Further, SWB has cross-situational consistency. Diener and Larsen (1984) found that average pleasant and unpleasant affect correlated 0.58 and 0.70, respectively, across social versus alone situations, and 0.70 and 0.74 across work versus recreation situations. They found that life satisfaction judgments on single occasions correlated 0.44 between social and alone situations, but 0.92 when they aggregated life satisfaction reports over time. Futhermore, Pavot, Diener, Colvin, and Sandvik (1991) found life satisfaction rating for a target person completed by family members correlated 0.54 with friends' assessments of the target's life satisfaction. This is impressive because the parents and friends observed the subjects in quite different situations. Further, the use of informants again rules out an explanation based on common self-report method variance. Thus, studying long-term levels of well-being is defensible because temporally stable and cross-situationally consistent levels of longer-term SWB clearly exist.

Psychometric Qualities of Self-Report Measures

Research on SWB has relied almost exclusively on self-report assessment. Empirical analyses of these measures reveal that they are somewhat valid and reliable. In the first place, the scales tend to converge with each other. For example,

Pavot et al. (1991) report that the Satisfaction with Life Scale (Diener, Emmons, Larsen, & Griffin, 1985) converges with the Life Satisfaction Index-A at r = 0.81, and Sandvik, Diener, and Seidlitz (1993) found that the single-item scales of Andrews and Withey and Fordyce correlated at 0.62. Encouragingly, Rodgers, Herzog, and Andrews (1988) estimate that half of the variance in happiness measures is due to the underlying well-being construct, and only about one tenth of the variance is normally due to method.

It is possible to measure subjective well-being with methods other than traditional self-report. For example, a person's well-being might be estimated by friends and measured with informant reports, or it might be measured with the coding of vocal tone and facial expressions during an interview. Several nonself-report measures of SWB will be described later in the paper. Self-report measures of subjective well-being display moderate convergence with nonself-report measures of well-being (e.g., Costa and McCrae, 1988; Jasper, 1930; Lawton, 1972; Lawton, Kleban, & DiCarlo 1984; Neugarten, Havighurst, & Tobin, 1961; Stones & Kozma, 1980; Washburne, 1941; Wood, Wylie, & Sheafor, 1969). For example, Sandvik et al. (1993) found that Andrews and Withey's D-T scale correlated 0.58 with informant reports of well-being. They report that daily reports of mood over a six week period correlated 0.66 with the D-T scale given at a prior time. They also found that the Affectometer correlated 0.80 with a factor score comprised of nontraditional measures of SWB, and the single item Fordyce scale correlated 0.68 with this factor. Furthermore, they found that the nonself-report measures converged with each other. For example, they report that an event memory measure (the number of good minus bad events recalled) correlated 0.34 with informant reports of well-being. Pavot et al. (1991) reported that peer estimated and self-reported life satisfaction correlated 0.54 and 0.64 in two studies, and that peer-related and self-related affect balance correlated 0.51 and 0.57 in the two studies. Despite this moderate convergence of self-report and nonself-report measures of SWB, it will be argued that the size of these correlations provides insufficient justification for using only self-report assessment in the future. The convergence of self-report and nonself-report measures is ample to suggest that these measures contain substantial amounts of common variance, which points to a coherent phenomenon, but are modest enough to indicate that the various types of measures also capture nonoverlapping aspects of SWB which need to be separately measured. In other words, self-reports of SWB are often likely to yield interesting theoretical results because they do partly reflect common aspects of global well-being. These self-report measures, however, are unlikely to fully capture SWB phenomena because they converge only moderately with measures which tap well-being via other methodologies.

As suggested earlier, SWB measures have moderate temporal reliabilities. In addition, the measures possess Cronbach alphas (Larsen et al., 1985) which indicate a good degree of internal consistency in the scales. For example, the alpha of the Satisfaction with Life Scale (Pavot & Diener, 1993b) is about 0.84. A related issue is the degree of factorial invariance of the scales. If the factor structure of the scales remains similar across very different groups of respondents, it suggests that the measures are assessing a psychological universal with general properties. Fortunately the scales have tended to show factorial invariance across groups (Lawrence & Liang, 1988; MacKinnon & Keating, 1989; Wilson, Elias, & Brownlee, 1985). For instance, a cross-cultural comparison of the Philadelphia Geriatric Center Morale Scale in Japan and the US revealed that the factor structure of the scale was similar in the two countries (Liang, Asano, Bollen, Kahana, & Maeda, 1987). Similarly, Andrews (1991) reports evidence showing that the structure of well-being measures has remained stable in the US from 1972 to 1988. Watson, Clark, and Tellegen (1984) and Balatsky and Diener (1993) both found that affect formed two clear global factors in different cultures. Nevertheless, Shao (1992) and Balatsky and Diener (1993) found that the alphas for the Satisfaction with Life Scale were much lower in China and Russia, respectively, than in the US. This suggests that the items do not cohere together in a unified whole as well in those cultures. The factorial invariance of SWB measures across cultures deserves greater research attention. Similarly the second order factor structure of subjective well-being measures over time (e.g. McCulloch, 1991) also deserves further study.

Despite adequate reliabilities of SWB scales, they appear to be sensitive to change (Horley & Lavery, 1991). For instance, Headey and Wearing (1989) found in a longitudinal study that favorable and adverse life events influenced SWB beyond the predictive effects of personality. Atkinson (1982) reported test-retest correlations of about 0.50 for respondents who reported no major life changes, but smaller stabilities for subjects reporting changes. Chamberlain and Zika (1992) found that current hassles predicted well-being in addition to past well-being. Pavot and Diener (1993a) review evidence suggesting that SWB measures improve for clients in therapy. Thus, despite the moderate temporal reliabilities of the scales, they do move in response to changed circumstances. These findings are important for two reasons. First, they indicate that subjective well-being measures are sensitive to change. Second, they indicate that subjective well-being is not identical to personality—it can be influenced by life events, especially recent ones.

A concern with all self-report instruments is whether the language used influences responding. Research among those with different languages within the same countries is encouraging in that few differences in reported well-being are found. For example, Flemish and French speaking Belgians, Swiss of different languages (Inglehart, 1977), and French and English speaking Canadians (Blishen & Atkinson, 1980) report similar levels of well-being when the same measure is translated into different languages. This is encouraging because it suggests that the specific words used do not have a substantial influence on the overall score. Nevertheless, the scales have been used in very similar cultures, so language comparability has not been strongly tested. What is needed is a demonstration that items cluster together in a similar manner across very different cultures. The issue is not only whether words can be adequately translated, but whether the concepts themselves are comparable across cultures.

Individual differences in social desirability in responding is a potential artifact (Carstensen & Cone, 1983) in interpreting SWB scores because the SWB measures correlate at moderate levels with desirability scales (e.g., Campbell et al., 1976; Kammann & Flett, 1983). Social desirability, however, is now seen as a substantive individual difference (Furnham, 1986; Hogan & Nicholson, 1988; Weinberger,

1990) and not necessarily as an artifact (Diener, Fujita, & Smith, 1993; McCrae & Costa, 1983). For example, "social desirability" scores may correlate with conformity and avoidance of thinking about unpleasant affect, both of which correlate with well-being. Thus, controlling individual differences in "social desirability" may not enhance the validity of SWB scales. This has been shown to be true in reference to well-being measures in several studies (e.g. McCrae, 1986). For example, Diener, Sandvik, Pavot, and Gallagher (1991) found that a measure which controlled for "social desirability" correlated more poorly with nonself-report measures of well-being. In addition, Diener, Colvin, Pavot, and Allman (1991) discovered that controlling for Crowne-Marlowe social desirability in the relationship between self-report and non-self report measures of well-being reduced the size of the correlations. Similarly, Kozma and Stones (1988) found that controlling social desirability in the correlation between SWB measures and an external criterion did not improve the zero-order correlations. Thus, individual differences in "social desirability" are related to personality content that is related to subjective well-being, and scoring high on "social desirability" does not indicate a threat to the validity of SWB scores. This does not mean that impression management does not decrease the validity of the SWB scales. What it does mean is that current social desirability scales do not correct for such impression management because they tap personality content which is actually related to SWB. Thus, controlling for social desirability scores may simultaneously reduce the effects of impression management and also substantive personality influences on well-being, with no net increase in validity.

An alternative method of assessing the effects of social desirability is to collect half of the data in face-to-face interviews and the other half of the data in anonymous or quasi-anonymous group settings. In the former setting, impression management should be magnified, whereas in the latter it should be reduced. Thus, the effects of impression management on responding can be assessed. It can be determined not only whether mean scores differ in the two conditions, but also standard deviations and validity coefficients can be examined. Fujita, Smith, and Diener (1993), using this strategy with American college students, found no differences in the validity of SWB measures when they were obtained in interviews versus in quasi-anonymous questionnaires. This method represents a powerful way of examining self-presentational difference between groups.

Conclusion

Self-report measures of well-being appear to possess adequate psychometric properties. The reader is referred to Andrews & Robinson (1991), Andrews and Withey (1976), and Sandvik et al. (1993) for further material on the psychometrics of SWB scales. Although the data are encouraging, several issues demand further study. For example, sophisticated multimeasure factor analytic studies are needed to separate true change in the latent constructs from unreliability due to error of measurement. Additional work is needed on factorial invariance across very different cultures. Finally, research on social desirability is needed which differentiates self-deception versus other-deception (e.g., Paulhus, 1988).

Correlates of SWB

Many demographic variables have been correlated with SWB, with the typical finding being that advantaged groups such as the wealthy are slightly happier than others (e.g., Diener, Horowitz, & Emmons, 1985; Diener, Diener, & Diener, 1993). For example, Campbell, Converse, and Rodgers reported that the unemployed were the unhappiest group they studied. Nevertheless, some advantaged groups such as men and the highly educated do not always report higher levels of well-being (e.g., Campbell et al., 1976; Diener, 1984). In general, resources such as health, income, and physical attractiveness have shown surprisingly small correlations with SWB, whereas personality variables have been much stronger predictors (Costa, McCrae, & Zonderman, 1987; Diener & Larsen, 1993). E. Diener, and M. Diener (1993) reported that self-esteem correlated about 0.53 with life satisfaction in eight western countries and an average of 0.47 across the 31 diverse countries they examined. Some correlates of subjective well-being such as being married (Glenn & Weaver, 1978) may be due to pre-existing personality differences rather than solely to the situation of marriage per se (Scott, Diener, & Fujita, 1992). A number of psychological characteristics such as maturity (Alker & Gawin, 1978) have proven to be strong correlates of SWB. Emmons (1986) found that past goal success predicted positive affect, ambivalence over one's strivings predicted negative affect, and that the importance of one's strivings predicted life satisfaction. Global subjective well-being usually correlates at moderate to high levels with satisfaction with particular aspects of one's life (Diener, 1984). For example, Campbell (1981) reported that life satisfaction correlated 0.55 with satisfaction with the self and 0.37 with work satisfaction. There are cross-cultural differences in happiness and life satisfaction (e.g., Balatsky and Diener, 1993; E. Diener, and M. Diener, 1993; E. Diener, M. Diener, & C. Diener, 1993; Shao, 1992) which are not completely explained by income differences (Diener, Suh, Smith, & Shao, 1995). Finally, differences in SWB covary with the discrepancies one perceives between what one has, what others have, and what one had in the past (Michalos, 1991). Thus, SWB scales show interesting theoretical patterns of relations to other variables.

More sophisticated analyses are desirable in examining the correlates of subjective well-being in order to determine the causal interconnections of variables. For example, certain life events such as divorce may be a hardship for some people and a blessing for others. Additional measures of the meaning of life events for each individual should provide more powerful insights into the genesis of subjective well-being. Longitudinal research can help disentangle whether subjective well-being is the cause or effect of predictor variables. For example, Scott et al. (1992) hypothesized that marriage might be an effect of high subjective well-being rather than simply a cause of it. Headey, Veenhoven, and Wearing (1991) used a longitudinal panel survey to examine the direction of influence between variables. Even experimental designs are sometimes possible (e.g. Kozma, Stone, Stones, Hannah, & McNeil, 1990; Pavot & Diener, 1993a). For instance, Fujita (1993) found in an experimental assignment of college roommates that social comparison did not influence satisfaction judgments. Thus, there are more powerful designs to determine the causes of subjective well-being than simple cross-sectional correlations, and these designs should be used more frequently.

Divergent Validity

The divergent validity of subjective well-being measures has been extensively explored at the single-measure level. For example, a meta-analysis by Okun and Stock (1987) showed that subjective well-being measures were moderately associated with adjustment (0.38), with neuroticism (0.33) with work satisfaction (0.33), and with family satisfaction (0.29), but were more substantially related to each other (0.52). Although SWB is highly related, as would be expected, with constructs such as optimism (Carver & Gaines, 1987) and self-esteem (Diener & Emmons, 1985; Fordyce, 1988), these correlations do not approach unity. For example, Marshall, Wortman, Kusulas, Hervig, and Vickers (1992) found an average correlation between optimism and positive affect of 0.35 and an average correlation between pessimism and negative affect of 0.27.

Another finding which points to the divergent validity of SWB scales is the fact that additional variables can predict subjective well-being beyond the predictive power of variables to which SWB might be seen as identical (E. Diener, and M. Diener, 1993). For example, extraversion and neuroticism are both predictors of SWB and might be viewed as the temperament underpinnings to a predilection towards positive and negative affect, respectively. Agreeableness and conscientiousness, however, predict SWB incrementally over the influence of E and N (McCrae & Costa, 1991). Furthermore, Costa and McCrae (1980) found that the average correlation between positive affect and extraversion was 0.20, while between negative affect and neuroticism it was 0.38. These findings suggest that extraversion and neuroticism, although correlates of SWB, cannot be seen as synonymous with SWB. The fact that subjective well-being reacts to life changes and life events (e.g., Atkinson, 1982; Ormel & Schaufeli, 1991; Tran, Wright, & Chatters, 1991) also indicates that it is not isomorphic with personality traits.

More sophisticated approaches to the divergent validity of SWB scales using multi-method matrices or confirmatory factor analyses are rare. Larsen and Diener (1985), using MTMM, found that hedonic level was independent of emotional intensity. Andrews and Withey (1976) found in several studies that global evaluations of one's life formed a core cluster which was separable from satisfaction with various life domains. Smith, Pope, Rhodewalt, and Poulton (1989) found, however, that the LOT measure of optimism correlated as strongly with negative affect as with an alternative measure of optimism. Fujita (1991) employed LISREL and found that extraversion and long-term positive affect were highly related constructs and found that long-term negative affect and neuroticism were not distinguishable. Similarly, Watson and Clark (1984) have argued that negative affectivity and neuroticism are the same thing. Positive and negative affect, however, each appear to make independent contributions to life satisfaction (Pavot & Diener, 1993b).

Clearly, a more systematic mapping of the interrelation of subjective well-being and related constructs is needed. Such a mapping must bebased on the use of multiple measures for each construct so that the effects of error can be assessed and the relation of both manifest variables and latent traits can be estimated. In addition, it would be valuable to explore the relation of personality measures such as extraversion, optimism, and neuroticism to both shorter- and longer-term measures of positive and negative affect because short-term measures of SWB may be more strongly affected by events, whereas longer-term measures may be more strongly tied to temperament.

Advancing Subjective Well-Being Measurement: Developments in Other Areas of Psychology

The evidence reviewed above indicates that coherent levels of longterm well-being exist, and that the typical self-report measurement of SWB produces psychometric indices that are as good or better than those in many areas. Nevertheless, recent advances in a number of subdisciplines of psychology indicate that the exclusive reliance on self-report measures of SWB has limitations. and that theoretical and empirical advances are probable if additional types of measures are employed.

The study of subjective well-being has its roots in survey research. One of the early scales simply asked respondents "how things are these days," and gave them three response choices: "very happy," "pretty happy," and "not too happy" (Gurin, Veroff, & Feld, 1960). Although recent scales such as the Satisfaction with Life Scale (Diener, Emmons, Larsen, & Griffin, 1985) tend to use more items, and offer more finely graded response options, they still rely on straightforward self-reports. Yet, in recent years progress in various areas such as emotion theory and cognitive psychology have important implications for the way SWB is conceived and for the self-report measurement of well-being. I review several of the relevant advances below, and explicate their implications for the measurement of well-being. Next, the ramifications of these findings for definitions and theory are discussed, and additional measurement method are described.

The Multiple Components of Emotion

The reader is referred to Frijda (1986), Lazarus (1991), and Oatley and Jenkins (1992) for more complete discussions of emotion. Emotion is defined here following Lazarus (1991), as organized psychophysiological reactions which occur because of self-relevant information in the environment (p. 38). It is now widely agreed that emotion is composed of behavioral, nonverbal, motivational, physiological, experimental, and cognitive components (Scherer, 1984). For example, Plutchik (1984) defines emotions as a response to a stimulus which involves experienced feeling, neural and autonomic arousal, goal directed behavior, expressive reactions, and appraisal.

Many emotions evidence typical facial expressions (Ekman, Friesen, & Ellsworth, 1972; Izard, 1971). Smiling for joy is a cultural universal (e.g., Ekman, 1984). Cacioppo, Petty, Losch, and Kim (1986) discovered that even when facial muscle movements are not visible, EMG activity occurs in the face in reaction to emotional stimuli. Emotions include nonobservable events such as subjective experience, as well as appraisal and coping processes (Lazarus, 1991). Emotions are also accompanied by action readiness (e.g., Frijda, 1986), a motor component (Zajonc, 1984a). For instance, angry persons show physical preparation for attack and fearful persons evidence a readiness to flee. The physiological component of emotion includes activation of the autonomic system, and emotional feelings are often accompanied by physiological reactions (Ekman, Levenson, & Friesen, 1983). Thus, emotion appears to be a complex process, with experience being only one component. Furthermore, there is now mounting evidence that although the various components of emotion do covary, they show some degree of independence (e.g., Frijda, 1986; Leventhal, 1984; Schwartz, 1982; Tyrer, 1976; Zajonc, 1984b). Therefore a measure of one component is not a sure indicator of other components of the emotion system. The self-reports of affective well-being which form the basis of the vast majority of SWB research rely almost totally on cognitive labelling of emotions, and thus largely ignore the remaining parts of the emotion system. Because the labelling of emotions reflected in self-reports do not give a complete view of the affective life of an individual.

Compounding the limitations of self-report, if respondents are asked to report their emotional well-being, the researcher depends on subjects labelling their emotions in the same way that the experimenter and other subjects do. This is not always a safe assumption (Kagan, 1984). For example, my mother claims never to have been unhappy in her life, although she will admit to being sad or fearful. Apparently she uses the word "unhappy" in a way that makes her self-reports not comparable to the reports of many other people. The issue is not whether she is right or wrong, but rather that individuals, cohorts, or other groups may not give the exact same meaning to words. Because it is likely that individuals, groups, and cultures use emotion labels differently (Russell, 1991) a total reliance on self-reports of emotion is risky.

Thus, if we are to validly assess the affective portion of SWB, we must examine more than the cognitive labels respondents give their emotions. In addition to the imprecision and variability of emotion words, the fact that emotion has a number of components which are only moderately correlated makes it imperative that we assess other emotion channels if we want to obtain a complete picture of people's affective well-being.

It might be argued that self-report is the only way to assess the experiential component of emotion, and that subjective well-being is most related to subjective experience. It is not self-evident, however, that self-reports are either direct measures of experience or the only measures of experience. For example, behavioral preferences and depth of processing memory measures might be just as valid measures of experience. Self-reports do not have privileged status as the only measures of experience, and researchers should creatively engineer additional ways to assess subjective experience. As Izard (1992) wrote, "feeling states must be studied by multiple methods that yield convergent data" (p. 563).

Denial

Related to the emotional labelling problem described above is the fact that individuals may deny or ignore their emotional reactions. A modular view of the
brain (Gazzaniga, 1985) suggests that the sub-cortical centers from which emotions emanate show some degree of independence from the verbal center of the
brain (MacLean, 1975; Panksepp, 1982). For example, Haggard and Isaacs (1966)
found that patients showed momentary facial expressions of which they were not
aware when discussing emotionally conflictual topics. The language centers in the
left cerebral hemisphere may be partly dissociated from the emotion centers in the
right cerebral hemisphere (Borod, 1992; Galin, 1974), thus making verbal reports
of emotions imperfect indicants of other types of emotional reactions.

There are individual differences in the degree to which the components of emotion are dissociated. Recent work shows that some individuals strongly deny or
avoid their emotional reactions (e.g., Bonanno & Singer, 1990; Gudjonsson, 1981;
Schwartz, 1983; Weinberger, 1990). These individuals either do not label unpleasant emotions, do not attend to their emotional reactions, or isolate emotional information from their left cerebral hemisphere (Davidson, 1983). Yet these same
people show evidence that they are experiencing emotional reactions in nonverbal channels. For example, although avoiders deny negative emotions, they show
greater speech disfluencies under stress (Weinberger, Schwartz, & Davidson, 1979),
evidence greater physiological reactivity (e.g., King, Albright, Taylor, Haskell, &
Debusk, 1986; Levenson & Mades, 1980), and are rated as having greater facial
anxiety (Asendorpf & Scherer, 1983).

Although repression is usually not conceptualized in Freudian terms by modern
emotion theorists, most would agree that individuals differ in the degree to which
they attend to their emotional reactions. An edited volume by Singer (1990) presents
an excellent overview of the effects of denial and repressive coping on the memory
for unpleasant affective experiences. For example, Davis reviews evidence showing
that individuals identified as repressors have a more difficult time retrieving emotional experiences from memory. She found that "repressors" were able to remember many fewer emotional memories in a free recall task, but were almost equal
to nonrepressors in a cued recall task. Davis concluded that "repressors may be
individuals with a propensity to engage in less elaborative processing of their own
emotional experiences, with a consequent reduction in the richness of associative
pathways among affect-related experiences stored in memory" (p. 402). This line of
research suggests that personality may influence subjective well-being, not simply in
terms of temperament propensities to experience specific types of affect, but also in
terms of certain individuals avoiding emotional reactions. Multi-channel emotional
assessment thus becomes imperative because the researcher otherwise cannot fully
understand the cause of self-reported levels of negative affect.

Assessing denial. There are a number of scales to assess individual differences in
denial of distress or the avoidance of emotional feelings (e.g., Weinberger, 1990).
Other measures have also been used to assess denial or avoidance of emotion:
The Crowne-Marlowe Scale of Social Desirability (usually in combination with

an anxiety scale), Byrne's Repression-Sensitization Scale, and a dichotic listening task (Bonanno & Singer, 1990). When used in conjunction with self-report SWB measures, these scales may help the researcher interpret the SWB responses. For example, subjective well-being may be interpreted in a different light for emotional avoiders versus nonavoiders. The subjective well-being of emotional avoiders may be accompanied by stress in other channels, for example in physiological reactions. In contrast, if an emotional nonavoider reports a high level of SWB, it is more likely that she will show a dearth of negative emotional reactions in other channels as well. Differences between self-report and reports by knowledgeable informants or behavioral information can also be employed to help infer the denial of negative emotions. Physiological recordings have also been used; if a person reacts in the physiological channel, but says he is not feeling emotional, denial might be inferred. Finally, emotionally avoidance may be present if a person denies feeling unpleasant emotions, but the presence of negative affect is evident in mood sensitive tasks. Discrepancies will sometimes be noted between self-reports and measures which depend more heavily on nonself-report channels. When self-reports yield less negative affect, the investigator might suspect emotional avoidance or denial. The inclusion of other scales such as those measuring avoidance or self-presentation (Paulhus, 1988) will also aid in diagnosing avoidance. Further, an anonymity-identifiability manipulation can also help separate self-presentation from emotional avoidance effects. If an anonymity manipulation has no influence on responses, emotional avoidance would be suspected in the case in which self-reports reveal less unpleasant affect than nonself-report items.

In order to fully understand the nature of a group's SWB, we need to understand the role that denial or avoidance coping plays in their emotional life. For example, Allman (1990) found that the SWB report of wheelchair-bound respondents correlated very highly with their Crowne-Marlowe scores, and this might indicate that repression of negative affect was integral to the happiness of the disabled subjects. At this time there appear to be two major approaches to assessing the denial of negative affect: direct measures of denial such as Weinberger's scales, and searching for a discrepancy between self-reports and other types of measures.

Conclusion. It is evident that scientists cannot gain a complete measure of people's emotional reactions only from self-report. Self-reported affect and reactions in other emotional channels show only moderate convergence. Certain people do not admit to emotional reactions, but may show motoric, physiological, and facial evidence of affective responses. Some individuals have a more difficult time retrieving emotional material from memory. Thus, researchers must employ additional measures besides self-reports to tap the nonverbal channels of emotion and to veridically assess emotional reactions across individuals.

Emotion is Multifaceted

In addition to the various response components of emotion described earlier, affect also varies in other ways besides simple hedonic level or valence. For example, there are a number of separate unpleasant emotions such as sadness, fear and anger

(Izard, 1972; Plutchik, 1980; Tomkins & McCarter, 1964), and describing the emotions only as "negative affect" may lose substantial information. Furthermore, in addition to mean hedonic level, we can also describe emotions in terms of peak amplitude and variability. For instance, two individuals who possess the same average hedonic level may differ greatly in emotional intensity (Larsen & Diener, 1987) or emotional variability (Diener & Larsen, 1986). Current measures of SWB fail to capture the full richness of emotional life. The following examination of the relation of the duration versus peak amplitude of emotion to SWB demonstrates that a more intricate conception of emotional life would be beneficial. Although aspects of emotion such as duration and intensity are not fully understood, ignoring these distinctions or lumping them together will hardly produce better understanding.

Time and intensity of emotions. Diener, Sandvik, and Pavot (1990) argue that the total amount of time a person experiences pleasant emotions versus unpleasant emotions (regardless of the peak intensity of emotions experienced) forms the basis of affective well-being. Diener et al. (1990) found that the relative frequency of pleasant affect was necessary and sufficient to produce high scores on both self-report and nonself-report well-being measures. In support of this conclusion, Andrews and Withey (1976) found that a question assessing the frequency of pleasant versus unpleasant emotions over time loaded most highly of 50 global well-being measures on the central component of subjective well-being.

In terms of evidence showing that peak intensity contributes little to global SWB as currently measured, Larsen and Diener (1985) discovered that emotional intensity was distinct from SWB in a multitrait-multimethod examination of long-term affect measures, and Larsen et al. (1985) found that emotional intensity and well-being measures loaded on two separate factors. Diener et al. (1990) offer a number of reasons why intense positive emotions are not as strongly related to well-being as are frequent positive experiences. Chief among these reasons is that intense positive emotions are very rare (thus contributing little to long-term well-being), and that intense positive emotions often have countervailing costs (Diener et al., 1991). Intense emotions are rare—extremely intense joy was virtually never reported by college age students (Diener et al., 1990). In contrast, some level of pleasant affect was reported by college students over 70% of the time. Thus, the amount of time one experiences pleasant affect can have a greater influence than the rare intense moments. In terms of countervailing costs, intense positive emotions often follow unpleasant emotional periods and often depend on psychological conditions which would have resulted in intense negative emotions had circumstances not turned out favorably. Thus, the long-run effect of intense pleasant emotions may not be that positive because their net effect may be slight when countervailing unpleasant emotions are also considered (see Diener et al., 1991, for a more thorough exposition).

Thus, a tenable hypothesis is that global emotional SWB can be defined as the proportion of time one experiences pleasant emotions. I note, however, that even if peak intensity does not strongly influence the level of SWB reported by a respondent, it is likely to influence the quality of the person's emotional life. Two people could be equally "happy," but might experience their happiness in different ways if one has low intensity emotions and the other has large mood swings. The evidence that SWB depends more directly on the time/duration of pleasant emotions than on their intensity is tentative. If, however, SWB researchers systematically assess various aspects of emotion such as duration, intensity, and variability, a more definitive conclusion can be reached regarding how various parameters of emotion influence SWB.

Positive and negative affect. In recent years it has become debatable whether one should combine pleasant and unpleasant emotions into a single valence score. An unexpected finding in mood research is that positive and negative emotions often form independent dimensions (Bradburn, 1969; Diener & Emmons, 1985; Zevon & Tellegen, 1982). In addition, a number of investigators have discovered different correlates for pleasant and unpleasant affect (Beiser, 1974; Costa and McCrae, 1980; Emmons & Diener, 1985; Headey, Holmstrom, & Wearing, 1985; Lawton, 1983). Baker, Cesa, Garz, and Mellins (1992) trace different environmental and genetic influences for positive and negative affect. Despite these findings, the independence of pleasant and unpleasant emotions is still a contentious issue (e.g., Diener & Emmons, 1985; Watson, 1988) and the empirical work is mixed. For example, several researchers have found a strong inverse correlation between positive and negative affect (e.g., Kammann, Christie, Irwin, & Dixon, 1979; Zautra, Guarnaccia, & Reich, 1988), whereas others have found tiny correlations between the two (e.g., Zevon & Tellegen, 1982).

How can we reconcile the discrepant findings on the relation of pleasant and unpleasant affect? Investigators have found that the relation between the two depends on the time frame sampled (Diener & Emmons, 1985; Staats, Partlo, & Adam, 1989), on the intensity of the emotions sampled (Diener & Emmons, 1985; Diener and Iran-Nejad, 1986; Watson, 1988), on the type of response scale used (Brenner, 1975; Warr, Barter, & Brownbridge, 1983), on the particular pleasant and unpleasant emotions sampled (Watson, 1988), on whether verbal or nonverbal measures are employed (Ketelaar, 1989), and on whether acquiescence response set is controlled (Lorr, Qing Shi, & Youniss, 1989). Therefore, a simple answer as to whether positive and negative affect are independent is not possible. Strict independence of positive and negative affect are found when a restricted set of mood adjectives is factor analyzed, and a varimax rotation is applied (which guarantees independence).

Diener and Iran-Nejad (1986) found that the relationship between positive and negative emotions is not homoscedastic. The relation between pleasant and unpleasant affect formed an L pattern rather than the "cigar" ellipse of homoscedastic correlations. The L pattern emerged because at a low level of intensity of one type of emotion, people could feel virtually any level of the other types of emotion, from very low to very high. Although low levels of the two types of emotion frequently occurred together, intense levels never occurred together. This pattern thus suggests that simple correlations and factor analysis might not fully capture the complex relation between the two types of emotion at varying levels of intensity.

Another problem is that factor analysis may be an inappropriate analytical tool because the trace line between mood adjective words and the underlying emotional feeling is not monotonic. For many mood words of intermediate intensity, a person may report feeling just as much of them when expressing a feeling a distance below that mood word as when he or she is the same distance above that mood word. For such data, Coombs's (1964) unfolding analysis might be a more appropriate statistical technique than is factor analysis.

Green, Goldman, and Salovey (1993) showed that measures of positive and negative affect varied inversely, but only at modest levels. When measurement error was controlled through a latent factor analysis based on multiple measures, however, the two correlated inversely at an extremely strong level. Diener, Fujita, and Smith (1993) followed up this lead by examining both discrete emotions and positive and negative affect using a LISREL analysis of multiple measures of each construct. They found that positive and negative affect were statistically separable into two factors even though they were strongly inversely correlated when measurement error was controlled. That is, positive and negative affect were clearly separable, although not orthogonal, thus suggesting that they should be measured separately. Furthermore, there were relations between specific discrete emotions which could not be accounted for by the general structure, indicating that for some purposes it will also be useful to separately assess specific emotions. They found, however, strong convergence between the positive emotions and between the negative emotions. This indicates that global positive affect and negative affect are useful categories and account for much of the variance in discrete emotions.

Conclusion. A simple self-report of mean hedonic level is unlikely to capture the full complexity of emotional well-being. Although positive and negative affect may not be entirely independent, it nevertheless seems desirable to separately assess each because they show some degree of autonomous variation, at least under certain measurement conditions. Furthermore, in many SWB studies, scientists can also assess specific emotions such as anger, fear, joy, and sadness because global pleasant and unpleasant emotion categories may not fully capture important differences between people in emotional experience. In addition, measurement methods which allow the assessment of dimensions such as peak intensity, emotional episode duration, and total time experiencing specific emotions will yield a much more unabridged picture of people's emotional lives. For this reason, experience sampling methods in which people's emotions are sampled over time will be described in future sections. Many previous measures of SWB give a single summary score of respondents' emotional lives. Clearly, such a single score is unlikely to capture the richness of a person's emotional well-being. At the same time, individuals in single session self-reports are unlikely to be able to accurately separate out and report complex facets of their emotional experiences. Thus, measures which validly capture additional emotions and dimensions seem desirable.

Cognitive Processing of Self-Report Items

The conventional view of SWB measures assumes that people simply access their state of morale from memory and then report it. But people must search for information in memory and perform computations on that information in order to give a report in acceptable form. Torangeau and Rasinski (1988), in discussing a model of attitudes which is applicable to well-being measurement, suggest that respondents must interpret attitude questions, search working and long-term memory for relevant information, and seek standards of comparison in order to present appropriate output. People must construct an answer to self-report measures based on information stored in memory. Because individuals rely on search, computational, and constructivist processes in order to arrive at the answer to self-report SWB items, scores are often influenced by situational factors which affect these processes.

Memory. In order to answer well-being questions, subjects must consult working and/or long-term memory and construct their report based on the material in consciousness. It is well known that people will often use heuristic shortcuts (Kahneman, Slovic, & Tversky, 1982) rather than thoroughly search their memory for answers to questions. Because the amount of information available on which well-being judgments can be made is enormous, the respondent is usually forced to take short-cuts. Whereas some information required is not easily available in memory or is stored in incomplete fashion, other information is readily available because it was recalled more recently (Wyer & Srull, 1989). For example, Skelton and Strohmetz (1990) demonstrated that priming can influence the reporting of physical symptoms. Larsen (1992) has shown that neuroticism influences the selective recall of physical symptoms compared to symptoms reported on a daily basis. A number of studies have shown that prior questions can influence responses to the subsequent well-being items (Schwarz and Strack, 1991; Sinclair, Mark, & Wellens, 1989; Wellens, Tanaka, & Panter, 1989), possibly because these questions make specific information more salient to the respondents.

Memory biases also depend on the dimensions of mood which are retrieved. Thomas and Diener (1990) found that subjects tend to overestimate their emotional intensity, but underestimate the frequency of their positive affect. They found that subjects were somewhat accurate at estimating the relevant frequency of their emotions, but very poor at estimating the intensity of their unpleasant emotions. Furthermore, negative intensity estimates were biased by the frequency of the emotions. Diener, Larsen, and Emmons (1984) found that happy individuals overestimated their average positive affect and that unhappy individuals overestimated their average negative affect.

Another type of memory bias revolves around subject's current mood. Because of state-dependent and mood-congruent effects (Blaney, 1986), people may recall more positive experiences when in a good mood, and may therefore overestimate their degree of long-term happiness if in that state. Similarly, people may be able to recall more negative experiences when in a bad mood, and therefore give a lower SWB estimate when in that state.

To further complicate matters, memory seems to be a constructive process rather than a retrieval of discrete information (Mandler, 1985). What this means is that the respondent will not simply recall an accurate picture of his past emotional life. The memories are constructed or reconstructed by subjects depending of their beliefs, and other material in consciousness at the time. Thus, single-occasion reports of long-term mood obviously do not perfectly reflect an individual's on-line affective reactions.

Controlling memory effects. One way to obtain memories which accurately represent the person's life is to lead respondents through a life review before presenting the well-being questions. Such a life review can decrease the chances that one salient memory will exert a disproportionate influence on the SWB report. Another alternative is to use experience sampling (e.g., Csikszentmihalyi and Larson, 1987), including audio tape or portable computer aided recording, to gain a relatively accurate picture of on-line mood. In experience sampling, the researcher relies on memory because she asks respondents how they feel at the moment. Similarly, we can obtain satisfaction ratings on a daily basis over a period of time to reduce recall biases (e.g., Pavot et al., 1991). Procedures which shorten the time period on which respondents report and which reinforce the subjects for systematically searching memory should enhance accuracy and thereby increase the validity of measures. If daily or moment reports are obtained over a long enough time period, an estimation of the subjects' long-term SWB can be made. Nevertheless, self-reports of emotion over time are still subject to some of the other artifacts mentioned above. Further, the reactive effects of experience sampling or daily recording (Hammen & Glass, 1975; Harmon, Nelson, & Hayes, 1980) have not yet been studied in depth.

Mood as information. Because a thorough memory search is so difficult and time-consuming, participants may simply consult their mood at the moment in order to determine their subjective well-being (Schwarz & Clore, 1983). Schwarz and Strack (1991) showed that both life satisfaction and happiness judgments can be affected by current moods (see also Kozma et al., 1990). Even seemingly trivial factors such as sunny weather or finding a dime in a phone booth can induce people to report higher life satisfaction scores! People can discount the effect of their current mood if attention is called to it, but otherwise use this easily available mood information to give a quick answer to well-being questions.

Diener et al. (1991) reasoned that in real testing situations current mood often is not a problem because it correlates moderately with enduring mood. They suggested that the correlation between long-term mood and current mood implies that the constant variance added by current mood is usually nonspurious, whereas the error variance would tend to be random because of the multiplicity of other factors influencing current mood. They examined the effects of current mood on SWB measures after controlling for the effects of long-term mood as measured by nonself-report measures such as peer reports. Diener et al. (1991) found that on one measurement occasion out of three, current mood added significantly to the prediction of happiness measures taken at that time, although the effect was modest. They concluded that the influence of current mood on happiness scales is often slight, but is certainly worth controlling and measuring.

Moods generated by the interview situation are of particular concern. For example, Schwarz and Strack (1991) report that individuals who were asked about a recent hospitalization thereafter reported less well-being. Similarly, Lehman, Wortman, and Williams (1987) found that people who lost a spouse or child in an auto accident many years earlier still reported being less happy. It could be, however, that the reminder of the loss by the interviewer created a negative mood which then influenced their well-being report. A related complication is that influences such as current mood could also affect the reporting of other variables such as life events (Cohen, Towbes, & Flocco, 1988). Thus, correlations might result from the influence of current mood on both well-being reports and on the independent variables.

Controlling current mood effects. We can infer the influence of current mood on global SWB reports by measuring both current mood and longer-term subjective well-being. If groups differ to a greater degree in standardized terms on current mood than they do on long-term well-being estimates, there is a chance that a current mood artifact could be operating. We can control the influence of current mood by assessing well-being on several occasions and by insuring that testing is conducted so that a population's current mood at the time of testing is likely to be similar to its long-term average. For example, if a researcher wanted to assess long-term mood, she would not want to study a group entirely on sunny spring days after a dreary winter, or after the local team won a championship. Finally, researchers must be alert to factors within the interview (e.g., prior questions) which could influence the mood of participants.

Scaling. A number of situational and individual difference variables can influence how subjects use response scales. Schwarz and Strack (1991) and Branscombe and Diener (1987) showed that moods and events can serve as contrast or assimilation anchors when well-being judgements are made. For example, people reporting a hospitalization in the distant past reported greater happiness because this unhappy event served as a contrast anchor (Schwarz and Strack, 1991). Similarly, when subjects heard another person tell of an unfortunate medical condition, they rated their own life satisfaction as higher. Finally, when a handicapped person was in their visual field, subjects also reported more happiness (Strack, Schwarz, Chassein, Kern, & Wagner, 1990). In contrast, reports of one's own *recent* hospitalization lowered well-being responses because of the information these reports contained on one's current life. In a similar vein, Dermer, Cohen, Jacobsen, and Anderson (1979) found that people rated their lives as worse or better depending on whether they had previously read descriptions which painted a favorable or unfavorable picture of past living conditions.

In addition to the contrast and assimilation effects noted above, there is the problem that individuals may use scale responses differently. For example, how can we be sure that one respondent's "4" is higher than another subject's "3," much less know the size of the interval between the two responses? Diener et al. (1990) contend that scales which measure the time people experience various types of affect are in principle of ratio quality. A person who experiences pleasant affect 80% of the time is twice as happy in a meaningful sense compared to a person who feels it 40% of the time. Therefore, if we can accurately assess frequency of pleasant and unpleasant affect (e.g., with the experience sampling method), strong scale properties might exist even across individuals. In contrast, scales which assess the intensity of affect might not even be ordinal. For instance, one person's "very intense" emotion may be less intense than another's "moderately intense" emotion.

Controlling scaling effects. Several procedures in psychometrics are utilized to reduce the scaling problems noted above. One is to provide subjects with concrete anchors for each choice so that responses are more likely to mean the same thing from time to time and across subjects. Another precaution is to use constant conditions in testing so that transitory effects are reduced. Although we can control situational influences on scaling in part by standardized testing conditions, we can also assess them by using repeated measurements under systematically varying conditions. Nevertheless, as long as we rely entirely on self-reports to assess SWB, we cannot be sure to what degree an adjustment of the response scale (Tversky and Griffin, 1991) has influenced the subject's responses.

Conclusion. Experimental work on memory and scaling clearly demonstrates that one-time self-reports of well-being are not simple readouts of people's underlying state of SWB. Situational factors can influence what participants recall and how they scale their responses, and thus can influence self-reports of SWB. These facts point to the desirability of more sophisticated measurement of well-being.

Communication Effects

The need to communicate the answer to well-being questions to the experimenter can influence the responses subjects furnish. For example, when respondents were interviewed by an attractive experimenter, life satisfaction judgements were higher than when made anonymously. But when interviewed by a disabled experimenter, subjects reported lesshappiness, apparently because they did not want to appear too happy (Strack, Schwarz, & Wanke, 1990).

Hogan (1983) suggests that reports to questionnaires are self-presentations which follow certain strategies and norms. As such, it would be naive to interpret them in a way that does not recognize their dramaturgical quality. It is well known that respondents may adjust their output to create a desired impression. What is less well known is that there are additional communication effects involved in subjects' interpretations of the questions posed by the researcher.

Interpretation of questions. The context for subjects' interpretation of questions is provided both by the interview situation and by other preceding questions (Strack et al., 1991). For instance, an experimenter might ask a subject how satisfied she is with her work, and then with her family. In another study, the order of questions might be about satisfaction with the marriage, and then satisfaction with the family. In the first study, the subject's satisfaction with the family is likely to include information about the marriage because the family includes the spouse. But in the second study, the subject may interpret the family question to mean the family other than the spouse because information on marriage satisfaction was already requested. Schwarz and Strack (1991) interpret SWB responses within a "Gricean" communication framework (Grice, 1975) which asserts that one of the norms of communication is that it should not be redundant. Thus, differences between the two hypothetical studies above could result from the contextual meaning of the question, *even if an identical question were used.* If the marriage is viewed quite positively, the second study might find lower family satisfaction, even if the actual satisfaction were identical for the groups, because subjects are likely to omit a positive component from their family satisfaction response.

Social desirability. Different groups may possess varying norms for how desirable it is to be happy or how undesirable it is to be unhappy (Sommers, 1984). Furthermore, groups and cultures may differ in how normative it is to express or admit these emotions. Taylor (1977, p. 33) wrote, "Some cultures place considerable value on portraying life as a pain in the neck. Six to 8% of the inhabitants of most modern countries admit to unhappiness but about half of Frenchmen do so." The implication is that the French appear more happy because of a norm which approves the expression of dissatisfaction with life. Such norms, however, might actually lead to experiencing more unpleasant emotions. Thus, we should investigate normative differences in terms of their producing both actual and artifactual differences in well-being. We can measure norms for happiness—the degree to which individuals believe that experiencing pleasant or unpleasant affect or specific emotions is appropriate and desirable. We can also assess the degree to which subjects believe that *expressing* certain emotions is desirable. Differences between groups in reported well-being can then be interpreted in light of group norms for experiencing or expressing positive and negative emotions. Ouweneel and Veenhoven (1991) and Diener et al. (1994) concluded that differences in desirability had little influence on reports of subjective well-being.

The effects of situational social desirability in terms of varying anonymity of responses is another potential problem. Because being happy is often considered normatively desirable (Sommers, 1984), people may report higher levels of happiness when queried in a face-to-face interview than on an anonymous questionnaire (King and Buchwald, 1982; Smith, 1979; Sudman, 1967), although studies on this issue are mixed (Fujita et al., 1993).

Conclusion. A variety of communication effects may influence self-reports of SWB and make them less reliable indicators of people's long-term emotional states. First, impression management effects are problematical in some testing situations. Furthermore, social desirability may differ from group to group and testing situation to testing situation. Finally, communication effects are not simply self-presentational; the interview situation can also influence the way subjects interpret questions.

Systematically varying anonymity can be used profitably to assess the degree to which group averages reflect a propensity on the part of respondents to appear happy to others. For example, King and Buchwald (1982) found that men and women both increased their happiness responses when interviewed nonanonymously, but that this difference was approximately equivalent for both sexes. This finding suggested that a desire to seem happy to others does not differentially influence the reports of men and women. Other ways of inferring self-presentational effects are through social desirability scales (e.g., Paulhus, 1988) and through the comparison of scores from traditional SWB scales with scores from scales which control social desirability (e.g., Sandvik et al., 1993). Finally, we can assess people's norms for being happy, and for communicating this to others. If people differ in their beliefs about the desirability of being happy or acting happy, their SWB responses can be interpreted in this light.

Advancing the Theoretical Definition of Subjective Well-Being

In light of the findings from other fields, we can now move forward in terms of defining and measuring subjective well-being. Recall that SWB was defined earlier as people's evaluations of their lives. These evaluations might be assessed both in terms of cognitive appraisals (satisfaction) and in term of affect (the pleasantness of one's moods and emotions resulting from the appraisals of ongoing events in the person's life). It is now possible to define SWB in more sophisticated and complex ways.

Cognition and Life Satisfaction

Compelling findings in cognitive psychology, especially from the laboratories of Fritz Strack and Norbert Schwarz, indicate that it may be incorrect to think that people usually simply recall a stored life satisfaction judgment and report it. Instead, people seem to form a life satisfaction judgment in response to the interview situation. Because they form the judgment at the moment, it can be influenced by the memories and life domains which are salient at the time, as well as by what comparison standards are particularly prominent. This reasoning suggests that life satisfaction for most people is not likely to be a Platonic form, stored in a discrete and simple way. Rather, it is a complex judgment which can be altered and updated. As such, it can be subject to the influence of current mood and of situational influences which make certain memories of life domains salient. At the same time, life satisfaction judgments are likely to show some stability because many people have made and stored judgments about specific aspects of their lives, and because the life circumstances on which life judgments rest tend to be stable.

The implications of conceptualizing life satisfaction as an ongoing judgment which is updated in terms of the immediate situation are manifold. First, it will not be possible to measure the exact level of life satisfaction because it is not an entity which is invariant. It is a judgment which will depend on how the respondent makes the valuation and under what circumstances. This means that many factors must be similar in order to compare life satisfaction judgments made in different studies. Further, it means that it will be desirable to measure life satisfaction on a number of occasions if the researcher is interested in obtaining a long-term stable average. On the other hand, differences in life satisfaction in various circumstances become the object of legitimate inquiry when life satisfaction is thought of in this way. Variations in life satisfaction judgments will not necessarily be conceived as arising entirely from measurement error, but may come about because of the situations in which the judgments are made.

Differences in comparison standards are one reason that life satisfaction judgments may vary. Such differences, however, need not be thought of narrowly in terms of the problem of inducing individuals to all use the same standards. People may actually compare their lives to different standards in different circumstances. They may use an absolute standard in terms of their ideals, to their goals, but people may also compare to other persons, to their ideals, to their past, and so forth. The differences in life satisfaction resulting from comparison to different standards need not be thought of as measurement error. Rather, these differences can be thought of as theoretically interesting variations in the way life judgments are made.

The need to communicate life satisfaction judgments to others may change the actual judgment made. It is not simply that respondent may retrieve a judgment, but alter it at output because he wants to regulate the impression made on the researcher. It may be that the respondent actually considers different information and constructs a different life satisfaction judgment depending on the specific interview situation. Once again, situational influences on satisfaction judgments are important to study.

What this line of reasoning suggests is the importance of examining the processes by which people make life satisfaction judgments. Rather than being seen as error, differences in life satisfaction judgments become the object of exciting scientific work. Of course, the baby must not be thrown out with the bath water. There are some long-term coherencies to life satisfaction judgments, and the source of these coherencies is a legitimate question for researchers. Although transient factors can influence life satisfaction judgments, it is also interesting to explore why there are stabilities in life satisfaction across many years and across situations.

Emotion and Hedonic Level

Subjective well-being theorists can also learn much from recent work on emotion. For example, it is now widely agreed that there are important discrete emotions such as fear, anger, sadness, and joy. It is still not agreed whether these discrete emotions have separate biological bases, or whether they rest on prototypical appraisals which are likely to be universal in all cultures. Nevertheless, both theoretical (e.g., Izard, 1971) and empirical (Shaver, Schwartz, Kirson, & O'Connor, 1987) work has arrived at the conclusion that there are a finite number of important emotions which are separable. This suggests that SWB researchers often should, when time permits, assess a number of specific emotions rather than global hedonic level. Individuals may arrive at the same hedonic level through different emotional paths. Thus, understanding the correlates of hedonic level will be aided by knowledge of the specific pleasant and unpleasant emotions which individuals experience. Furthermore, subjective well-being can now be defined more specifically as comprising certain emotions which are unpleasant (e.g., sadness, jealousy, and fear) and certain ones which are pleasant (e.g., affection and joy).

Similarly, defining and appraising subjective well-being can be improved by considering long-term emotion to have more facets than simple hedonic level, which is the average pleasantness level of a person's affect over time. Parameters such as a person's emotional intensity (Larsen & Diener, 1987), emotional range (Larsen & Cutler, 1992), and mood variability (Diener & Larsen, 1986) are also necessary to fully describe a person's affective life and subjective well-being. Two persons might have the same average hedonic level, but one may experience many varied and intense positive and negative emotions, whereas the other might experience a few mild emotions. Although their subjective well-being would be equivalent in terms of the average pleasantness of their affect, their quality of experience would be quite different. Furthermore, the antecedents and consequences of their emotions would likely be different. Thus, research on emotions suggests that a more complex assessment of long-term affect would benefit our understanding of subjective well-being.

A final way that advances in the field of emotion can contribute to our understanding of subjective well-being is by indicating which are the key components of emotion: action readiness, conscious experience, physiological reactions, nonverbal reactions such as vocal and facial parameters, and cognitive appraisals and labelling of emotions. The one-time measures of subjective well-being are like to heavily tap cognitive labelling aspects of emotion, and to some degree emotional experience. Other facets of emotion are less likely to be directly reflected in SWB self-report measures. Under most circumstances there will be incomplete agreement between measures of various emotional channels. For example, some individuals may deny negative emotions and not label them, even though they show signs of emotion in terms of action readiness or nonverbal behavior. Self-reports may be the best single measure of emotional experience, but they are limited in terms of the channels of emotion they are likely to accurately capture. Therefore, assessing additional emotional channels will help SWB researchers to determine the genesis of self-reports of affect, and yield a broader understanding of the emotional differences between individuals.

Time Frame and SWB Reports

Measures of subjective well-being can be phrased so that they reflect different time frames. For example, the SWLS item, "If I could live my life over, I would change almost nothing," is likely to elicit responses referring to a large segment of the person's life. In contrast, the SWLS item, "I am satisfied with my life," might draw responses which refer to the respondent's entire life or only to the person's present life. The causes and consequences of SWB measured in terms of different time frames are likely to differ. For example, temperament is likely to have a bigger influence on measures that have a longer-frame, and recent daily hassles will have a greater influence on measures which reflect a shorter time-frame. Although SWB researchers are interested in reactions which are not merely momentary mood, there is not a time frame which is "correct." Instead, different time frames all fall within the boundaries of subjective well-being and can produce interesting findings. But researchers should be aware that the time frame of their measures is likely to influence the correlations of SWB they uncover.

An additional issue about time is the fact that measures will differ in terms of accurately reflecting on-line experience. More reconstructive and judgmental processes will be involved for questions tapping long periods of time, whereas measures which rely on the experience sampling method will more accurately reflect on-line experience. Either variable might be of interest to the researcher, but she should understand the limitations of the measures used in terms of each phenomenon. Global measures given at a single session are unlikely to accurately reflect on-line emotional experiences, and are likely to be biased by memory heuristics as well as by the respondent's beliefs about his or her emotions. If the researcher desires to assess the respondent's construction of his or her emotions, the global measure is likely to be valuable. On the other hand, if the researcher uses an experience sampling or daily recording method, more fidelity is likely in the measure in reference to on-line emotional experience. But the measure is less likely to capture respondents' meta-moods—their conceptualization of their emotions.

The Satisfaction and Hedonic Level Relation

Finally, advances in the field of cognition, emotion, and personality suggest ways of conceptualizing the relation between life satisfaction and long-term affect. Just as life satisfaction arises from a judgment by the person of his or her life, affect also arises from cognitive appraisals. In the case of emotion, however, the appraisals are ongoing reactions to events. Thus, the emotion system produces hedonic level which is much more reactive to short-term life events. In contrast, life satisfaction judgments may take a more Olympian perspective and are more likely to involve a big picture of the person's life. Hassles or uplifts during the past week may have less impact on a life satisfaction judgment, whereas they may impact hedonic level substantially. In contrast, the fact that a person won the Nobel prize many years ago may substantially increase her life satisfaction, but may have little impact on her hedonic level over the last week. The relation between life satisfaction and hedonic level is likely to be substantial, but is unlikely to have one set value. The size of the relation will depend on the time frame of the affect and satisfaction questions, on the degree to which the person's conscious and unconscious motives differ, and on numerous other factors. Life satisfaction is dependent on global appraisals of life, appraisals which are guided to some extent by the immediate situation and current mood. Hedonic level, in contrast, is dependent on the on-line, often unconscious, appraisals the person makes of ongoing events. Such a conceptualization should aid SWB researchers in exploring the covariation between the two in a more theoretical way.

Contributions in other areas of psychology lead us to conceive of subjective well-being in a more differentiated, less monolithic way. The goal will then be, not to discover *the* cause of SWB, but rather to understand the antecedents of various types of SWB parameters. Subjective well-being cannot be considered to be a brute, incontrovertible fact, but will, like all scientific phenomena, depend on the types of measures used to assess it.

Developing New Measures

The evidence indicates that self-report measures of SWB are psychometrically adequate. At the same time, there are reasons to believe that the typical one-time self-reports of well-being, including my Satisfaction with Life Scale, have a host of potential shortcomings (e.g., see Diener & Fujita, 1994). We can greatly reduce the spurious influences on self-reports of SWB described earlier by using latent variables which depend on maximally different measures of the construct. It is also likely that multiple sources of nonself-report data such as those recommended below will better integrate the study of subjective well-being with basic psychological knowledge about emotion and cognition. Finally, the inclusion of additional types of measures in SWB batteries will yield a more complete picture of the various components of emotion. Thus, although self-report is usually the measure of choice if only one method of assessment can be used, additional types of measurement can help investigators triangulate and better understand the phenomenon. Below I describe a variety of new, nontraditional methods of SWB assessment:

a. Recording of nonverbal behaviors, either in natural settings or in reaction to stimuli sampled from the subjects' lives, can supplement self-reports. Paravo-cal, gestural, postural, and facial assessment can all give valuable information about subjects' emotions. For example, subjects could be videotaped while they are interviewed about their lives. Their micromomentary facial expressions and vocal tone could then be scored for emotional reactions, in addition to the verbal content of their answers. Some of the nonverbal channels such as vocal tone are less controllable than self-report (Babad, Bernieri, & Rosenthal, 1989; DePaulo & Rosenthal, 1979) and these are less likely to be contaminated by impression management. Further, these recordings will reflect emotional components which are not directly mediated by language.

b. Reports by significant other have potential as sources of information about well-being, although they have several inherent limitations. For example, because in-formants are not directly privy to their acquaintance's feelings, they must infer these from outward behaviors. Thus, their reports are more likely to be based on nonverbal behaviors and what the acquaintance says about his or her experiences. Further-more, informants may skew their reports so as to be positive about their friend. Finally, informants often see their acquaintance in only one setting, and thus may not know their friend's full range of emotions. Despite these limitations, informant reports are valuable because they provide another source of data with-out compounding the errors of self-report, and because they are likely to reflect a different mix of emotional components than self-report measures. Although these reports tend to primarily assess external manifestations of well-being, they are not subject to some of the same sources of error as self-report and are therefore complementary to it. Sandvik et al. (1993) found that when a number of infor-mant reports were aggregated, they converged substantially with other measures of SWB.

c. Although still in its infancy, the measurement of hormones and other physio-logical indices has promise. For example, electromyographic facial recording while a subject watches slides of her life and her close associates is a potential source of information. Similarly, cortisol, norepinephrine, and so forth could pro-vide alternative sources of information about a subject's emotional well-being. Vitaliano, Paulsen, Russo, and Bailey (1993) offer an excellent example of how life satisfaction may be related to heart rate reactivity and recovery. Physiological measures are not without flaws, but they have strengths which are complementary to those of self-report. For example, many physiological measures are unlikely to be altered by self-presentation effects.

d. Cognitive measures such as depth of processing have thus far received little attention in assessing well-being. We find that memory production measures of happy and unhappy events can provide valuable information about subjects' happiness (Sandvik et al., 1993; Seidlitz & Diener, 1993) while being much less subject to some sources of error (e.g., self-presentational style) which are problematical for self-report. People high and low in subjective well-being are likely to differ in their chronically accessible constructs. Therefore, memory, priming, and attentional paradigms borrowed from experimental cognitive psychology offer promise as alternative measures of SWB.

e. Behavioral information (e.g., crying, sleep disturbances, alcohol consumption, activity level, and lack of appetite) offers another form of information about well-being.

f. Moods can be assessed on-line in the behavioral sampling technique pioneered by Csikszentmihalyi (e.g., Csikszentmihalyi, Larson, & Prescott, 1977). For a discussion of the validity and reliability of this technique, see Csikszentmihalyi and Larson (1987) and Hormuth (1986). Because people are "beeped" at random moments, and record their current moods immediately, there is much less chance for memory distortion than there is when one asks subjects to summarize information from long periods of time. An extension of this technique is to require respondents to write down their moods each evening for that particular day. Despite the obvious strengths of the experience sampling technique, problems such as reactivity have not been thoroughly explored. Nevertheless, the experience sampling method seems to be a more accurate way of assessing mood than requesting global self-reports.

g. The recording of cognitive content (e.g., thoughts about self-worth, goals, helplessness, and success) can provide additional information about SWB beyond emotion based self-reports. For example, people's thoughts can be sampled when they are beeped at random moments, and these cognitions can be coded for rumination, and so forth. Appraisals of important life situations by the respondent would also be a valuable method for gaining a more complete assessment of respondents' SWB.

h. In-depth interviews about people's lives can provide qualitative information (Thomas and Chambers, 1989; Wood and Johnson, 1989) on well-being which is not subject to number use artifacts. Another advantage of such data is that they can be customized to a specific respondent's life. In addition, qualitative material can then be rated by coders and such ratings may be more resistant to idiosyncratic differences in scaling between subjects.

i. Mood sensitive tasks are available (Clark, 1983; Friswell & McConkey, 1989; Goodwin & Williams, 1982; Hama & Tsuda, 1989; Ketelaar, 1989; Mayer, Mamberg, & Volanth, 1988) which could be used as indicants of a person's moods, especially when repeated over time. If mood sensitive tasks are used

on several occasions and indicate that a person is depressed or elated, a measure
of SWB is obtained which does not share many of the pitfalls of self-report. At
this time, it is not yet clear what types of mood sensitive tasks perform robustly
across age groups, and which tasks show mood effects which are not swamped
by stable individual differences in reaction time and so forth.
j. Tversky and Griffin (1991) remind us that economists rely on choice behavior as
   their major dependent variable, as a reflection of quality of life. SWB researcher
   also could use choice as a reflection of life satisfaction. For example, rather than
   simply obtain self-reports of satisfaction, a researcher could ask subjects which
   aspect of their lives they would choose to change and not change if they could do
   so. These descriptions could then be coded by raters for the degree of change the
   person would like in her life.

Clinical psychologists have long been wary of an uncritical acceptance of self-
reports, and therefore have often sought additional information about their clients in
behavioral measures, in nonverbal signs of emotion, and in the reports of significant
others. It is time that SWB researchers adopt such a catholic approach to assessment.
Where the measures converge, greater confidence can be placed in the results. If the
measures diverge, the researcher can gain greater insights into how and why groups
and individuals differ in SWB. Although additional measures can be expensive and
time-consuming, their use seems imperative if we are to truly understand the SWB
differences between groups.

Applied Research: The Survey Practitioner

What recommendations can be given to the survey researcher who has limited time
with each respondent and who cannot use intrusive methods (e.g., physiological
recording)? Survey field workers can systematically introduce a number of factors into the assessment session to increase the validity of their measures. Interviewers can allow adequate time for subjects to consider their responses, can reinforce careful responding, and can repeat wording and give very explicit instructions
(Stimson, 1988). Naturally, it is desirable to keep these behaviors constant across
interviews.

Survey researchers should consider measuring at least the three major components of well-being: satisfaction, positive affect, and negative affect, and measures
of specific moods and emotions may be desirable as well. In addition, a measure
of current momentary mood is very desirable in survey situations because it will
allow the researcher to infer the influence of temporary mood states on the SWB
measures.

Survey researchers also should carefully consider the context in which the well-
being questions are asked. For example, the effects of question order must be considered. Instituting certain safeguards such as repeating the well-being questions at
both the beginning and end of the interview will pay dividends in terms of more

reliable measurement and as a check on contextual effects. When possible, researchers can administer well-being questions on two occasions in order to achieve a
more stable judgment. Finally, survey researchers can sometimes include brief alternative measures of well-being: (a) ratings of subjects' affective facial expressions,
(b) ratings of paravocal factors (for example, based on a tape recording), (c) memory
production measures of good and bad events or factors in the subjects' lives, and (d)
the questioning of informants.

Future Research

The issues outlined in this paper present exciting opportunities for study and theory
building. For instance, the new measures of well-being proposed above will require
much development and testing. There are many questions for future research, for
example:

a. Given the diversity of emotion theories, can we develop a common set of emotions which broadly reflect affective well-being across cultures? Will the pleasantness value of various emotions have to be assessed on an individual basis, or
   will it be possible to develop universal pleasantness or unpleasantness values for
   the basic emotions?
b. What is the relation of life satisfaction to emotional well-being? How do happiness and life satisfaction interrelate?
c. What factors influence emotional well-being as consciously labelled by the individual, and what factors influence emotional reactions which are not labelled?
d. To what degree does the pleasantness of an emotion covary with its degree of
   judged desirability or normativeness in a culture, and what factors influence this
   relation?
e. What is the influence of one's beliefs about happiness and of emotional self-
   presentation on happiness reports? To what degree is this influence spurious, and
   to what degree do these factors influence actual subjective well-being?
f. Can we develop an assessment battery which will reflect each of the components of affect and satisfaction, and optimally protect against likely self-report
   artifacts?

Conclusion

The study of subjective well-being is growing into a major area in the social sciences. It is imperative that we build this area on a solid measurement foundation.
The major message is simply this: SWB measures are good, but they can be better. Measures of subjective well-being often simply ask respondents how happy
or satisfied they are. These existing measures served surprisingly well during the

initial stages of study in this field. But measurement should be an increasingly sophisticated enterprise in any scientific area. Therefore, increasing the quality of well-being measures and theoretical definitions of well-being offers an important vehicle for the field to progress.

The theory and measurement of subjective well-being were not well connected in the past with related areas of psychology such as emotion and cognition. The present paper begins constructing bridges to these areas by discussing well-being measurement in terms of the components of emotion, the concept of emotional avoidance, and the role of memory and judgment in making satisfaction judgments. Because measurement is so intertwined with theory, it is natural that conceptual bridges between SWB and other areas of psychology begin in this area. Several major conclusions can be drawn from the material reviewed in this paper.

1. Whenever possible, researchers should use multiple measures of SWB, both to reduce and assess error of measurement, but also to assess the multiple components of SWB. Self-reports of subjective well-being are adequate in a traditional psychometric sense. If one could choose only one type of SWB measure, in most cases it would be a self-report instrument because such measures have shown acceptable levels of validity and reliability. Nevertheless, measurement of SWB can be improved considerably by the addition of other methods of measurement such as experience sampling. Self-report measures covary strongly enough with other types of measures to indicate that they are tapping some common SWB variance, but moderately enough to indicate that other types of measures will yield additional information.

2. A single score is likely to over-simplify the phenomenon of SWB. Multiple scores which capture multiple aspects of SWB such as various discrete emotions, emotional intensity, and life satisfaction are likely to lead to more sophisticated theories and understanding. Although positive and negative affect are not strictly independent in many measurement situations, they show enough unique variation and differing patterns of correlations with other variables to recommend that they be assessed separately.

3. Memory, judgment, and attentional processes must be considered in order to understand how respondents create their responses to SWB measures. Variations in these processes under varying measurement conditions can produce error variance in the measures which hitherto has been overlooked by researchers. Furthermore, understanding these processes will lead to a better theoretical understanding of subjective well-being.

4. Subjective well-being should not be reified as a concrete thing. There are clearly aspects of SWB which are often stable and consistent, and these coherencies are of deep scientific interest. Yet, it must be remembered that SWB is composed of a number of types of ongoing reactions in the individual, and these reactions will best be understood as processes, not as entities. At the same time, there are long-term stabilities and cross-situational consistencies in these processes which make the study of long-term well-being a defensible endeavor.

5. Researchers have often exclusively emphasized the negative reactions of individuals. Positive reactions in terms of pleasant affect and life satisfaction are of equal theoretical importance and should be afforded equal scientific attention.

In every area of the psychological sciences, concepts are originally conceived in relatively simple terms. Over time more complex views of these phenomena emerge, and measurement methods are created which reflect the more complex theoretical approach. The area of subjective well-being has been served by a relatively rudimentary concept of well-being, and the resulting measures have been extremely simple. Enough knowledge has now been accumulated, however, to indicate the needed advances in the concept of subjective well-being, and in this paper I recommend new measurement methods which reflect a more refined theory of what constitutes subjective well-being.

References

Alker, H. A., & Gawin, F. (1978). On the intrapsychic specificity of happiness. *Journal of Personality, 46,* 311–322.

Allman, A. L. (1990). *Subjective well-being of people with disabilities: Measurement issues.* Unpublished masters thesis, University of Illinois.

Andrews, F. M. (1991). Stability and change in levels and structure of subjective well-being: USA 1972 and 1988. *Social Indicators Research, 25,* 1–30.

Andrews, F. M., & Robinson, J. P. (1991). Measures of subjective well-being. In J. P. Robinson, P. Shaver, & L. Wrightsman (Eds.), *Measures of personality and social psychological attitudes* (pp. 61–114): San Diego: Academic Press.

Andrews, F. M., & Withey, S. B. (1976). *Social indicators of well-being: America's perception of life quality.* New York: Plenum.

Asendorpf, J. B., & Scherer, K. R. (1983). The discrepant repressor: Differentiation between low anxiety, high anxiety, and repression of anxiety by autonomic-facial-verbal patterns of behavior. *Journal of Personality and Social Psychology, 45,* 1334–1346.

Atkinson, T. (1982). The stability and validity of quality of life measures. *Social Indicators Research, 10,* 113–132.

Babad, E., Bernieri, F., & Rosenthal, R. (1989). Nonverbal communication and leakage in the behavior of biased and unbiased teachers. *Journal of Personality and Social Psychology, 56,* 89–94.

Baker, L. A., Cesa, I. L., Garz, M., & Mellins, C. (1992). Genetic and environmental influences on positive and negative affect: Support for a two-factor theory. *Psychology and Aging, 7,* 158–163.

Balatsky, G., & Diener, E. (1993). Subjective well-being among Russian students. *Social Indicators Research, 28,* 225–243.

Beiser, M. (1974). Components and correlates of mental well-being. *Journal of Health and Social Behavior, 15,* 320–327.

Blaney, P. H. (1986). Affect and memory: A review. *Psychological Bulletin, 99,* 229–246.

Blishen, B., & Atkinson, T. (1980). Anglophone and francophone differences in perceptions of the quality of life in Canada. In A. Szalai & F. M. Andrews (Eds.), *The quality of life: Comparative studies.* London: Sage.

Bonanno, G. A., & Singer, J. L. (1990). Repressive personality style: Theoretical and methodological implications for health and pathology. In J. L. Singer (Ed.), *Repression and dissociation: Implications for personality theory, psychopathology, and health* (pp. 455–470). Chicago: University of Chicago Press.

Borod, J. C. (1992). Interhemispheric and intrahemispheric control of emotion: A focus on unilateral brain damage. *Journal of Consulting and Clinical Psychology, 60,* 339–348.

Bradburn, N. M. (1969). *The structure of psychological well-being.* Chicago: Aldine.

Branscombe, N. R., & Diener, E. (1987). *Consequences of priming of emotions: contrast and assimilation effects.* Paper presented at the 95th Annual Meeting of the American Psychological Association, New York.

Brenner, B. (1975). Quality of affect and self-evaluated happiness. *Social Indicators Research, 2,* 315–331.

Cacioppo, J. T., Petty, R. E., Losch, M. E., & Kim, H. S. (1986). Electromyographic activity over facial muscle regions can differentiate the valence and intensity of affective reactions. *Journal of Personality and Social Psychology, 50,* 260–268.

Campbell, A. (1981). *The sense of well-being in America.* New York: McGraw Hill.

Campbell, A., Converse, P. E., & Rodgers, W. L. (1976). *The Quality of American Life.* New York: Russell Sage Foundation.

Carstensen, L. L., & Cone, J. D., (1983). Social desirability and the measurement of psychological well-being in elderly persons. *Journal of Gerontology, 38,* 713–715.

Carver, C. S., & Gaines, J. G., (1987). Optimism, pessimism, and post-partum depression. *Cognitive Therapy and Research, 11,* 449–462.

Chamberlain, K. (1988). On the structure of well-being. *Social Indicators Research, 20,* 581–604.

Chamberlain, K., & Zika, S. (1992). Stability and change in subjective well-being over short time periods. *Social Indicators Research, 26,* 101–117.

Clark, D. M. (1983). On the induction of depressed mood in the laboratory: Evaluation and comparison of the Velten and musical procedures. *Advances in Behavioral Research and Therapy, 5,* 27–49.

Cohen, L. H., Towbes, L. C., & Flocco, R. (1988). Effects of induced mood on self-reported life events and perceived and received social support. *Journal of Personality and Social Psychology, 55,* 669–674.

Coombs, C. H. (1964). *A theory of data.* New York: Wiley.

Costa, P. T., & McCrae, R. R. (1980). Influence of extraversion and neuroticism on subjective well-being: Happy and unhappy people. *Journal of Personality and Social Psychology, 38,* 668–678.

Costa, P. T., & McCrae, R. R. (1988). Personality in adulthood: A six-year longitudinal study of self-reports and spouse ratings on the NEO personality inventory. *Journal of Personality and Social Psychology, 54,* 853–863.

Costa, P., McCrae, R., & Zonderman, A. (1987). Environmental and dispositional influences on well-being: Longitudinal follow-up of an American national sample. *British Journal of Psychology, 78,* 299–306.

Csikszentmihalyi, M., & Larson, R. (1987). Validity and reliability of the experience-sampling method. *Journal of Nervous and Mental Disorders, 175,* 526–536.

Csikszentmihalyi, M., Larson, R., & Prescott, S. (1977). The ecology of adolescent activity and experience. *Journal of Youth and Adolescence, 6,* 281–294.

Davidson, R. J. (1983). Affect, repression, and cerebral asymmetry. In L. Temoshok, C. VanDyke, & L. S. Zegans (Eds.), *Emotions in health and illness* (pp. 123–135). New York: Grune & Stratton.

Davis, P. J. (1990). Repression and the inaccessibility of emotional memories. In J. L. Singer (Ed.), *Repression and dissociation: implications for personality theory, psychopathology and health* (pp. 387–404). Chicago: University of Chicago Press.

DeHaes, J. C., Pennink, B. J. W., & Welvaart, K. (1987). The distinction between affect and cognition. *Social Indicators Research, 19,* 367–378.

DePaulo, B. M., & Rosenthal, R. (1979). Ambivalence, discrepancy, and deception in nonverbal communication. In R. Rosenthal (Ed.), *Skill in nonverbal communication* (pp. 204–248). Cambridge, MA: Oelgeschlager, Gunn & Hain.

Dermer, M., Cohen, S. J., Jacobsen, E., & Anderson, E. A. (1979). Evaluative judgments of aspects of life as a function of vicarious exposure to hedonic extremes. *Journal of Personality and Social Psychology, 37,* 247–260.

Diener, E. (1984). Subjective well-being. *Psychological Bulletin, 95*, 542–575.

Diener, E., Colvin, C. R., Pavot, W., & Allman, A. (1991). The psychic costs of intense positive emotions. *Journal of Personality and Social Psychology, 61*, 492–503.

Diener, E., & Diener, M. (1993). *Self-esteem and life satisfaction across 31 countries.* Sixth Meeting of the International Society for the Study of Individual Differences, Baltimore.

Diener, E., Diener, M., & Diener, C. (1993). *Factors predicting the subjective well-being of nations.* Manuscript submitted for publication.

Diener, E., & Emmons, R. (1985). The independence of positive and negative affect. *Journal of Personality and Social Psychology, 47*, 1105–1117.

Diener, E., Emmons, R. A., Larsen, R. J., & Griffin, S. (1985). The satisfaction with life scale. *Journal of Personality Assessment, 49*, 71–75.

Diener, E., & Fujita, F. (1994). Methodological pitfalls and solutions in satisfaction research. In A. C. Samli & M. J. Sirgy (Eds.), New dimensions in marketing/*quality-of-life interface.* Westport, Connecticut: Quorum Books.

Diener, E., Fujita, F., & Smith, H. (1993). *The death of social desirability: An empirical demonstration.* Unpublished manuscript, University of Illinois.

Diener, E., Horwitz, J., & Emmons, R. A. (1985). Happiness of the very wealthy. *Social Indicators Research, 16*, 263–274.

Diener, E., & Iran-Nejad, A. (1986). The relationship in experience between various types of affect. *Journal of Personality and Social Psychology, 50*, 1031–1038.

Diener, E., & Larsen, R. J. (1984). Temporal stability and cross-situational consistency of affective, behavioral, and cognitive responses. *Journal of Personality and Social Psychology, 47*, 871–883.

Diener, E., & Larsen, R. J. (1986). *The emotionally reactive individual: Intensity, variability, and stimulus responsivity.* Unpublished manuscript.

Diener, E., & Larsen, R. J. (1993). The experience of emotional well-being. In M. Lewis & J. M. Haviland (Eds.), *Handbook of emotions* (pp. 405–415). New York: Guilford.

Diener, E., Larsen, R. J., & Emmons, R. A. (1984). Person X situation interactions: Choice of situations and congruence response models. *Journal of Personality and Social Psychology, 47*, 580–592.

Diener, E., Larsen, R. J., Levine, S., & Emmons, R. A. (1985). Intensity and frequency: Dimensions underlying positive and negative affect. *Journal of Personality and Social Psychology, 48*, 1253–1265.

Diener, E., Sandvik, E., & Pavot, W. (1990). Happiness is the frequency, not the intensity, of positive versus negative affect. In F. Strack, M. Argyle, & N. Schwarz (Eds.), *Subjective well-being: An interdisciplinary perspective* (pp. 119–136). New York: Pergamon.

Diener, E., Sandvik, E., Pavot, W., & Gallagher, D. (1991). Response artifacts in the measurement of subjective well-being. *Social Indicators Research, 24*, 35–56.

Diener, E., Sandvik, E., Seidlitz, L., & Diener, M. (1992). The relationship between income and subjective well-being. Social *Indicators Research, 28*, 195–223.

Diener, E., Smith, H., & Fujita, F. (1993). *The structure of long-term affect.* Manuscript in preparation, University of Illinois.

Diener, E., Suh, E., Smith, H., & Shao, L. (1995). National differences in reported subjective well-being: Why do they occur? *Social Indicators Research, 34*, 7–32.

Ekman, P. (1984). Expression and the nature of emotion. In K. R. Scherer & P. Ekman (Eds.), *Approaches to emotion* (pp. 319–344). Hillsdale, NJ: Lawrence Erlbaum.

Ekman, P., Friesen, W. V., & Ellsworth, P. (1972). *Emotion in the human face: Guidelines for research and an integration of findings.* New York: Pergamon Press.

Ekman, P., Levenson, R. W., & Friesen, W. V. (1983). Autonomic nervous system activity distinguishes between emotions. *Science, 221*, 1208–1210.

Emmons, R. A. (1986). Personal strivings: An approach to personality and subjective well-being. *Journal of Personality and Social Psychology, 51*, 1058–1068.

Emmons, R. A., & Diener, E. (1985). Personality correlates of subjective well-being. *Journal of Personality and Social Psychology, 11*, 89–97.

Fordyce, M. W. (1988). A review of research on the happiness measures: A sixty second index of happiness and mental health. *Social Indicators Research, 20*, 355–381.

Frijda, N. H. (1986). *The emotions.* Cambridge: Cambridge University Press.

Friswell, R., & McConkey, K. M. (1989). Hypnotically induced mood. *Cognition and Emotion, 3*, 1–26.

Fujita, F. (1991). *An investigation of the relationship between extraversion, neuroticism, positive affect and negative affect.* Unpublished Masters Thesis, University of Illinois.

Fujita, F. (1993). *The effects of naturalistic social comparison on satisfaction.* Doctoral dissertation, University of Illinois.

Fujita, F., Smith, H., & Diener, E. (1993). *Variations in anonymity and the validity of well-being reports.* Manuscript submitted for publication.

Furnham, A. (1986). Response bias, social desirability, and dissimulation. *Personality and Individual Differences, 7*, 385–400.

Galin, D. (1974). Implications for psychiatry of left and right cerebral specialization. *Archives of General Psychiatry, 31*, 572–583.

Gazzaniga, M. S. (1985). *The social brain: Discovering the networks of the mind.* New York: Basic Books.

George, L. K., & Bearon, L. B. (1980). *Quality of life in older persons: Meaning and measurement.* New York: Human Sciences Press.

Glenn, N. D., & Weaver, C. N. (1978). A multivariate, multisurvey study of marital happiness. *Journal of Marriage and the Family, 40*, 269–281.

Goodwin, A. M., & Williams, M. G. (1982). Mood induction research – Its implications for clinical depression. *Behavior Research and Therapy, 20*, 373–382.

Green, D. P., Goldman, S., & Salovey, P. (1993). Measurement error masks bipolarity in affect ratings. *Journal of Personality and Social Psychology, 64*, 1029–1041.

Grice, H. P. (1975). Logic and conservation. In P. Cole & J. L. Morgan (Eds.), *Syntax and semantics: Speech acts* (pp. 41–58). New York: Academic Press.

Gudjonsson, G. H. (1981). Self-reported emotional disturbance and its relation to electrodermal reactivity, defensiveness and trait anxiety. *Personality and Individual Differences, 2*, 47–52.

Gurin, G., Veroff, J., & Feld, S. (1960). *Americans view their mental health.* New York: Basic Books.

Haggard, E. A., & Isaacs, K. S. (1966). Micromomentary facial expression as indicators of ego mechanisms in psychotherapy. In L. A. Gottschalk & A. H. Auerbach (Eds.), *Methods of research in psychotherapy.* New York: Appleton-Century-Crofts.

Hama, H., & Tsuda, K. (1989). *Analysis of emotions evoked by schematic faces and measured with clynes' sentograph.* Paper presented at the Fourth International Meeting of the International Society for Research on Emotions, Paris, France.

Hammen, C., & Glass, D. R. (1975). Activity, depression, and evaluation of reinforcement. *Journal of Abnormal Psychology, 84*, 718–721.

Harmon, T. M., Nelson, R. O., & Hayes, S. C. (1980). Self-monitoring of mood versus activity by depressed clients. *Journal of Consulting and Clinical Psychology, 48*, 30–38.

Headey, B., Holmstrom, E., & Wearing, A. (1985). Models of well-being and ill-being. *Social Indicators Research, 17*, 211–234.

Headey, B., Veenhoven, R., & Wearing, A. (1991). Top-down versus bottom-up theories of subjective well-being. *Social Indicators Research, 24*, 81–100.

Headey, B., & A. Wearing, (1989). Personality, life events, and subjective well-being: Toward a dynamic equilibrium model. *Journal of Personality and Social Psychology, 57*, 731–739.

Hogan, R. (1983). A socioanalytic theory of personality. In M. M. Page (Ed.), *Personality – Current Theory and Research: 1982 Nebraska Symposium on Motivation* (pp. 621–626). Lincoln, Nebraska: University of Nebraska Press.

Hogan, R., & Nicholson, R. A. (1988). The meaning of personality test scores. *American Psychologist, 43*, 621–626.

Horley, J., & Lavery, J. J. (1991). The stability and sensitivity of subjective well-being measures. *Social Indicators Research, 24*, 113–122.

Horley, J., & Little, B. R. (1985). Affective and cognitive components of global subjective well-being measures. *Social Indicators Research, 17*, 189–197.

Hormuth, S. E. (1986). The sampling of experiences in situ. *Journal of Personality, 54*, 262–293.

Inglehart, R. (1977). *The silent revolution: Changing values and political styles among western publics*. Princeton, NJ: Princeton University Press.

Izard, C. E. (1971). *The face of emotion*. New York: Appleton-Century-Crofts.

Izard, C. E. (1972). *Patterns of Emotions: A new analysis of anxiety and depression*. New York: Academic Press.

Izard, C. E. (1992). Basic emotions, relations among emotions, and emotion-cognition relations. *Psychological Review, 99*, 561–565.

Jasper, H. H., (1930). The measurement of depression-elation and its relation to a measure of extraversion-introversion. *Journal of Abnormal and Social Psychology, 25*, 307–318.

Jones, H. M. (1953). *The pursuit of happiness*. Cambridge, MA: Harvard University Press.

Judge, T. (1990). Job satisfaction as a reflection of disposition: Investigating the relationship and its effects on employee adaptive behaviors. (Doctoral dissertation, University of Illinois).

Kagan, J. (1984). The idea of emotion in human development. In C. E. Izard, J. Kagan, & R. B. Zajonc (Eds.), *Emotions, cognition, and behavior*. Cambridge: Cambridge University Press.

Kahneman, D., Slovic, P., & Tversky, A. (Eds.). (1982). *Judgment under uncertainty: Heuristics and Biases*. New York: Cambridge University Press.

Kammann, R., Christie, D., Irwin, R., & Dixon, G. (1979). Properties of an inventory to measure happiness (and psychological health). *New Zealand Psychologist, 8*, 1–9.

Kammann, R., & Flett, R. (1983). *Coursebook for measuring well-being with the affectometer 2*. Dunedin, New Zealand: Why Not? Foundation.

Ketelaar, T. (1989). *Examining the dimensions of affect in the domain of mood-sensitive tasks*. Unpublished master's thesis, Purdue University, West Lafayette, IN.

King, A. C., Albright, C. L., Taylor, C. B., Haskell, W. L., & Debusk, R. F. (1986). *The repressive coping style: A predictor of cardiovascular reactivity and risk*. Presented at the annual meeting of the Society of Behavioral Medicine, San Francisco.

King, D. A., & Buchwald, A. M. (1982). Sex differences in subclinical depression: Administration of the Beck Depression Inventory in public and private disclosure situations. *Journal of Personality and Social Psychology, 42*, 963–996.

Kozma, A., Stone, S., Stones, M. J., Hannah, T. E., & McNeil, K. (1990). Long- and short-term affective states in happiness: Model, paradigm, and experimental evidence. *Social Indicators Research, 22*, 119–138.

Kozma, A., & Stones, M. J. (1988). Social desirability in measures of subjective well-being: Age comparisons *Social Indicators Research, 20*, 1–14.

Kushman, J., & Lane, S. (1980). A multivariate analysis of factors affecting perceived life satisfaction and psychological well-being among the elderly. *Social Science Quarterly, 61*, 264–277.

Larsen, R. J. (1992). Neuroticism and selective encoding and recall of symptoms: Evidence from a combined concurrent-retrospective study. *Journal of Personality and Social Psychology, 62*, 480–488.

Larsen, R. J., & Cutler, S. E. (1992). *The complexity of individual emotional lives: A process analysis of affect structure*. Manuscript submitted for publication, University of Michigan.

Larsen, R. J., & Diener, E. (1985). A multitrait-multimethod examination of affect structure: Hedonic level and emotional intensity. *Personality and Individual Differences, 6*, 631–636.

Larsen, R. J. & Diener, E. (1987). Emotional response intensity as an individual difference characteristic. *Journal of Research in Personality, 21*, 1–39.

Larsen, R. J., Diener, E. & Emmons, R. A. (1985). An evaluation of subjective well-being measures. *Social Indicators Research, 17*, 1–18.

Lawrence, R. H., & Liang, J. (1988). Structural integration of the Affect Balance Scale and the Life Satisfaction Index A: Race, sex, and age differences. *Psychology and Aging, 3*, 375–384.

Lawton, M. P., (1972). The dimensions of morale. In D. P. Kent, R. Kastenbaum, & S. Sherwood (Eds.), *Research, planning and action for the elderly*. New York: Behavioral Publications.

Lawton, M. P., (1983). The varieties of well-being. *Experimental Aging Research, 9*, 65–72.

Lawton, M. P., Kleban, M. H., & DiCarlo, E. (1984). Psychological well-being in the aged. *Research on Aging, 6*, 67–97.

Lazarus, R. S., (1991). *Emotion and adaptation*. New York: Oxford University Press.

Lehman, D. R., Wortman, C. B., & Williams, A. F. (1987). Long-term effects of losing a spouse or child in a motor vehicle crash. *Journal of Personality and Social Psychology, 52*, 218–231.

Levenson, R. W., & Mades, L. L. (1980). *Physiological response, facial expression, and trait anxiety: Two methods for improving consistency*. Paper presented at the Society for Psychophysiological Research, Vancouver, British Columbia.

Leventhal, H., (1984). A perceptual motor theory of emotion. In K. R. Scherer & P. Ekman (Eds.), *Approaches to emotion* (pp. 271–292). Hillsdale, NJ: Lawrence Erlbaum.

Liang, J. (1985). A structural integration of the Affect Balance Scale and the Life Satisfaction Index A. *Journal of Gerontology, 40*, 552–461.

Liang, J., Asano, H., Bollen, K. A., Kahana, E. F., & Maeda, D. (1987). Cross-cultural comparability of the Philadelphia Geriatric Center Morale Scale: An American–Japanese comparison. *Journal of Gerontology, 42*, 37–43.

Lorr, M., Qing Shi, A., & Youniss, R. P. (1989). A bipolar multifactor conception of mood states. *Personality and Individual Differences, 10*, 155–159.

MacKinnon, N. J., & Keating, L. J. (1989). The structure of emotions: Canada-United States comparisons. *Social Psychology Quarterly, 52*, 70–83.

MacLean, P. D. (1975). Sensory and perceptive factors in emotional functions in the triune brain. In L. Levi (Ed.), *Emotions: Their parameters and measurement*. New York: Raven Press.

Mandler, G. (1985). Cognitive psychology: An essay in cognitive science. Hillsdale, NJ: Erlbaum.

Marshall, G. N., Wortman, C. B., Kusulas, J. W., Hervig, K. L., & Vickers, R. R. (1992). Distinguishing optimism from pessimism: Relations to fundamental dimensions of mood and personality. *Journal of Personality and Social Psychology, 62* 1067–1074.

Mayer, J. D., Mamberg, M. H., & Volanth, A. J. (1988). Cognitive domains of the mood system. *Journal of Personality, 56*, 453–486.

McConville, C., & Cooper, C. (1992). The structure of moods. *Personality and Individual Differences, 8*, 909–919.

McCrae, R. R. (1986). Well-being scales do not meassure social desirability. *Journal of Gerontology, 41*, 390–392.

McCrae, R. R., & Costa, P. T. (1983). Social desirability scales: More substance than style. *Journal of Consulting and Clinical Psychology, 51*, 882–888.

McCrae, R. R., & Costa, P. R. (1991). Adding liebe and arbeit: The full five-factor model and well-being. *Personality and Social Psychology Bulletin, 17*, 227–232.

McCulloch, B. J. (1991). A longitudinal investigation of the factor structure of subjective well-being: The case of the Philadelphia Geriatric Center Morale Scale. *Journal of Gerontology, 46*, 251–258.

McKennell, A. (1974). Surveying subjective welfare: Strategies and methodological considerations. In B. Strumpel (Ed.), *Subjective elements of well-being* (pp. 45–72). Paris: Organization for Economic Development and Cooperation.

McNeil, J. K., Stones, M. J., & Kozma, A. (1986). Subjective well-being in later life: Issues concerning measurement and prediction. *Social Indicators Research, 18*, 35–70.

Michalos, A. (1991). *Global report on student well-being: Volume 1, Life satisfaction and happiness*. New York: Springer Verlag.

Neugarten, B. L., Havighurst, R. J., & Tobin, S. S. (1961). The measurement of life satisfaction. *Journal of Gerontology, 16*, 134–143.

Nydegger, C. N. (Ed.) (1977). Measuring morale: A guide to effective assessment. Washington, DC: Gerontological Society.

Oatley, K., & Jenkins, J. M. (1992). Human emotions: Function and dysfunction. *Annual Review of Psychology, 43*, 55–85.

Okun, M. A., & Stock, W. A. (1987). A construct validity study of subjective well-being measures: An assessment via quantitative research syntheses. *Journal of Community Psychology, 15*, 481–492.

Ormel, J., & Schaufeli, W. B. (1991). The stability and change in psychological distress and their relationship with self-esteem and locus of control: A dynamic equilibrium model. *Journal of Personality and Social Psychology, 60*, 288–299.

Ouweneel, P., & Veenhoven, R. (1991). Cross-national differences in happiness: Cultural bias or societal quality. In N. Bleichrodt & P. J. D. Drenth (Eds.), *Contemporary issues in cross-Cultural psychology* (pp. 168–184). Amsterdam: Swets & Zeitlinger.

Panksepp, J. (1982). Toward a general psychobiological theory of emotions. *The Behavioral and Brain Sciences, 5*, 407–467.

Paulhus, D. L. (1988). *Assessing self deception and impression management in self-reports: The balanced inventory of desirable responding.* Department of Psychology, University of British Columbia, Vancouver, BC, Canada V6T 1Y7.

Pavot, W., & Diener, E. (1993a). The affective and cognitive context of self-reported measures of subjective well-being. *Social Indicators Research, 28*, 1–20.

Pavot, W., & Diener, E. (1993b). A review of the satisfaction with life scale. *Psychological Assessment, 5*, 164–172.

Pavot, W., Diener, E., Colvin, C. R., & Sandvik, E. (1991). Response artifacts in the measurement of subjective well-being. *Social Indicators Research, 24*, 35–56.

Plutchik, R. (1980). *Emotion: A psychoevolutionary synthesis.* New York: Harper & Row.

Plutchik, R. (1984). Emotions: A general psychoevolutionary theory. In K. R. Scherer & P. Ekman (Eds.), *Approaches to emotion* (pp. 197–219). Hillsdale, NJ: Erlbaum.

Rodgers, W. L., Herzog, A. R. & Andrews, F. M. (1988). Interviewing older adults: Validity of self-reports of satisfaction. *Psychology and Aging, 3*, 264–272.

Russell, J. A. (1991). Culture and the categorization of emotions. *Psychological Bulletin, 110*, 426–450.

Sandvik, E., Diener, E., & Seidlitz, L. (1993). The assessment of well-being: A comparison of self-report and nonself-report strategies. *Journal of Personality, 61*, 317–342.

Scherer, K. R. (1984). On the nature and function of emotion: A component process approach. In K. R. Scherer & P. Ekman (Eds.), *Approaches to emotion* (pp. 293–318). Hillsdale, NJ: Lawrence Erlbaum.

Schwartz, G. E., (1982). Psychophysiological patterning of emotion revisited: A systems perspective. In C. E. Izard (Ed.), *Measuring emotions in infants and children* (pp. 67–93). Cambridge: Cambridge University Press.

Schwartz, G. E. (1983). Disregulation theory and disease: Applications to the repression/cerebral disconnection/cardiovascular disorder hypothesis. *International review of applied psychology, 32*, 95–118.

Schwarz, N., & Clore, G. (1983). Mood, misattribution, and judgments of well-being: Informative and directive functions of affective states. *Journal of Personality and Social Psychology, 45*, 513–523.

Schwarz, N., & Strack, F. (1991). Evaluating one's life: A judgment model of subjective well-being. In F. Strack, M. Argyle, & N. Schwarz (Eds.), *Subjective well-being: an interdisciplinary perspective* (pp. 27–48). Oxford: Pergamon.

Scott, C., Diener, E., & Fujita, F. (1992). *Personality versus the situational effect in the relation between marriage and subjective well-being.* Unpublished manuscript, University of Illinois.

Seidlitz, L., & Diener, E. (1993). Memory for positive versus negative life events: Theories for the differences between happy and unhappy persons. *Journal of Personality and Social Psychology, 64*, 654–664.

Shao, L. (1992). *Multilanguage comparability of life satisfaction and happiness measures in Mainland Chinese and American students.* Unpublished Master Thesis, University of Illinois.

Shaver, P., Schwartz, J., Kirson, D., & O'Connor, C. (1987). Emotional knowledge: Further exploration of a prototype approach. *Journal of Personality and Social Psychology, 52*, 1061–1086.

Sinclair, R. C., Mark, M. M., & Wellens, T. R. (1989). *Administration of the Beck Depression Inventory on self-Report of mood state: A case in contrast.* Paper presented at the Midwest Psychological Association Meeting, Chicago.

Singer, J. L. (Ed.): (1990). *Repression and dissociation: Implications for personality theory, psychotherapy, and health.* Chicago: University of Chicago Press.

Skelton, J. A., & Strohmetz, D. B. (1990). Priming symptom reports with health related cognitive activity. *Personality and Social Psychology Bulletin, 16,* 449–464.

Smith, T. W. (1979). Happiness: Time trends, seasonal variations, intersurvey differences, and other mysteries, Social Psychology Quarterly, 42, 18–30.

Smith, T. W., Pope, M. K., Rhodewalt, F., & Poulton, J. L. (1989). Optimism, neuroticism, coping and symptom reports: An alternative interpretation of the Life Orientation Test. *Journal of Personality and Social Psychology, 56,* 640–648.

Sommers, S. (1984). Reported emotions and conventions of emotionality among college students. *Journal of Personality and Social Psychology, 46,* 207–215.

Staats, S., Partlo, C., & Adam, N. (1989). *When time frame makes a difference.* Paper presented at the 61st Annual Meeting of the Midwestern Psychological Association, Chicago.

Stimson, R. J. (1988). Problems of research on spatial behavior in large scale urban environments: Methodological issues in minimizing error and bias to produce valid and reliable data. Paper presented at the 24th International Congress of Psychology, Sydney, Australia.

Stock, W. A., Okun, M. A., & Benin, M. (1986). Structure of subjective well-being among the elderly. *Psychology and Aging, 1,* 91–102.

Stones, M. J., & Kozma, A. (1980). Issues relating to the usage and conceptualization of mental health constructs employed by gerontologists. *International Journal of Aging and Human Development, 11,* 269–281.

Strack, F., Schwarz, N., Chassein, B., Kern, D., & Wagner, D. (1990). Salience of comparison standards and the activation of social norms: Consequences for judgments of happiness and their communication. *British Journal of Social Psychology, 29,* 303–314.

Strack, F., Schwarz, N., & Wanke, M. (1991). Semantic and pragmatic aspects of context effects in social and psychological research. *Social Cognition, 9,* 111–125.

Sudman, S. (1967). Reducing the cost of surveys. *NORC monographs in social research.* Chicago: Aldine.

Tatarkiewicz, W. (1976). *Analysis of happiness.* The Hague, Netherlands: Martinus Nijhoff.

Taylor, C. (1977). Why measure morale?. In C. Nydegger (Ed.), Measuring morale: A guide to effective assessment (pp. 30–33). Washington, DC: Gerontological Society.

Thomas, D., & Diener, E. (1990). Memory accuracy in the recall of emotions. *Journal of Personality and Social Psychology, 59,* 291–297.

Thomas, L. E., & Chambers, K. D. (1989). Phenomenology of life satisfaction among elderly men: Quantitative and qualitative views. *Psychology and Aging, 4,* 284–289.

Tomkins, S. S., & McCarter, R. (1964). What and where are the primary affects? Some evidence for a theory. *Perceptual and Motor Skills, 18,* 119–158.

Torangeau, R., & Rasinski, K. A. (1988). Cognitive processes underlying context effects of attitude measurement. *Psychological Bulletin, 103,* 299–314.

Tran, T. V., Wright, R., & Chatters, L. (1991). Health, stress, psychological resources, and subjective well-being among older blacks. *Psychology and Aging, 6,* 100–108.

Tversky, A., & Griffin, D. (1991). Endowment and contrast in judgments of well-being. In F. Strack, M. Argyle, & N. Schwarz (Eds.), *Subjective well-being: An interdisciplinary perspective* (pp. 101–118). New York: Pergamon.

Tyrer, P. (1976). *The role of bodily feelings in anxiety.* New York: Oxford Press.

Veenhoven, R.: (1984), Conditions of Happiness (D. Reidel, Dordrecht).

Vitaliano, P. P., Paulsen, V. M., Russo, J., & Bailey, S. L. (1993). *Cardiovascular recovery: Biopsyosocial concomitants in older adults.* Manuscript submitted for publication, University of Washington, Seattle.

Warr, P., Barter, J., & Brownbridge, G. (1983). On the independence on negative and positive affect. *Journal of Personality and Social Psychology, 44,* 644–651.

Washburne, J. N., (1941). Factors related to the social adjustment of college girls. *Journal of Social Psychology, 13*, 281–289.

Watson, D. (1988). The vicissitudes of mood measurement: Effects of varying descriptors, time frames, and response formats on measures of positive and negative affect. *Journal of Personality and Social Psychology, 55*, 128–141.

Watson, D., & Clark, L. A. (1984). Negative affectivity: The disposition to experience aversive emotional states. *Psychological Bulletin, 96*, 465–490.

Watson, D., Clark, L. A., & Tellegen, A. (1984). Cross-cultural convergence in the structure of mood: A Japanese replication and comparison with U.S. findings. *Journal of Personality and Social Psychology, 47*, 127–144.

Weinberger, D. A. (1990). The construct validity of the repressive coping style. In J. L. Singer (Ed.), *Repression and dissociation: Implications for personality theory, psychopathology, and health* (pp. 337–386). Chicago: University of Chicago Press.

Weinberger, D. A., Schwartz, G. E., & Davidson, R. J. (1979). Low-anxious, high-anxious, and repressive coping styles: Psychometric patterns and behavioral and physiological responses to stress. *Journal of Abnormal Psychology, 88*, 369–380.

Wellens, T. R., Tanaka, J. S., & Panter, A. T. (1989). *The role of item order in the assessment of dysphoric affect.* Paper presented at the Midwest Psychological Association Meeting, Chicago.

Wessman, A. E., & Ricks, D. F. (1966). *Mood and personality.* New York: Holt.

Wilson, G. A., Elias, J. W., & Brownlee, L. J. (1985). Factor invariance and the life satisfaction index. *Journal of Gerontology, 40*, 344–346.

Wood, L. A., & Johnson, J. (1989). Life satisfaction among the rural elderly: What do the numbers mean?. *Social Indicators Research, 21*, 379–408.

Wood, V., Wylie, M. L., & Sheafor, B. (1969). An analysis of a short self-report measure of life satisfaction: Correlation with rater judgments. *Journal of Gerontology, 24*, 465–469.

Wyer, R. S., & Srull, T. K. (1989). *Memory and cognition in its social context.* Hillsdale, NJ: Erlbaum.

Zajonc, R. B. (1984a). The interaction of affect and cognition. In K. R. Scherer & P. Ekman (Eds.), *Approaches to emotion* (pp. 239–246). Hillsdale, NJ: Lawrence Erlbaum.

Zajonc, R. B. (1984b). On the primacy of affect. In K. R. Scherer & P. Ekman (Eds.), *Approaches to emotion* (pp. 259–270). Hillsdale, NJ: Lawrence Erlbaum.

Zautra, A. J., Guarnaccia, C. A., & Reich, J. W. (1988). Factor structure of mental health measures for older adults. *Journal of Consulting and Clinical Psychology, 56*, 514–519.

Zevon, M. A., & Tellegen, A. (1982). The structure of mood change: An idiographic/nomothetic analysis. *Journal of Personality and Social Psychology, 43*, 111–122.

The Evolving Concept of Subjective Well-Being: The Multifaceted Nature of Happiness

Ed Diener, Christie Napa Scollon, and Richard E. Lucas

Abstract Subjective well-being, or what is popularly often called "happiness," has been of intense interest throughout human history. We review research showing that it is not a single factor, but that subjective well-being is composed of a number of separable although somewhat related variables. For example, positive feelings, negative feelings, and life satisfaction are clearly separable. In understanding the various types of subjective well-being, it is important to remember that appraisals move from immediate situations to a later recall of feelings, and then to global evaluations of life. At each stage, from momentary feelings to large global life evaluations, somewhat different processes are involved in what is called "happiness." In order to understand how to measure subjective well-being, one must understand the time course and components of the phenomenon in question, and be clear about what is most important to assess. On-line feelings are very different from global evaluations of life, although both have been studied under the rubric of subjective well-being. Although debate has focused on which type of subjective well-being should be called "true happiness," the goal of scientists is to understand each type, their relations with each other, and their causes. The future of the field depends on understanding the differences between various types of well-being, and the different and similar causes of each.

Evolving Conceptions of Subjective Well-Being: The Multifaceted Nature of Happiness

Subjective well-being (SWB) is the field in the behavioral sciences in which people's evaluations of their lives are studied. SWB includes diverse concepts ranging from momentary moods to global judgments of life satisfaction, and from depression to euphoria. The field has grown rapidly in the last decade, so that there are now thousands of studies on topics such as life satisfaction and happiness. Scientists who

E. Diener (✉)
Department of Psychology, University of Illinois, Champaign, IL 61820, USA
e-mail: ediener@s.psych.uiuc.edu

E. Diener (ed.), *Assessing Well-Being: The Collected Works of Ed Diener,*
Social Indicators Research Series 39, DOI 10.1007/978-90-481-2354-4_4,
© Springer Science+Business Media B.V. 2009

study aging have shown particular interest in SWB, perhaps because of concern that declines in old age could be accompanied by deteriorating happiness. In this chapter we touch upon age trends in SWB, but our major goalis to alert researchers to the intriguing multi-faceted nature of this concept that has emerged in recent years.

Concern About Happiness and the Good Life Throughout History

A widely presumed component of the good life is happiness. Unfortunately, the nature of happiness has not been defined in a uniform way. Happiness can mean pleasure, life satisfaction, positive emotions, a meaningful life, or a feeling of contentment, among other concepts. In fact, for as long as philosophers have been discussing happiness, its definition has been debated. One of the earliest thinkers on the subject of happiness, the pre-Socratic philosopher Democritus, maintained that the happy life was enjoyable, not because of what the happy person possessed, but because of the way the happy person reacted to his/her life circumstances (Tatarkiewicz, 1976). Incorporated in Democritus's definition of happiness were ideas about disposition, pleasure, satisfaction, and subjectivity. However, this view was buried for centuries as Socrates, Plato, and Aristotle championed the eudemonia definition of happiness in which happiness consisted of possessing the greatest goods available (Tatarkiewicz, 1976).

Although there was little agreement among classical thinkers as to what the highest goods were, for Aristotle, they involved realizing one's fullest potential (Waterman, 1990). Most important, this view defined happiness according to objective standards, and pleasure was not considered central to this definition. In contrast, Aristippus advanced an extreme form of hedonism, the unrestrained pursuit of immediate pleasure and enjoyment (Tatarkiewicz, 1976). Happiness, for hedonists, was simply the sum of many pleasurable moments. This form of hedonism, of course being undesirable and impractical, led to a more moderate form of hedonism when the Epicureans sought to maximize pleasures, but with some degree of prudence. Stoics, on the other hand, sought to minimize pains.

Jeremy Bentham's term "utility," also with its roots in hedonism, later widened the meaning of pleasure to include "benefits, advantages, profits, good or happiness ... [and the absence of] failure, suffering, misfortune or unhappiness" (Tatarkiewicz, 1976, p. 322). Happiness, for utilitarians, was thus equated with both the presence of pleasure and absence of pain. Borrowing from Bentham, modern economists believe that people make choices designed to maximize utility.

Because of the multiplicity of meanings that happiness holds, researchers in this field often avoid the term. However, the term happiness has such currency in public discourse that it is often difficult to dodge. Some researchers prefer to use the term "subjective well-being" (SWB), although happiness is sometimes used synonymously with SWB as well. Echoing the beliefs of Democritus, the term subjective well-being emphasizes an individual's own assessment of his or her own life—not the judgment of "experts"—and includes satisfaction (both in general and satisfaction with specific domains), pleasant affect, and low negative affect.

In the 20th Century psychologists and other scientists became interested in studying happiness, answering the questions—What is happiness? Can it be measured? And what causes happiness?—with empiricalmethods. In a landmark paper, Jahoda (1958) called for the inclusion of positive states in definitions of well- being, which sparked a paradigmatic shift in conceptions of mentalhealth. No longer was the absence of mental illness sufficient for mental health; happiness became important as well.

Wessman and Ricks (1966) conducted early intensive personality work on happy people. Like many of the early SWB researchers, they were interested in the characteristics of a happy person. Is the happy person well-liked, balanced, et cetera? However, the scientific study of happiness still generated a bit of doubt. When Wilson (1967) wrote about "avowed happiness," his discussion hedged on whether it was real happiness that scientists were measuring, although he did not fully define the state.

A watershed finding in SWB research came when Bradburn discovered that positive affect (PA) and negative affect (NA) are independent (Bradburn, 1969). By demonstrating that positive and negative emotions form separate factors that are influenced by different variables, Bradburn's findings lent empirical support to Jahoda's notion of mentalhealth. In addition, the independence of PA and NA became important to the study of happiness because it suggested that happiness is not unidimensional, but instead is at least two-dimensional. In other words, PA and NA are not simply polar ends of a single continuum, and thus need to be measured separately. Andrews and Withey's (1976) contribution to the science of SWB was to include the third, cognitive component of life satisfaction. At the same time, Campbell, Converse, and Rodgers (1976) were exploring a fourth form of SWB, domain satisfaction.

In 1984, Diener reviewed the field of SWB, including the various theories and known characteristics of happy individuals at the time. Large national studies of SWB concluded that most Americans were indeed happy, regardless of age, race, sex, income, or education level (Myers & Diener, 1995). Since 1990 there has been an explosion of research in the field, with a large number of SWB studies now occurring in the area of gerontology as well. Neugarten, Havighurst, and Tobin (1961), for example, developed a scale that measures life satisfaction specifically among the elderly.

Chapter Overview

Why is SWB important? First, high SWB leads to benefits (see Lyubomirsky, King, & Diener, 2002 for a review), not the least of which include better health and perhaps even increased longevity (Danner, Snowden, & Friesen, 2001). Second, people the world over think SWB is very important. In a survey of college students from 17 countries, Diener (2000) found that happiness and life satisfaction were both rated well above neutral on importance (and more important than money) in every country, although there was also variation among cultures. Furthermore, respondents from all samples indi- cated that they thought about happiness from time to time. Thus, even those from relatively unhappy societies value happiness to some extent. Third, SWB represents a major way to assess quality of life in addition to economic and social indicators such as GNP and levels of health or crime (Diener & Suh, 1997). In fact, SWB captures aspects of nationalconditions that the other measures cannot. Thus, when used in conjunction with the objective measures, SWB provides additionalinformation necessary to evaluate a society. Fourth, SWB is frequently assessed as a major outcome variable in research on the elderly (George, 1986), and on other target groups. SWB is an important indicator of quality of life and functioning in old age.

The present chapter will review several key areas. However, we will also discuss how the field is moving in new directions. Formerly researchers were searching for the core of SWB, but it is clear that there are multiple components that combine in complex ways, and that no single one of them reflects "true happiness." Instead, SWB must be studied as a multi-faceted phenomenon. People combine the basic building blocks of SWB in different ways.

Some of the topics and questions we will address are as follows:

1. Structure: What are the major components under the umbrella of SWB, and how do they relate to one another?
2. Frequency vs. intensity: Is it the frequency, duration, or intensity of good feelings and cognitions that compose SWB?
3. Temporalsequence and stages: The picture of SWB changes depending on whether one examines moments or longer time frames, such as lifetimes.
4. Stability and consistency: Is there enough temporal stability in people's feelings, and consistency across situations, to consider SWB a personality characteristic? Or is SWB entirely situational?
5. Affect vs. cognition: SWB includes both affective evaluations of one's life (e.g. pleasant feelings, enjoyment, etc.), but also a cognitive evaluation (e.g. satisfaction, meaning, etc.). Which is more important?
6. The functioning mood system: Even happy people experience unpleasant emotions, and the picture of SWB we are advocating does not equate happiness with uninterrupted joy. Adaptive emotions involve being able to react to events, and not being stuck in happy or sad moods.
7. Tradeoffs: Although happiness is desirable, people want to feel happy for the right reasons. Additionally, there are times when people are willing to sacrifice fun and enjoyment for other values.
8. Implications for measurement and research with the elderly: Given the multi-faceted nature of SWB, various measures cannot be assumed to be substitutes for one another.

Different measures may provide divergent conclusions about the well-being of the elderly. Thus, the choice of measures should be an informed decision.

Hierarchical Structure: The Components of SWB

In this section, we review the components that make up the domain of subjective well-being. We present these components as a conceptual hierarchy with various levels of specificity (see Fig. 1). At the highest level of this hierarchy is the concept of SWB itself. At this level, SWB reflects a general evaluation of a person's life, and researchers who work at this level should measure various components from lower levels in the hierarchy to get a complete picture of an individual's overall well- being. At the next highest level are four specific components that provide a more precise understanding of a person's SWB. These components—positive affect, negative affect, satisfaction, and domain satisfactions—are moderately correlated with one another, and they are all conceptually related. Yet, each provides unique information about the subjective quality of one's life. Finally, within each of these four components, there are more fine-grained distinctions that can be made. Some researchers, for example, may want to focus on specific negative emotions or satisfaction with specific life domains.

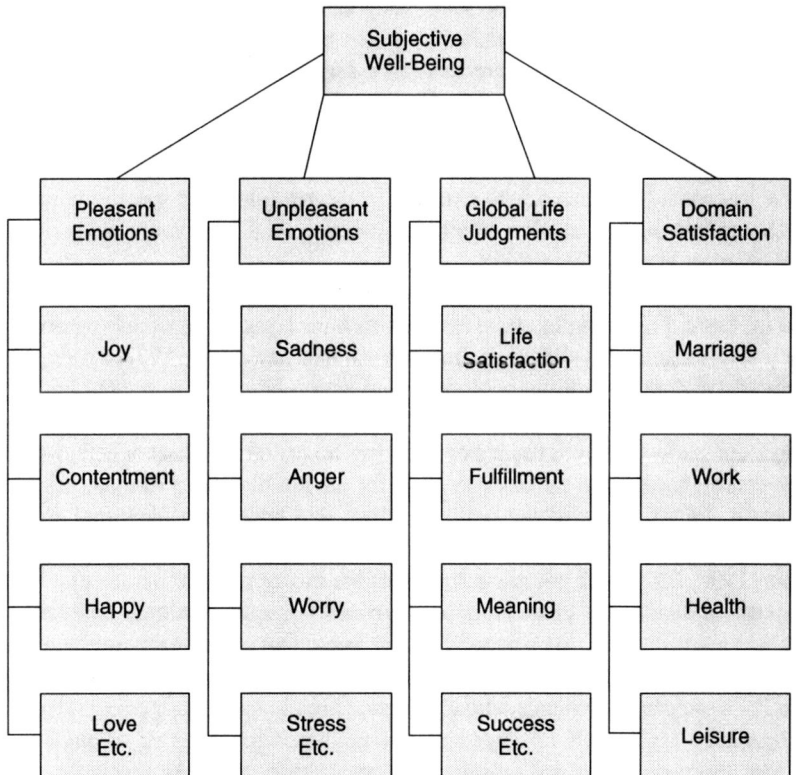

Fig. 1 A hierarchical model of happiness

Positive and Negative Affect

Pleasant and unpleasant affect reflect basic experiences of the ongoing events in people's lives. Thus, it is no surprise that many argue that these affective evaluations should form the basis for SWB judgments (Frijda, 1999; Kahneman, 1999). Affective evaluations take the form of emotions and moods. Although there are debates about the nature of and relation between these two constructs (Morris, 1999), emotions are generally thought to be short-live reactions that are tied to specific events or externalstimuli (Frijda, 1999), whereas moods are thought to be more diffuse affective feelings that may not be tied to specific events (Morris, 1999). By studying the types of affective reactions that individuals experience, researchers can gain an understanding of the ways that people evaluate the conditions and events in their lives.

Much research on affective evaluations has been focused on the ways that emotions and moods can be categorized, and there are two generalapproaches to this issue. Some researchers focus on determining whether there are a small number of basic emotions. Researchers who work from this perspective generally try first to identify the basic features of emotions. They can then go on to examine variations in these features in order to determine which emotions are basic. Frijda (1999), for example, argued that there are five basic features of emotions. First, emotions involve affect, meaning that they are associated with a feeling of pleasure or pain. Second, emotions include an appraisal of an object or event as good or bad. Third, the elicitation of an emotion is generally associated with changes in behavior toward the environment (or at least with changes in the readiness for specific behaviors). Fourth, emotions often involve autonomic arousal. And finally, emotions often involve changes in cognitive activity.

By examining variation in these features, researchers can classify which emotions are basic. For example, some researchers have argued that a basic emotion will have a distinct action readiness or motivationalproperty (Izard, 1977; Frijda, 1986). Seemingly different emotions with the same action tendency may then be seen as variations of the same basic emotion. Other researchers have avoided analyzing the component parts of emotions, instead relying on criteria such as whether there is a universally recognized facial expression for the emotion (e.g. Ekman, Friesen, & Ellsworth, 1972). Some of the basic emotions that have been identified are listed under the Positive and Negative Affect headings in Fig. 1 (though see Ortony & Turner, 1990, for a more complete review of the basic emotion literature).

An alternative to the basic emotion approach is the dimensional approach. Researchers working from this perspective have noted that certain emotions and moods tend to be highly correlated both between individuals and within individuals over time. For example, individuals who experience high levels of sadness are also likely to experience high levels of other negative emotions such as fear or anxiety. The fact that these emotions are correlated suggests that they may result from some of the same underlying processes. Thus, according to the dimensional approach, it should be possible to identify certain basic dimensions that underlie the covariation among the various emotions and moods that people experience. Research into the causes and outcomes of emotionalexperience can then progress by focusing on these underlying dimensions rather than on the individual emotions themselves. Subjective well-being researchers often focus on emotional dimensions rather than specific emotions, because over long periods of time, distinct emotions of the same valence are moderately to strongly correlated (Zelenski & Larsen, 2000).

Most dimensional models of emotions have focused on two underlying dimensions. Russell (1980), for example, argued that the orthogonal dimensions of pleasantness and arousal can be used to describe the variation in emotional experience. According to this model, each emotion can be described by noting the extent to which it is a pleasant emotion and the extent to which it is an aroused emotion. An emotion like excitement, for example, would be a pleasant, highly aroused emotion; whereas an emotion like contentment would be pleasant but much lower in arousal. By plotting emotions on these two dimensions, researchers have developed circumplex models of emotional structure, with most emotions located somewhere on the outer circle formed by orthogonal pleasantness and arousal axes (see Larsen & Diener, 1992, for a discussion of circumplex models; see Fabrigar, Visser, & Browne, 1997 and Watson, Wiese, Vaidya, & Tellegen, 1999 for recent evidence on the circumplex structure).

Other researchers have argued that although pleasantness and arousal are useful dimensions in a descriptive sense, these axes do not reflect the underlying systems that are responsible for the affect that individuals experience. Watson and Tellegen (1985), for example, argued that the pleasantness and arousal dimensions should be rotated 45° to form separate activated positive and negative affect dimensions. Positive affect is a combination of arousal and pleasantness, and it includes emotions such as active, alert, and excited; negative affect is a combination of arousal and unpleasantness, and it includes emotions such as anxious, angry, and fearful. Like other researchers before him (e.g. Costa & McCrae, 1980), Tellegen (1985) noted that the positive affect dimension is closely aligned with the broad personality trait of extraversion, whereas negative affect is closely aligned with the broad personality trait of neuroticism. Tellegen (1985) argued that together, these extraversion/positive affect and neuroticism/negative affect dimensions reflect two underlying personality systems that are responsible for many of the individual differences in affect and behavior. Thus, he argued, studying these rotated dimensions (rather than arousal and pleasantness) is more likely to prove fruitful when attempting to understand the basic processes underlying personality and emotion.

The disagreements about the structure of affect have led to a sometimes confusing debate about whether positive and negative affect are really separable and independent dimensions (as we have suggested in Fig. 1). Part of the confusion regarding this issue has to do with the fact that the dimensions that are most likely to be independent the activated positive and negative affect dimensions in Watson & Tellegen's (1985) model) were given names that suggest bipolarity. Watson et al. (1999) recently renamed these constructs as positive activation and negative activation to emphasize the activated nature of these dimensions and to avoid some of this confusion. Yet, the debate is not simply semantic, and there are many unresolved issues regarding the independence of positive and negative affect. Some researchers have suggested that at any given moment, positive and negative affect are bipolar, whereas when aggregated over time they become independent (Diener & Emmons, 1985). According to this view people cannot experience positive and negative emotions simultaneously (Diener & Iran-Nejad, 1986), but over time, people could experience high levels of both. Other researchers have suggested that positive and negative emotions can, in unusualcircumstances, be experienced at the same time (Larsen, McGraw, & Cacioppo, 2001). Whatever the final outcome of this debate, it seems wise to separately assess positive and negative affect, especially in light of the fact that there are often different correlates of the two.

Frequency and Intensity of Positive and Negative Affect

A final issue that arises when assessing affective components of well-being is what type of emotional experience we should measure. At any given moment a person may experience either high or low intensity emotions. Is the person who experiences intense positive emotions better off than the person who is only mildly happy most of the time, or is the frequency with which an individual experiences positive emotions the most important factor in determining overall affective well-being? Research shows that the intensity with which one feels emotions is not the same thing as the frequency with which he or she feels these emotions, and these two aspects of emotional experience have distinct implications for well-being.

Schimmack and Diener (1997) used experience sampling methods to demonstrate that emotional intensity can be separated from frequency. Specifically, by assessing moods and emotions repeatedly over time, researchers can assess frequency by summing the number of times a person reports experiencing an emotion. Intensity can be determined by examining the average intensity of that emotion when a person reports feeling it. The importance and validity of these two components can then be determined by comparing these scores with other measures of well-being.

In their investigation of this issue, Diener, Sandvik, and Pavot (1991) suggested that frequency of emotional experience was more important for overall well-being than was intensity. Specifically, they argued that there were both theoretical and empirical reasons for focusing on frequency information. First, at a theoretical level, it seems as though the processes that lead to intense positive emotions are likely often to lead to intense negative emotions, and thus very intense emotions often cancel each other out. Laboratory studies show, for instance, that people who use dampening or amplifying strategies with emotion are likely to use the same strategies with both positive and negative affect (Larsen, Diener, & Cropanzano, 1987; Diener, Colvin, Pavot, & Allman, 1992). Thus, people who experience positive emotions intensely will likely experience negative emotions intensely, a finding that is supported by research on individual differences in affect intensity (Larsen & Diener, 1987).

A second theoretical reason why intensity should not affect overall levels of well-being is that very intense emotional experiences are very rare. Diener et al. (1991) reviewed evidence showing that extremely intense positive and negative emotions (those that get the highest scores on emotion scales) are very rare when emotions are sampled repeatedly over time. Thus, if these events occur infrequently, they are unlikely to influence overall levels of well-being.

A third reason why researchers might focus on frequency information is that frequency-based measures appear to have better psychometric characteristics. Kahneman (1999), for instance, argued that it is not difficult to determine whether one is feeling positive or negative at any given moment. Reports based on this type of question are likely to be valid and to have a similar meaning across respondents. On the other hand, it is difficult to accurately report how intensely positive or negative one is feeling, and the meaning of an intensity scale may vary across individuals. Intensity reports may mean different things for different people. Research on this issue does suggest that frequency-based measures have more validity than intensity based measures. For example, Thomas and Diener (1990) and Schimmack and Diener (1997) both found that people could recall frequency information better than intensity information. It is not surprising that Diener et al. (1991) and Schimmack and Diener (1997) both found that frequency reports were more strongly related to global well-being measures.

To determine people's general level of affective well-being, frequency measures appear to be theoretically and empirically more desirable than intensity measures. Yet, there are cases where intensity information can be important. Wirtz, Kruger, Scollon, and Diener (2003), for example, found that when people's emotions were sampled multiple times over the course of a spring break vacation, the intensity of their emotions was a better predictor of desire to go on another similar vacation than was the frequency of their emotions. In addition, research suggests that the intensity of emotions may be related to specific personality traits. Eid and Diener (1999) found that intra- personal variability in emotion was related to neuroticism and lower levels of overall happiness. Thus, intensity information can be useful for examining certain questions about emotional well-being.

Recommendations

Although debates about the nature of affective well-being continue, researchers interested in SWB can confidently tap the emotional well-being components by assessing a broad range of positive and negative emotions. Researchers who are interested in recording a general sense of a person's affective well-being will want to examine the separable positive and negative affect dimensions. Researchers who are interested in specific emotions should consider the debates about basic emotions and insure that they include multiple-item measures of these more specific components. We should note, however, that the study of emotions can occur at even more specific levels. Researchers can assess specific emotions, but they can also go on to examine specific situations in which these emotions can be elicited. For example, some individuals may feel anger in some situations but not in others. Researchers must tailor their emotion assessment strategies to the specific research questions in which they are interested. If separate emotions do not produce different results, they can be aggregated. Although the frequency of emotions appears to be more related to long-term happiness, the intensity of emotions will certainly be of interest for many research questions.

Affect reflects a person's ongoing evaluations of the conditions in his or her life. It is easy to see why these dimensions make up an important part of the general subjective well-being construct. It would be hard to imagine a person saying he or she has high well-being if that person experiences high levels of negative affect and low levels of positive affect. Yet, we must caution that affective well-being, alone, does not appear to be sufficient for most people when they provide an overall evaluation of their lives. People do not seem to want purely hedonistic experiences of positive affect. Instead, people want these experiences to be tied to specific outcomes that reflect their goals and values, as we will discuss later in the section on Trade-offs. Thus, domains beyond affective well-being must be assessed to gain a complete understanding of a person's well-being.

Life Satisfaction

The affective components of well-being described above reflect people's ongoing evaluations of the conditions in their lives. We can contrast this type of evaluation with global judgments about the quality of a person's life. Presumably, individuals can examine the conditions in their lives, weigh the importance of these conditions, and then evaluate their lives on a scale ranging from dissatisfied to satisfied. We refer to this global, cognitive judgment as life satisfaction. Because we assume that this judgment requires cognitive processing, much research has focused on the way that these judgments are made.

After years of research, we now know quite a bit about how life satisfaction judgments are made. For example, it appears as though most individuals do not (and perhaps cannot) examine all aspects of their lives and then weight them appropriately. Instead, because this task is difficult, people likely use a variety of shortcuts when coming up with satisfaction judgments (Robinson & Clore, 2002; Schwarz & Strack, 1999). Specifically, people are likely to use information that is salient at the time of the judgment. For example, Schwarz and Clore (1983) showed that seemingly irrelevant factors such as the weather at the time of judgment can influence ratings of life satisfaction. This research suggests that current mood can influence ratings of life satisfaction, even if that current mood is not indicative of one's overall levels of affective well-being.

Yet, even with the use of these shortcuts, there is substantial temporal stability in people's life satisfaction judgments (Magnus & Diener, 1991; Ehrhardt, Saris, & Veenhoven, 2000). This is because much of the information that is used in making satisfaction judgments appears to be chronically accessible. In other words, people's satisfaction judgments are based on the information that is available at the time of the judgment, but much of that information remains the same over time. If there are domains in people's lives that are extremely important to them, this information is likely to come to mind when people are asked to make judgments about their life satisfaction. In fact, there is evidence that people seem to know what type of information they use when they make life satisfaction judgments. Schimmack, Diener, and Oishi (2002), for example, found that those domains that people said were important in making life satisfaction judgments were more strongly correlated with life satisfaction than domains that were rated as being less important. So although the processes by which satisfaction judgments are made can often lead to what may be thought of as mistakes, in many cases people use relevant and stable information, resulting in stable and meaningful satisfaction judgments.

The research on the processes of satisfaction judgments has led to a greater understanding of the relation between affective and cognitive well-being. It appears that people do use their affective well-being as information when judging their life satisfaction, but this is only one piece of information. The weight that this information is given varies across individuals and cultures. Suh, Diener, Oishi, and Triandis (1998), for example, found that participants from individualistic cultures relied on their affective well-being to a greater extent than participants from collectivist cultures when judging life satisfaction. Collectivists, in contrast, relied more on whether or not significant others thought their life was on the right track. Additional information beyond affective well-being is used when constructing life satisfaction judgments. Thus, the association between affective and cognitive well-being will not be perfect, and will vary across samples. Even within a culture, individual differences can moderate what type of information is included in global judgments. For example, the daily experience of pleasure is a greater predictor of life satisfaction for individuals high in sensation seeking than for those low in sensation seeking (Oishi, Schimmack, & Diener, 2001).

Other sources of information that people may use include comparisons with important standards. Campbell et al. (1976) argued that individuals look at various important life domains and compare these life domains to a variety of comparison standards. For example, an individual may compare her income to the income of those around her, to the income she had in the past, or to the income she desires for the future. Interestingly, just as people seem to be very flexible in the type of information that they use when making satisfaction judgments, they also seem flexible in the way they use this information. Diener and Suh (1997) noted, for example, that social comparison effects are not always consistent across studies or across individuals. Sometimes people may look at individuals who are better off and see these individuals as inspirations (resulting in positive well-being), whereas at other times this type of comparison would lead to a negative comparison and lower levels of well-being.

The advantage of life satisfaction as a measure of well-being is that this type of measure captures a global sense of well-being from the respondent's own perspective. People seem to use their own criteria for making this judgment, and research has begun to identify what these criteria are and how they vary across individuals. Yet, the processes that allow for these individual differences also allow for irrelevant information to be included in satisfaction judgments. People often use whatever information is at hand at the time of judgment, and sometimes this can lead to unreliable or less valid measures. However, on average, the research suggests that although experimental studies can demonstrate the errors that people make, most information that is used in satisfaction judgments is information that is chronically accessible and, presumably, important to the individual.

Domain Satisfactions

The fourth component that is included in our hierarchical model of SWB is domain satisfaction. Domain satisfaction reflects a person's evaluation of the specific domains in his or her life. Presumably, if we were able to assess all the important domains in a person's life, we would be able to reconstruct a global life satisfaction judgment using a bottom-up process. But, as we noted above, the process by which the domain satisfaction judgments are aggregated, and the weight that is given to each domain may vary by individuals. Diener, Lucas, Oishi, and Suh (2002), for example, found that happy individuals were more likely to weight the best domains in their life heavily, whereas unhappy individuals were more likely to weight the worst domains in their life heavily. Thus, domain satisfaction scores do not simply reflect the component parts of a life satisfaction judgment, and they can provide unique information about a person's overall well-being.

More importantly, domain satisfaction will be important for researchers interested in the effects of well-being in particular areas. For example, if a researcher is trying to foster increased well-being at work, job satisfaction may provide a more sensitive measure of these effects than any global well-being scale will. Similarly, researchers who work with certain populations may want to separately assess domain satisfactions that are particularly relevant for that group. Students may be very concerned about grades and learning, whereas the elderly may be more concerned about health and social support. Thus, domain satisfaction scores can provide information about the way individuals construct global well-being judgments; but they can also provide more detailed information about the specific aspects of one's life that are going well or going poorly.

Convergent and Discriminant Validity of SWB Components

Conceptually, each of the components of well-being represents a distinct way of evaluating one's life. Positive and negative affect reflect the immediate, on-line reactions to the good and bad conditions of one's life. Domain satisfactions reflect the cognitive evaluation of specific aspects of one's life. Life satisfaction reflects a global judgment that is constructed through somewhat idiosyncratic processes across individuals, but which provides useful information about a person's satisfaction with life as a whole. Research on the discriminant validity of these constructs shows that they are not only theoretically distinct, but also empirically separable. Lucas et al. (1996), for instance, used self- and informant-reports of well-being constructs to examine the convergent and discriminant validity of positive affect, negative affect, and life satisfaction. Different methods of measuring the same construct tended to converge, and the correlations across methods of measuring the same construct were usually stronger than the correlations between measures of different constructs. Thus, the empirical evidence suggests that positive affect, negative affect, and life satisfaction are empirically distinct constructs.

Summary

There are a number of separable components of SWB. To obtain a complete picture of an individual's evaluation of his or her life, more than one component must be measured. For researchers who are interested in attaining a complete evaluation, we recommend that they assess positive affect, negative affect, satisfaction with important domains, and life satisfaction. Depending on the specific research question, additional components may be needed. For example, researchers who are interested in specific emotions like anxiety, anger, joy, or love should make sure to administer reliable and valid measures of these emotions. These researchers may want to focus on the basic emotion literature when choosing measures; whereas researchers who want a general understanding of affective well-being can focus more on the broad affective dimensions. Furthermore, researchers need to consider the time-frame of their measures, an issue to which we now turn.

Temporal Sequence and Stages

In this section we describe the multifaceted nature of SWB with an emphasis on the unfolding of different stages or components over time. These components, ranging from external events to global judgments of one's life, are depicted in Fig. 2. In particular, we highlight the transition between the stages and the divergences among measures of the different stages. Although convergence of measurement is often regarded as the ideal, we will see that discrepancies are also interesting and can inform a theory of SWB.

Our conceptualization begins with two basic premises. First, we have organized our model in terms of sequential stages that unfold over time. Thus, the temporal stages are seen as alternative facets of SWB, and are not identical to one another. Second, no one stage or component can be considered "true" happiness. For instance, both momentary affect and memory for emotions are important to SWB.

At step one, events happen to people, but their effects on long-term well-being are weak (Suh, Diener, & Fujita, 1996). In fact, all demographics account for less than 20% of variance in SWB (Campbell et al., 1976). Because there are many intervening steps between an event and the construction of a global life satisfaction judgment, events can only have a distal effect on SWB. On the other hand, according to our model, events are expected to have greater influence on online emotional reactions. For example, daily events such as health, family, and social interactions, have an impact on the daily mood of nursing home patients (Lawton, DeVoe, & Parmelee, 1995), but we would not expect daily events to influence global

E. Diener et al.

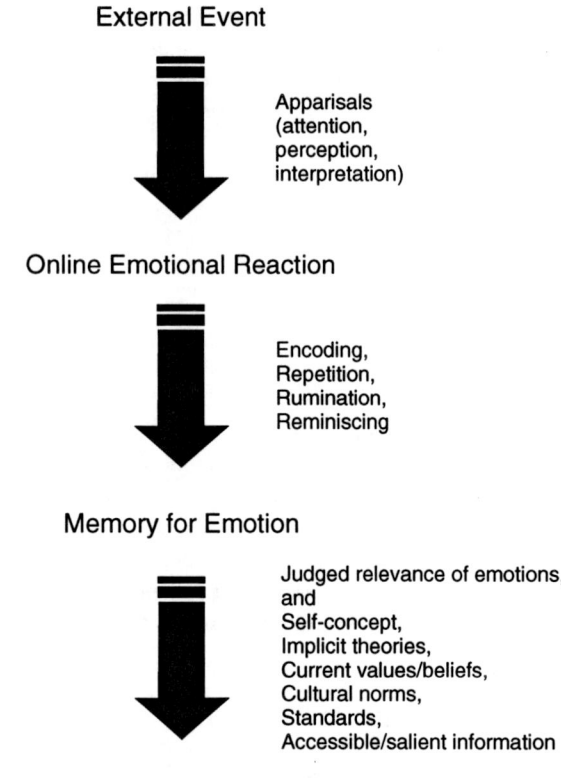

External Event

Apparisals
(attention,
perception,
interpretation)

Online Emotional Reaction

Encoding,
Repetition,
Rumination,
Reminiscing

Memory for Emotion

Judged relevance of emotions,
and
Self-concept,
Implicit theories,
Current values/beliefs,
Cultural norms,
Standards,
Accessible/salient information

Fig. 2 A temporal stage
model of subjective
well-being

Global SWB Judgment

judgments as strongly. In addition, the emotional impact of events will depend largely on people's appraisals, that is, individual differences in attention, perception, and interpretation of the event. Lazarus (1982, 1984) has written extensively on the subject of appraisals, therefore, we will not go into much detail here. For our model, it is sufficient to say that the transition from an event to one's emotional reaction involves evaluating whether the event is good or bad for one's goals and whether one has the resources necessary to cope with the event. Obviously not everyone will react the same way to the same events because events hold different meanings for different people.

The next stage, the on-line emotional reaction, is itself complex and multifaceted. The many aspects of a single emotional experience include physiological responses, nonverbal or behavioral expressions, and the verbal labeling of emotions. Even among these subcomponents of a single temporal stage there are sometimes discrepancies. For instance, a "repressor" might deny feelings of anxiety while showing increased perspiration, heart rate, and so forth (e.g. Weinberger, Schwartz, & Davidson, 1979). The verbal on-line measures are postulated to relate to memory for emotions, the next phase, but less so to global evaluations. On-line emotions become encoded in memory by a number of processes, including repetition of emotional information, rumination, and reminiscing, which can influence the degree of relation between on- line experience and the recall of that experience.

Once the on-line emotions are encoded in memory, they do not remain static. Instead, the memory is constantly reconstructed, and this is a critical feature of our model. We treat memory as a separate phenomenon from on-line experience. Some factors involved in the transition from on-line emotion to memory for emotion—that is, factors responsible for the discrepancy between the two stages—include self-concept (Diener, Larsen, & Emmons, 1984; Feldman Barrett, 1997), current beliefs (Levine, Prohaska, Burgess, Rice, & Laulere, 2001), implicit theories (Ross,1989), and cultural norms (Oishi, 2000). To illustrate, when McFarland, Ross, and DeCourville (1989) asked women to recall their mood during menstruation, they found that women recalled more negative emotion than they previously reported on-line. Furthermore, the amount of negative emotion remembered was moderated by the women's implicit theories about the relation between menstruation and mood. Similarly, Feldman Barrett (1997) found that individuals who scored high on trait measures of neuroticism overestimated in retrospect the amount of negative emotion they experienced online, while individuals high in trait extraversion overestimated the amount of on-line positive emotion. In describing the discrepancy between on-line emotions and memory, Robinson and Clore (2002) noted that two strategies of retrieval can guide recall. Recollections over a wide time frame (e.g. over the past month or year) rely on heuristic information, such as the self-concept. For narrower time frames (e.g. the past hour or day), people use a "retrieve and aggregate" strategy. That is, they recall specific instances of felt emotion and aggregate them to form their retrospective reports. In support of this notion and our model, Scollon, Diener, Oishi, and Biswas-Diener (2002) found that recalled reports were predicted by self-concept measures above and beyond on-line emotion.

At the broadest stage are global constructions, including life satisfaction. This stage is influenced by all the previous stages, but again, the degree to which depends on proximity. Thus, on-line experiences can influence global constructions. For example, someone who constantly experiences unpleasant mood would probably evaluate his/her life as unsatisfactory. However the extent to which on-line emotions influence global constructions depends on people's memory for emotions. In support of this, Schimmack et al. (2002) found that not only did hedonic memories correlate with life satisfaction judgments, but changes in memories correlated with life satisfaction as well. In addition to affective information, life satisfaction judgments incorporate several other sources that vary across cultures and individuals. As discussed earlier, these include cultural norms (Suh et al., 1998), and irrelevant but salient information (Schwarz and Clore, 1983). In some sense, global judgments such as life satisfaction, meaning in life, and fulfillment, capture the non-hedonistic meanings of happiness that were advanced by Democritus and Aristotle (even though the global judgments are subjective).

The current picture of SWB is more complex than any one stage can capture. Although each component is influenced by the previous stages, the stages are uniquely influenced by additional factors such as self-concept. Furthermore, there is evidence that the various stages converge moderately, but there are also processes that lead to differences between the stages. Likewise, the different stages of SWB are expected to predict different outcomes. For example, two studies indicate that recalled emotion is a better predictor of behavioral choices than on-line emotion. Wirtz et al. (2003) had students record their on-line emotions during a vacation and found that the degree to which students wanted to take a similar vacation later was strongly predicted by how much fun and enjoyment participants recalled, more so than the amount of fun and enjoyment they reported during the vacation. Similarly, in a study of dating couples, Oishi (2002) found that couples who misremembered interactions with their romantic partner as being more pleasant than in on-line reports were more likely to have intact relationships six months later.

In terms of practical application, the emerging evidence in support of a multicomponential approach to SWB raises new concerns about the measurement of SWB among the elderly. For instance, how should researchers measure the SWB of an elderly person with memory loss? The meaning of global or retrospective measures might be challenged because recollections about past emotions incorporate self- concept information, perhaps to an even greater degree than actual experience. And as memory loss becomes more severe, we predict, the recall of emotions will be more strongly influenced by self-concept. If researchers only rely on retrospective reports, they may be learning more about the self-concept of the elderly than about moment- to-moment experiences.

Philosophically, reconstructive memory also poses an intriguing question: Is happiness the *experience* or the *memory* of pleasant emotions? According to our model, no one measure deserves elevated status. Both the experience and memory (which includes some self-concept information), along with other components, are important. Nor can the different measures be considered substitutes for one another. Often researchers measure a single component or several components to see what correlates most highly with a given outcome measure. Such a practice belies the complexity and inter-relatedness of the different levels of SWB.

What the multi-component approach to SWB suggests is that measures at each stage provide interesting information, but researchers need to understand and specify the components of SWB they are measuring. In some ways, each stage of SWB reflects a different philosophical tradition of happiness. For example, on-line emotion is related to hedonistic views of happiness, whereas global judgments are more closely related to eudaimonia or Democritus's ideas. In the measurement section, we will discuss what researchers need to consider in order to assess SWB. For instance, most researchers would prefer to measure only the recall or global stages of SWB, and we will discuss how valid this practice seems to be.

Stability and Consistency of SWB

Subjective well-being variables are thought to reflect the actual conditions in a person's life. Thus, when these conditions change, reports of SWB should change accordingly. Yet, because there is some degree of stability in these conditions, we should also expect SWB measures to be relatively stable over time. Furthermore,

SWB constructs are influenced by a variety of stable personality factors, a finding that supports the notion that SWB should be relatively stable (Diener & Lucas, 2000), because adult personality is very stable (Costa & McCrae, 1988). In fact, in the literature, there are even debates about whether SWB should be considered a trait or a state (Veenhoven, 1994, 1998; Stones, Hadjistavopoulo, Tuuko, & Kozma, 1995; Lykken & Tellegen, 1996; Ehrhardt et al., 2000). In this section, we review the evidence regarding the stability and consistency of well-being constructs.

There is considerable evidence that SWB variables do exhibit some degree of stability. Magnus and Diener (1991), for example, found that life satisfaction scores exhibited stability coefficients of 0.58 over a 4-year period. Even when different methods of assessment were used to measure life satisfaction (e.g. self- and informant-reports), stability was high ($r = 0.52$). Ehrhardt et al. (2000) examined life satisfaction reports in a large, nationally representative German panel study, and they found stability coefficients of 0.27 across 10 years. For the purposes of this chapter, we reanalyzed this data set (with an additional 5 years of satisfaction reports; see Lucas, Clark, Georgellis, & Diener, 2003) and found that stability coefficients did not drop off as the length of the study increased. The correlation between life satisfaction in the first year of the study and life satisfaction in the 15th year was still 0.28. We should also note that this satisfaction measure is a single-item scale, and thus, it probably does not have ideal psychometric characteristics. Across those 15 years, stable between-person variance accounted for 44% of the total amount of variance in these measures. Thus, there is considerable stability in life satisfaction scores over long periods of time; though there are also changes that occur within persons over time.

Additional research shows that positive and negative affect scores are also somewhat stable over time. Watson and Walker (1996), for example, found 6- to 7- year stability coefficients in the range of 0.36–0.46 for positive affect and negative affect in a student sample, and Costa and McCrae (1988) found 6-year stability coefficients in the 0.50 range in an adult sample. Costa and McCrae's findings are particularly impressive given that these stability coefficients compared self-reports of affect with spouse ratings of affect. Thus, like Magnus and Diener's (1991) longitudinal study of life satisfaction, stability cannot be explained solely by stability of self-concept or by response artifacts.

The stability of well-being measures does not mean, however, that these measures are insensitive to changing life circumstances. On the contrary, Lucas et al. (2003) and Clark, Georgellis, Lucas, and Diener (2002) used the 15-year German panelstudy described above to show that life satisfaction scores increased following marriage and decreased following widowhood or unemployment. Thus, life circumstances do influence life satisfaction scores, as we would expect. Interestingly, in both the Lucas et al. study and the Clark et al. study, satisfaction scores were very stable from the periods before an event to the periods after the event, suggesting that relative satisfaction scores are stable even in the face of changing life circumstances (also see Costa, McCrae, & Zonderman, 1987) that can influence mean levels.

A different way to examine the stability of SWB constructs is to look within persons across situations. If well-being reflects a person's evaluation of his or her life as a whole, we would not expect scores to be completely determined by changing situationalfactors. Diener and Larsen (1984) examined this question by asking participants to complete mood reports multiple times a day for multiple days. They found that positive affect, negative affect, and life satisfaction were very stable even across diverse situations. For example, positive affect in work situations correlated 0.70 with positive affect in recreation situations, and negative affect in work situations correlated 0.74 with negative affect in recreation situations (similar correlations were found across social vs. alone situations and across novel vs. typical situations). Correlations were even higher for life satisfaction scores, often around 0.95. Thus, well-being is not completely determined by situational factors. A substantialproportion of the variance in well-being reports is stable across situations and even over long periods of time.

We should also note that, to some extent, the consistency of well-being may vary across cultures. Oishi, Diener, Scollon, Biswas-Diener (2002), for example, showed that there is less consistency in affect in samples from Japan than there is in samples from the United States. In other words, people's affect varies to a greater extent across situations in Japan than it does in the United States. Thus, the notion of a happy person may be less meaningful in Japan because there is less person-level variance in SWB scores. Clearly more research is needed, but we recommend that researchers interpret the stability and consistency data cautiously until we can determine the factors that moderate the extent to which people are stable over time and across situations.

Affect vs. Cognition

SWB includes both an affective (i.e. on-going evaluations of one's life) and a cognitive component (i.e. life satisfaction). Theorists have long debated the degree to which affect and cognition are related (see Zajonc, 1980; Lazarus, 1982, 1984). This controversy bears particular relevance to the study of SWB because it highlights the dependence, and yet separability, of the two systems, suggesting a need to measure affect and cognition separately (even though they are not entirely independent) in order to gain a more complete picture of SWB.

On the one hand, researchers such as LeDoux (2000) argue that some simple emotions such as fear can occur without complex cognitive processing, or as a result of unconscious processing (Zajonc, 1980). Similarly, some people have been shown to deny their subjective feelings, despite showing a physiological reaction to events (Shedler, Mayman, & Manis, 1993). Both lines of evidence suggest that non-verbal, non-cognitive measures (e.g. eyeblink startle and cortisol) might detect reactions that self-report measures do not.

On the other hand, cognitive appraisals play an important role in shaping our reactions to events. For example, if a student feels responsible for getting a good grade on an exam (appraisal), then she will feel happy about it. As well, cultural norms provide a frame for interpreting events. That is, the emotions a person feels will tend to fit into his or her worldview. Returning to our example, the student who feels responsible for the event of making a good grade on an exam might not label her feeling as pride if her culture regards pride as a sinful emotion. Indeed, cultural norms for emotions are strongly related to reports of subjective experience (see Eid & Diener, 2001), and the rank ordering of societies on measures such as life satisfaction bear considerable resemblance to the rank ordering of societies on emotion norms (see Diener, Scollon, Oishi, Dzokoto, & Suh, 2000). Thus, self-report measures will detect what individuals label about their subjective feelings, although this is only one aspect of the emotional experience.

An added complication to the affect–cognition debate stems from disagreements about what constitutes cognition (Mathews & MacLeod, 1994). Some theorists argue that cognition includes only higher-order processing; other definitions include lower-order processes such as attention. Although we recognize the importance of attention in affect regulation (see Mathews & MacLeod, 1994; Segerstrom, 2001), of central importance to the present discussion of SWB are the higher-order conscious processes such as cognitive judgments or global evaluations of one's life.

By treating affect and cognition as partially separable constructs, we invite the possibility that one can be satisfied with one's life, and yet experience little pleasant affect, and vice versa. To illustrate, let us consider the SWB of a spouse and caretaker of an Alzheimer's patient. Narrative accounts of individuals who have cared for family members with Alzheimer's disease (e.g. Bayley, 1999) suggest a caretaker's daily life is fraught with frustration and difficulty, with brief and infrequent joys. Despite a preponderance of negative affect, however, the caretaker might still evaluate his overall life positively. This discrepancy between affect and cognitive judgments can occur for several reasons.

First, as discussed in the previous section, people rely on different sources of information when constructing global judgments. Even though enjoyment in a domain tends to correlate with satisfaction in that domain, affective information might be highly important for some people, but irrelevant for others (e.g. Oishi et al., 2001). One possibility is that with certain life tasks such as caregiving or with certain life stages, affect is given less weight in judgments of life satisfaction (cf. Carstensen, 1995), although this remains an empirical question. Second, the individual's culture will provide a framework for interpreting the importance of affect. As noted earlier, cultures differ in the degree to which they rely on affective information in life satisfaction constructions (Suh et al., 1998). But the impact of culture extends further because cultures also clearly differ in what they consider normative tasks. Thus, in a culture in which caring for the elderly is expected, the caretaker might derive a sense of satisfaction from doing the "right thing" and following cultural norms, even though the caretaking is unpleasant.

Third, the works of LeDoux (2000) and Shedler et al. (1993) suggest that the caretaker may be unable or unwilling to articulate his subjective emotional experience. Physiological measures might indicate a different picture, again underscoring the need for multiple measures, including non-cognitive ones.

Finally, people may rely on different standards in judging life satisfaction than in evaluating specific events. For example, daily affect may be determined by whether one is meeting one's lower-level goals, whereas global judgments may be determined by higher-level, more abstract goals. This allows for one's moment-to-moment affect to be quite negative while the bigger picture might reveal a sense of satisfaction for fulfilling some larger goal. Unfortunately, these questions have not yet been empirically tested, and it remains for future research to uncover which standards influence the different types and levels of SWB.

The Functioning Mood System

Although negative emotions are usually unpleasant, theorists have recognized their functionality. For example, fear can motivate us to avoid danger, anger can push us to correct an injustice, and sadness can make us withdraw so that we can renew our resources and make new plans of action after loss. Volumes have been written on the adaptive functions of negative emotions, but much less on the positive side. Recently, Fredrickson (1998, 2001) outlined a "broaden and build model" explaining that the function of positive emotions is to lead to sociability, play, and exploration. Thus, positive emotions help us build our social and material resources, and help us learn new behaviors for the future. Positive emotions occur when things are going well, and when we have the time to engage in actions that will benefit us later.

If emotions are, in many cases, functional and adaptive, and the emotion system has come to us through evolution to guide behavior, it would seem dysfunctional never to experience any negative emotions. In other words, it would also be maladaptive to chronically experience high positive moods all of the time, regardless of the circumstances. After all, the adaptiveness of the emotion system depends on its ability to provide calibrated feedback about one's relation to the environment, and chronic states of any valence would fail to serve that purpose because they are unresponsive to events. Berenbaum, Raghavan, Le, Vernon, and Gomez (2002) have similarly noted that there is nothing inherently good or bad about emotions of either valence, but rather excesses of either happiness or sadness present problems. A person who can only feel happy would not be able to avoid danger or other bad situations; such a person would be overly expansive and take on new goals even when it is not appropriate. This kind of behavior can best be seen in manics. In extreme form, manics start more projects than they can finish, and they do not exercise caution and good judgment in planning. This is not the picture of happiness that we are advancing. Happiness is not to be equated with mania or uninterrupted ecstasy. Instead, the adaptable happy person should have moods that fluctuate to some degree in reaction to good and bad events.

Indeed the data support both of these notions. First, in studies of thousands of people, we have found that it is very rare for people to be at a 10 on a 10-point scale, or to be at the very top of the Satisfaction With Life Scale (SWLS: Diener, Emmons, Larsen, & Griffin, 1985). Furthermore, even when people rate themselves as extremely satisfied, we find in follow-up that they are usually not at the top of the scale two years later. That is, people might occasionally move up to a euphoric state, but they do not stay there for long (Diener & Seligman, 2002).

Second, even happy people have pleasant and unpleasant moods. An investigation of 22 individuals who scored in the top 10% on various SWB measures revealed that even these people, although extremely satisfied with life, occasionally had unpleasant affect. Diener and Larsen (1984) found that although people have stable and consistent average moods, their momentary moods fluctuate. Thus, it is possible for happy people to react to events but still maintain an average positive level around which their moods fluctuate. This allows even happy people to react to negative events and not be stuck in a high happy mood.

But clearly chronic unrelieved negative emotion is undesirable and unhealthy. For one thing, people usually do not function well under conditions of severe and prolonged negative affect (Headey & Wearing, 1989; Hays, Wells, Sherbourne, Rogers, & Spritzer, 1995; Hammen, 2002). This state is very unpleasant, and prolonged NA can interfere with quality of life as well as produce a greater likelihood of negative life events. Thus, whereas temporary experiences of negative affect are normal and can be functional, prolonged negative affect is often very dysfunctional.

Tradeoffs

Just as the above conception of happiness is not the picture of uninterrupted ecstasy, we believe that people, moreover, do not desire a life of unvariegated joys, at least not without some qualifications. First, people want their happy feelings to be justified. This view marks a clear departure from hedonistic philosophy in which personal enjoyment was considered the ultimate goal (Tatarkiewicz, 1976). Robert Nozick's (1974) philosophical idea of an "experience machine" provides a good example of why good feelings alone are not enough. Nozick (1974) imagines an experience machine that would create the subjective feeling of being engaged in fun, exciting, pleasant activities of one's choosing—for instance, writing a novel, making a new friend, feasting on a fine dinner, or lounging on a tropical beach. The experience machine would provide all the sensations that would ordinarily accompany the activity, but in actuality, the person would be lying in a laboratory hooked up to a computer.

Certainly few people would choose to plug in to the experience machine, even though the feelings it provides are desirable. As Nozick (1974) points out, there is more that matters than people's experiences from the inside. In fact, when we asked college students to rate some hypothetical scenarios and varied aspects of each scenario (such as whether the event occurred in reality or was the product of an experience machine), we found that the reality of events was extremely important, even for intensely pleasant and joyous activities. In particular, when the event involved achievement, momentary pleasure and memory of the event were secondary, but reality was essential. In other words, it would be pointless to plug in to the experience machine to feel as if one has won the Nobel Prize, when, in fact, one has not.

The second limitation on a hedonistic view of happiness is that people are willing, at times, to sacrifice momentary positive affect for other goals that they value. For example, Kim-Prieto (2002) found that Asian and Asian American students were more likely to choose tasks that met their parents' approval or tasks that would lead to achievement over other tasks that were described as fun and personally enjoyable. Thus, some individuals or groups may choose to maximize the non-hedonistic meanings of subjective well-being. Interestingly, Caucasian students preferred tasks that were fun or that maximized personal enjoyment. Other evidence comes from studies of self-improvement. Oishi and Diener (2001) found that when Caucasians were not good at a particular activity, they would switch to a different activity when given the opportunity. On the other hand, Asian Americans often pursued the activity they were not good at, but switched to a different activity if they were good at the first one. Such a strategy might improve one's skills, but would certainly not maximize immediate enjoyment (see also Heine et al., 2001).

Implications for Measurement

Subjective well-being measures should tap well-being from a respondent's own perspective. For this reason, most studies of SWB have relied on self-report measures of the constructs. However, there are many reasons to be cautious in our interpretation of results based solely on self-report measures. Various response sets and response styles may influence people's ratings. Certain people may appear to be happier than others simply because they use high numbers on a response scale or because they want to look favorable in the eyes of the experimenter. Thus, although self-reports play a central role in SWB research, they must be supplemented with additional measurement techniques to obtain a complete understanding of the construct. In this section, we discuss the theoretical and methodological issues involved in selecting and using SWB measures (for a more detailed discussion, see Larsen & Fredrickson, 1999; Larsen, Diener, & Lucas, 2002; Lucas, Diener, & Larsen, 2003).

Self-reports of SWB vary considerably in their complexity. A number of studies have shown that even the simplest of these—the single-item measures—can exhibit some degree of reliability and validity. Diener, Nickerson, Lucas, and Sandvik (2002), for instance, showed that a single item measure ("cheerfulness") could predict criterion variables 18 years later. In a separate investigation of this single-item measure, Diener et al. found that it correlated between 0.73 and 0.89 with a multiple-item measure of positive emotions that was assessed multiple times over a 3-month period. Similarly, Lucas et al. (2003) showed that a single-item measure of life satisfaction was relatively stable over time and was sensitive to changes in life events. Thus, if the focus of one's research is to get a relatively reliable and valid measure of well-being and one cannot afford to include a variety of self-report indicators, one can confidently assess these constructs using single-item measures. Of course, multiple item measures will increase reliability and breadth of coverage, and therefore, they are more desirable when one can afford to include them.

There are a number of reliable and valid measures of well-being constructs (see MacKay, 1980; Larsen, Diener, & Emmons, 1985; Andrews & Robinson, 1991; Stone, 1995; Lucas et al., 2003 for reviews). Most measure one or more well-being constructs using items with clear face validity. For example, life satisfaction scales may ask respondents the extent to which they agree with statements like: "I am satisfied with my life" or "In most ways my life is close to my ideal" (Diener, 1985). Positive and negative affect scales may ask people to indicate the extent to which they experience a series of emotions like "happiness," "sadness," "anger," "affection," or "fear." As indicated in our discussion of the structure of well-being, the different components of well-being can be exhibited in different ways. One could experience a high frequency of positive affect without experiencing affect intensely at any particular moment. Thus, it is often useful to separate frequency from intensity when asking about SWB variables. Similarly, because affect does change from moment to moment, it is important to specify the time frame of well-being reports. If one is interested in relatively short term variation in well-being, one can choose emotion questionnaires that ask only about the past hour, the past day, or the past week. Researchers interested in longer term mood levels, on the other hand, may want to choose scales that ask about mood over the past month, year, or affect in general.

A desirable alternative to asking people to retrospectively judge their happiness is to assess SWB using experience sampling methods (ESM; also known as ecological momentary assessment, Stone, Shiffman, & DeVries, 1999). In ESM, participants report their mood multiple times over a relatively long period of time. For example, in some studies, participants may be asked to carry handheld computers that signal an alarm five times a day for seven days. Each time the alarm sounds, the participant completes an emotion report. By using ESM techniques, researchers can study affect as a state and a trait. For example, within-person analyses can elucidate within-person emotional processes. At the same time, an individual's entire set of emotion reports can be averaged to create a reliable trait measure of his or her well-being. Using this type of aggregation process eliminates the need for participants to recall and attempt to derive an overall emotion report. Kahneman (1999) reviewed evidence that individuals have difficulty remembering and aggregating across multiple occasions, and a number of studies have now shown that ESM reports often give different information about a person's overall well-being than do global reports.

The difficulties that people have in accurately recalling their affective experiences suggest that alternative measures should be used when possible. One easily administered alternative to self-report is the informant- or observer-report technique. Although informants may have their own set of biases and response sets, these are likely to be different than the biases and response sets of the target person, and together self- and informant-reports can provide valid information about a person's well-being.

There are two general types of observer reports. In the known-informant approach, friends and family members rate a target person's well-being. Presumably, these known-informants see the target exhibiting well-being relevant behaviors in his or her life, and thus, they should be able to provide information about how happy that target individual is. In general, these informant reports show moderate to substantial convergence with self-report measures (McCrae & Costa, 1989; Diener, Smith, & Fujita, 1995; Lucas et al., 1996). An alternative to the known-informant approach is the expert-rater approach. Informants who do not know the target can be trained to interpret specific signals of emotional experience (Krokoff et al., 1989; Gottman, 1993). Raters can even be trained to interpret facial expressions of emotions. For example, in the Facial Action Coding System (FACS; Ekman & Friesen, 1975, 1978 in refs), raters are trained to recognize specific muscle movements that usually co-occur with emotional responses. The expert-rater approach has an important advantage over self-report and the known-informant reports: This technique can be used to attain relatively objective measures of a person's emotional response.

Along the same lines, researchers have looked beyond facial muscle movements to examine other physiological correlates of emotional feelings. Variables such as heart rate, heart rate acceleration, blood pressure, bodily temperature, finger temperature, respiration amplitude, and skin conductance have all been used to measure emotional response (Cacioppo et al., 2000). Other researchers have noted that activity in certain brain regions seems to be associated with both individual differences in emotional levels as well as within-person changes in emotional experience (Davidson, 1992). Thus, electro-encephalograms, PET scans and functional MRIs can be used to measure this differential activity. These measures, like the Facial Action Coding System, can provide relatively objective measures of well-being. However, much more research is needed before these measures can tap the subtle features that can be picked up in self-report measures. For example, many of the objective indicators of emotion seem to be able to distinguish positive emotions from negative emotions (and sometimes certain negative emotions from one another), but distinctions beyond these basic categories are difficult.

A final technique that researchers have used to measure well-being is to examine people's responses to emotion sensitive tasks. Seidlitz and Diener (1993), for example, asked people to recall as many happy experiences from their lives as they could in a short amount of time. Because performance on this task is correlated with well-being measures, it can be used as an alternative measure that is less susceptible to response styles and demand characteristics. Other researchers have exposed participants to word-completion tasks or word recognition tasks (for a review of these cognitive tasks, see Rusting, 1998). Happy people are more likely than unhappy people to complete word stems using positive words and they are quicker to recognize positive words. When social desirability, demand characteristics, or other measurement issues are a concern, these emotion sensitive tasks can provide a useful alternative to self-report measures.

Self-report measures of SWB are likely to remain the most frequently used measures of the constructs. These measures are quick and easy, they are sensitive enough to capture the subtle differences between the various components of well-being, and they have substantial reliability and validity. Yet, they are imperfect. Researchers should use additional methods of measurement when possible. In addition, researchers who are interested in determining the way that people construct these judgments will need to use multiple self- and non-self-report techniques to under- stand these processes. Whatever the goalof the research, however, we recommend that people assess the multiple components of well-being separately when possible.

Implications for Research on Aging

Research on SWB over the lifespan offers a unique opportunity for psychologists interested in the processes underlying SWB judgments. SWB judgments are thought to reflect the conditions in one's life, and many of these conditions deteriorate in old age. Thus, studies of aging can provide a useful test of SWB theories. Yet when we examine the empirical evidence regarding age-related changes in SWB, there is somewhat of a paradox (Kunzmann et al., 2000). On the one hand, the objective conditions in one's life do seem to deteriorate. Income levels often decrease and the frequency of negative events including the death of one's spouse and friends and the experience of health problems often increase. Most research finds, however, that SWB levels remain stable over time, and sometimes these levels even increase (see Diener & Suh, 1998; Mroczek & Kolarz, 1998; Kunzmann, Little, & Smith, 2000; Lucas & Gohm, 2000; Lawton, 2001; Pinquart, 2001).

For example, Diener and Suh (1997) examined age differences in well-being in a sample of approximately 60,000 respondents from 43 nations. They found that life satisfaction increased very slightly, positive affect decreased slightly, and negative affect decreased from age 20 to 60, but then increased slightly among the oldest individuals in their sample. Lucas and Gohm (2000) showed that this effect did not vary substantially when the different nations were studied individually. A number of researchers have replicated these findings, showing little change in life satisfaction, slight declines in positive affect (correlations in the range of -0.05 to -0.12), and initial declines followed by a leveling effect or even subsequent increases in negative affect (Carstensen, Pasupathi, Mayr, & Nesselroade, 2000; Kunzmann et al., 2000). In a recent meta-analysis, Pinquart (2001) found that the average correlations between positive affect and age and between negative affect and age were both negative, but very small: $r = -0.03$ for positive affect and $r = -0.01$ for negative affect. There were also significant quadratic effects: Positive affect decreased more quickly and negative affect began to increase among the very old.

Diener and Suh (1998) suggested that some of the decrease in both positive and negative affect might be due to the measurement of high arousal positive and negative emotions. For example, older adults may feel as much pleasantness, but they may do so with less intensity, or they may be less likely to experience high arousal emotions such as excitement or energy. Pinquart's (2001) meta-analysis supported this hypothesis. Declines in the experience of emotions were greater among high arousal emotion scales than among low arousal emotion scales. Thus, when assessing emotions in older adults, researchers should tap a broad range of high arousal and low arousal positive and negative emotions.

We should also caution that much of the evidence for age changes in subjective well-being comes from cross-sectional studies. Both Kunzmann et al. (2000) and Pinquart (2001) noted that the size of age effects often varies depending on whether cross-sectional or longitudinal methods are used. Because cross-sectional studies conflate age effects with cohort effects, the interpretation of the correlations in these studies is somewhat unclear. Pinquart found that the decline in positive affect was steeper in longitudinal studies than in cross-sectional studies, whereas the decline in negative affect was less steep in longitudinal studies than in cross-sectional studies. Given that these differences across methodologies exist, researchers must be careful in interpreting evidence from cross-sectional studies. However, we should also note that in their examination of a large German panel study, Ehrhardt et al. (2000) found that people responded to the questionnaire differently after repeated measurements. Thus, age-related changes in longitudinal studies may be confounded with practice effects.

A final measurement issue regarding SWB over the life-span is the extent to which changes reflect true differences over time versus changes in the self-concept. Most research that examines age-related changes in SWB relies upon global, retrospective measures. As we noted in the section on measurement, the global measures require participants to be able to accurately remember and aggregate across many moments and many life domains. Older individuals may have a more stable sense of self-concept than younger individuals, and self-reports of emotional experience may reflect this stable self-concept. Similarly, older individuals may not be able to remember and aggregate across multiple experiences as well as younger individuals. Only a few studies have used experience sampling methods to examine the effects of memory on SWB reports of older people. For example, Carstensen et al. (2000) asked participants ranging in age from 18 to 94 years old to complete emotion reports multiple times a day. They found that, consistent with existing literature, reports of negative affect declined until about age 60, and then leveled off after that. Positive affect, in their study, did not show any significant changes across the different age groups.

Although questions about the influence of measurement issues remain, evidence from a variety of methodologies suggests that SWB does not decline very much over time. Thus, we must ask why SWB does not seem to change, even when external life circumstances are declining (Kunzmann et al., 2000). A number of theories have suggested that changes in life circumstances are balanced by changes in emotion regulation. Specifically, research suggests that as individuals mature, they are better able to regulate their emotions (e.g. Gross et al., 1997) or are more motivated to regulate their emotions. Carstensen (1995), for example, argued that as one ages, he or she monitors the amount of time he or she has left before death. This monitoring, in turn, leads to changes in goals. As one becomes more aware of (and closer to) one's mortality, he or she should place a higher premium on experiencing pleasant emotional states. Thus, emotion regulation theories suggest that SWB may, in fact, increase with age, even in the face of declining life circumstances.

Increasingly, researchers are focusing on the functional nature of SWB (Fredrickson, 1998, 2001; Lyubomirsky et al., 2002; Lucas & Diener, 2003). Researchers should keep this in mind when examining the SWB of older adults. If older adults do experience lower levels of well-being, this may not necessarily signal poor functioning. Instead, it may signal a functional response to real problems. Similarly, although some individuals may place a higher premium on experiencing positive emotions as they age (as Carstensen, 1995, suggested), others may be willing to trade positive well-being for other goals. Thus, researchers must examine changes in well-being within the context of the changing goals that individuals are likely to have as they age.

Conclusions: The Take-Home Message(s) and Directions for Future Research

From the early philosophical treatments of happiness to the modern science of subjective well-being, the concept of happiness has evolved considerably. Although subjective well-being can be defined simply as the way that people evaluate their lives, this simple definition belies the complex and multi-faceted nature of the construct. SWB is not a unitary dimension, and there is no single index that can capture what it means to be happy. Instead, SWB reflects a broad collection of distinct components, and to get a complete picture of one's well-being, researchers must understand the various ways that people can evaluate their lives. For example, an older individual may experience more health problems or financial difficulties than a younger individual, and these stressors may cause anxiety and negative emotions on a day-to-day basis. Yet, at the same time, the older individual may have a strong sense of satisfaction with the things he or she has accomplished over the course of an entire lifetime. Researchers who only focus on one component of well-being will not be able to capture the complex nature of these phenomena. A multi-faceted approach to SWB not only suggests the necessity of multiple measures, but the choice of measures should be theoretically meaningful. For example, if researchers are interested in making predictions about people's choices, then they might measure recalled emotions, rather than on-line experiences (Wirtz et al., 2003). Similarly, life events may have small effects on global evaluations, but rather larger effects on daily affect (e.g. Lawton et al., 1995).

Naturally, thorough SWB assessments are time-consuming, and this might discourage some researchers, but the payoff can be great in terms of understanding. Just as we do not assess intelligence, mental illness, creativity, or the Big Five with a few quick questions, we cannot expect to measure SWB with a five-minute global assessment. This is not to say that global assessments are useless, because they can provide valid and meaningful information. But they are very incomplete. To be thorough requires more in-depth measurement.

It is not solely for the sake of completeness, however, that we emphasize the multi-faceted nature of well-being. There are also many theoretical reasons for studying the components of well-being separately. We know, for instance, that the different components have different correlates. These findings have led researchers to suggest that distinct processes underlie the various components. Therefore, to develop a theory of these processes, researchers will need to understand the various components separately. Furthermore, although it may seem intuitive that the various components would tap into the same underlying constructs, oftentimes different measures of well-being do not completely converge. Divergent measures need not be cause for despair. Instead, studying the reasons for these divergences can elucidate the processes that lead to the various well-being judgments.

One of the strongest recommendations we can make to SWB researchers and gerontologists is to examine low vs. high intensity emotions separately. If intense emotions are assessed such as PANAS PA (e.g. "active" from Watson, Clark, & Tellegen, 1988) or Bradburn PA items (e.g. "on top of the world"), then the elderly might appear lower in PA. But if low arousal words, such as contentment or happy, are assessed, then we might not see a decline in PA with age (Lawton, Kleban, Rajagopal, & Dean 1992; Lawton, 2001). Likewise, there might be no decline in frequency of emotions with age, but a decline in intensity. That is, people might experience anger with the same frequency, but with age, they may experience it less intensely. A similar argument can be applied to the valence of affect, highlighting the need to measure PA and NA separately.

More research on the elderly is needed, and this research should include at least two important aims. First, the structure of SWB needs to be more clearly identified among the elderly (e.g. Lawton, Kleban, Dean, Rajagopal, & Parmelee, 1992). In fact, more research on many specific populations is needed in order to understand the structure of SWB in various groups (e.g. ethnic/cultural groups). Second, future studies should examine the multi-components of SWB and explore the steps involved in the emotion sequence.

Finally, the evolving conception of SWB suggests that ideal SWB is not to be equated with uninterrupted euphoria. Such a view would place too great an emphasis on hedonism when there are clearly non-hedonistic aspects of SWB as well (e.g. global judgments such as life satisfaction, meaning, and fulfillment). Furthermore, we should consider what is functional, and this includes some negative feelings from time to time. Although pleasant emotions may be desirable, happiness is not the ultimate goal at all times. Rather, individual and cultural differences in the valuing of enjoyment suggest that people are willing to sacrifice feeling happy for other goals. And even when people do seek enjoyment, they want to feel good for the right reasons. Thus, we need to understand people's goals, and consider their feelings within the context of their values.

References

Andrews, F. M., & Robinson, J. P. (1991). Measures of subjective well-being. In J. P. Robinson, P. R. Shaver, & L. S. Wrightsman (Eds.), *Measures of personality and social psychological attitudes* (pp. 61–114). San Diego: Academic Press.

Andrews, F. M., & Withey, S. B. (1976). *Social indicators of well-being: America's perception of life quality*. New York: Plenum Press.

Bayley, J. (1999). *Elegy for Iris*. St. New York: Martin's Press.

Berenbaum, H., Raghavan, C., Le, H.-N., Vernon, L. L., & Gomez, J. J. (2002). *A taxonomy of emotional disturbances*. Manuscript submitted for publication, University of Illinois, Urbana-Champaign.

Bradburn, N. M. (1969). *The structure of psychological well-being*. Chicago: Aldine.

Cacioppo, J. T., Berntson, G. G., Larsen, J. T., Poehlmann, K. M., & Ito, T. A. (2000). The psychophysiology of emotion. In M. Lewis & J. M. Haviland-Jones (Eds.), *Handbook of emotions* (2nd ed., pp. 173–191). New York: Guilford.

Campbell, A., Converse, P. E., & Rodgers, W. L. (1976). *The quality of American life*. New York: Russell Sage Foundation.

Carstensen, L. L. (1995). Evidence for a life-span theory of socioemotional selectivity. *Current Directions in Psychological Science, 4*, 151–156.

Carstensen, L. L., Pasupathi, M., Mayr, U., & Nesselroade, J. R. (2000). Emotional experience in everyday life across the adult life span. *Journal of Personality and Social Psychology, 779*, 644–655.

Clark, A. E., Georgellis, Y., Lucas, R. E., & Diener, E. (2002). *Unemployment alters the set-point for life satisfaction*. Unpublished manuscript.

Costa, P. T., & McCrae, R. R. (1980). Influence of extraversion and neuroticism on subjective well-being: Happy and unhappy people. *Journal of Personality and Social Psychology, 38*, 668–678.

Costa, P. T., & McCrae, R. R. (1988). Personality in adulthood: A six-year longitudinal study of self-reports and spouse ratings of the NEO Personality Inventory. *Journal of Personality and Social Psychology, 54*, 853–863.

Costa, P. T., McCrae, R. R., & Zonderman, A. (1987). Environmental and dispositional influences on well-being: Longitudinal follow-up of an American national sample. *British Journal of Psychology, 78*, 299–306.

Danner, D. D., Snowden, D. A., & Friesen, W. V. (2001). Positive emotions in early life and longevity: Findings from the Nun Study. *Journal of Personality and Social Psychology, 80*, 801–813.

Davidson, R. J. (1992). Anterior cerebralasymmetry and the nature of emotion. *Brain and Cognition, 20*, 125–151.

Diener, E. (2000). Subjective well-being: The science of happiness, and a proposal for a national index. *American Psychologist, 55*, 34–43.

Diener, E., Colvin, C. R., Pavot, W. G., & Allman, A. (1992). The psychic costs of intense positive affect. *Journal of Personality and Social Psychology, 52*, 492–503.

Diener, E., & Emmons, R. A. (1985). The independence of positive and negative affect. *Journal of Personality and Social Psychology, 47*, 1105–1117.

Diener, E., Emmons, R. A., Larsen, R. J., & Griffin, S. (1985). The satisfaction with life scale. *Journal of Personality Assessment, 49*, 71–75.

Diener, E., & Fujita, F. (1997). Social comparisons and subjective well-being. In B. Buunk & R. Gibbons (Eds.), *Health, coping, and social comparison* (pp. 329–357). Mahwah, NJ: Erlbaum.

Diener, E., & Iran-Nejad, A. (1986). The relationship in experience between various types of affect. *Journal of Personality and Social Psychology, 50*, 1031–1038.

Diener, E. & Larsen, R. J. (1984). Temporalstability and cross-situationalconsistency of affective, behavioral, and cognitive responses. *Journal of Personality and Social Psychology, 47*, 871–883.

Diener, E., Larsen, R. J., & Emmons, R. A. (1984). Person Â situation interactions: Choice of situations and congruence response models. *Journal of Personality and Social Psychology, 47*, 580–592.

Diener, E., & Lucas, R. E. (2000). Subjective emotional well-being. In M. Lewis & J. M. Haviland-Jones (Eds.), *Handbook of emotions* (2nd ed., pp. 325–337). New York: Guilford.

Diener, E., Lucas, R. E., Oishi, S., & Suh, E. M. (2002). Looking up and down: Weighting good and bad information in life satisfaction judgments. *Personality and Social Psychology Bulletin, 28*, 437–445.

Diener, E., Nickerson, C., Lucas, R. E., & Sandvik, E. (2002). Dispositional affect and job outcomes. *Social Indicators Research, 59*, 229–259.

Diener, E., Sandvik, E., & Pavot, W. (1991). Happiness is the frequency, not the intensity, of positive versus negative affect. In F. Strack, M. Argyle, & N. Schwarz (Eds.), *Subjective well-being: An interdisciplinary perspective. International Series in Experimental Social Psychology* (pp. 119–139). Oxford, England: Pergamon Press.

Diener, E., Scollon, C. K., Oishi, S., Dzokoto, V., & Suh, E. M. (2000). Positivity and the con-struction of life satisfaction judgments: Global happiness is not the sum of its parts. *Journal of Happiness Studies, 1*, 159–176.

Diener, E., & Seligman, M. E. P. (2002). Very happy people. *Psychological Science, 13*, 81–84.

Diener, E., Smith, H., & Fujita, F. (1995). The personality structure of affect. *Journal of Personality and Social Psychology, 50*, 130–141.

Diener, E., & Suh, E. (1997). Measuring quality of life: Economic, social and subjective indicators. *Social Indicators Research, 40*, 189–216.

Diener, E., & Suh, E. M. (1998). Subjective well-being and age: An international analysis. In K. W. Schaie & M. P. Lawton (Eds.), *Annual review of gerontology and geriatrics* (Vol. 8, pp. 304–324). New York: Springer.

Ehrhardt, J. J., Saris, W. E., & Veenhoven, R. (2000). Stability of life-satisfaction over time: Anal-ysis of change in ranks in a nationalpopulation. *Journal of Happiness Studies, 1*, 177–205.

Eid, M., & Diener, E. (1999). Intraindividual variability in affect: Reliability, validity, and person-ality correlates. *Journal of Personality and Social Psychology, 76*, 662–676.

Eid, M., & Diener, E. (2001). Norms for experiencing emotions in different cultures: Inter- and intra-national differences. *Journal of Personality and Social Psychology, 81*, 869–885.

Ekman, P., & Friesen, W. (1978). *Facial action codingsystem.* Palo Alto, CA: Consulting Psychol-ogists Press.

Ekman, P., Friesen, W., & Ellsworth, P. (1972). Emotion in the human face: Guidelines for research and an integration of findings. New York: Pergamon Press.

Fabrigar, L. R., Visser, P. S., & Browne, M. W. (1997). Conceptualand methodologicalissues in testing the circumplex structure of data in personality and social psychology. *Personality and Social Psychology Review, 1*, 184–203.

Feldman Barrett, L. (1997). The relationships among momentary emotion experiences, personality descriptions, and retrospective ratings of emotion. *Personality and Social Psychology Bulletin, 23*, 1100–1110.

Fredrickson, B. L. (1998). What good are positive emotions? *Review of General Psychology, 2*, 300–319.

Fredrickson, B. L. (2001). The role of positive emotions in positive psychology: The broaden-and-build theory of positive emotions. *American Psychologist, 56*, 218–226.

Frijda, N. H. (1986). *The emotions.* New York: Cambridge University Press.

Frijda, N. H. (1999). Emotions and hedonic experience. In D. Kahneman, E. Diener, & N. Schwarz (Eds.), *Well-being: The foundations of hedonic psychology* (pp. 190–210). New York: Russell Sage Foundation.

George, L. K. (1986). Life satisfaction in later life. *Generations, 10*, 5–8.

Gottman, J. M. (1993). Studying emotion in socialinteraction. In M. Lewis & J. M. Haviland (Eds.), *Handbook of emotions* (pp. 475–487). New York: Guilford.

Gross, J. J., Carstensen, L. L., Pasupathi, M., Tsai, J., Skorpen, C. G., & Hsu, A. Y. C. (1997). Emotion and aging: Experience, expression, and control. *Psychology and Aging, 12*, 590–599.

Hammen, C. (2002). Context of stress in families of children with depressed parents. In S. H. Goodman & I. H. Gotlib (Eds.),*Children of depressed parents: Mechanics of risk and implications for treatment* (pp. 175–199). Washington, DC: American Psychological Association.

Hays, R. D., Wells, K. B., Sherbourne, C. D., Rogers, W., & Spritzer, K. (1995). Functioning and well-being outcomes of patients with depression compared with chronic general medical illnesses. *Archieves of General Psychiatry, 52*, 11–19.

Headey, B., & Wearing, A. (1989). Personality, life events, and subjective well-being: Toward a dynamic equilibrium model. *Journal of Personality and Social Psychology, 57*, 731–739.

Heine, S. J., Kitayama, S., Lehman, D. R., Takata, T., Ide, E., Leung, C., et al. (2001). Divergent consequences of success and failure in Japan and North America. An investigation of self-improving motivations and malleable selves. *Journal of Personality and Social Psychology, 81*, 599–615.

Izard, C. E. (1977). *Human emotions*. New York: Plenum.

Jahoda, M. (1958). *Current conceptions of positive mental health*. New York: Basic Books.

Kahneman, D. (1999). Objective happiness. In D. Kahneman, E. Diener, & N. Schwarz (Eds.), *Well-being: The foundations of hedonic psychology* (pp. 3–25). New York: Russell Sage Foundation.

Kim-Prieto, C. Y. (2002). *What's a wonderful life? The pursuit of personal pleasure versus in-group desires*. Unpublished master's thesis, University of Illinois, Urbana-Champaign.

Krokoff, L. J., Gottman, J. M., & Hass, S. D. (1989). Validation of a global rapid couples interaction scoring system. *Behavioral Assessment, 11*, 65–79.

Kunzmann, U., Little, T. D., & Smith, J. (2000). Is age-related stability of subjective well-being a paradox? Cross-sectional and longitudinal evidence from the Berlin Aging Study. *Psychology and Aging, 15*, 511–526.

Larsen, R. J., & Diener, E. (1987). Emotional response intensity as an individual difference characteristic. *Journal of Research in Personality, 21*, 1–39.

Larsen, R. J., & Diener, E. (1992). Promises and problems with the circumplex model of emotion. In M. S. Clark (Ed.), *Review of personality and social psychology: emotion* (Vol. 13, pp. 25–59). Newbury Park, CA: Sage.

Larsen, R. J., Diener, E., & Cropanzano, R. S. (1987). Cognitive operations associated with individual differences in affect intensity. *Journal of Personality and Social Psychology, 53*, 767–774.

Larsen, R. J., Diener, E., & Emmons, R. A. (1985). An evaluation of subjective well-being measures. *Social Indicators Research, 17*, 1–17.

Larsen, R. J., Diener, E., & Lucas, R. E. (2002). Emotion: Models, measures, and individual differences. In R. G. Lord, R. J. Klimoski, & R. Kanfer (Eds.), *Emotions in the workplace* (pp. 64–106). San Francisco: Jossey-Bass.

Larsen, R. J., & Fredrickson, B. L. (1999). Measurement issues in emotion research. In D. Kahneman, E. Diener, & N. Schwarz (Eds.), *Well-being: The foundations of hedonic psychology* (pp. 40–60). New York: Russell Sage Foundation.

Larsen, J. T., McGraw, A. P., & Cacioppo, J. T. (2001). Can people feel happy and sad at the same time? *Journal of Personality and Social Psychology, 81*, 684–696.

Lawton, M. P. (2001). Emotion in later life. *Current Directions in Psychological Science, 10*, 120–123.

Lawton, M. P., DeVoe, M. R., & Parmelee, P. (1995). Relationship of events and affect in the daily life of an elderly population. *Psychology and Aging, 10*, 469–477.

Lawton, M. P., Kleban, M. H., Dean, J., Rajagopal, D., & Parmelee, P. A. (1992). The factorial generality of brief positive and negative affect measures. *Journal of Gerontology, 47*, 228–237.

Lawton, M. P., Kleban, M. H., Rajagopal, D., & Dean, J. (1992). Dimension of affective experience in three age groups. *Psychology and Aging, 7*, 171–184.

Lazarus, R. S. (1982). Thoughts on the relations between emotion and cognition. *American Psychology, 37*, 1019–1024.

Lazarus, R. S. (1984). On the primacy of cognition. *American Psychology, 39*, 124–129.

LeDoux, J. E. (2000). Emotion circuits in the brain. *Annual Review of Neuroscience, 23*, 155–184.

Levine, L. J., Prohaska, V., Burgess, S. L., Rice, J. A., & Laulere, T. M. (2001). Remembering past emotions: The role of current appraisals. *Cognition and Emotion, 15*, 393–417.

Lucas, R. E., Clark, A. E., Georgellis, Y., & Diener, E. (2003). Reexamining adaptation and the set point model of happiness: Reactions to changes in marital status. *Journal of Personality and Social Psychology, 84*, 527–539.

Lucas, R. E., & Diener, E. (2003). The happy worker: Hypotheses about the role of positive affect in worker productivity. In M. R. Barrick & A. M. Ryan (Eds.), *Personality and work: Reconsidering the role of personality in organizations* (pp. 30–59). San Francisco: Jossey Bass. (The organizational frontiers series).

Lucas, R. E., Diener, E., & Larsen, R. J. (2003). Measuring positive emotions. In S. J. Lopez & C. R. Snyder (Eds.), *Positive psychological assessment: A handbook of models and measures* (pp. 201–218). Washington, DC: American Psychological Association.

Lucas, R. E., Diener, E., & Suh, E. M. (1996). Discriminant validity of subjective well-being measures. *Journal of Personality and Social Psychology, 71*, 616–628.

Lucas, R. E., & Gohm, C. L. (2000). Age and sex differences in subjective well-being across cultures. In E. Diener & E. M. Suh (Eds.), *Culture and subjective well-being* (pp. 291–317). Cambridge, MA: MIT Press.

Lykken, D., & Tellegen, A. (1996). Happiness is a stochastic phenomenon. *Psychological Science, 7*, 186–189.

Lyubomirsky, S., King, L., & Diener, E. (2002). *Is happiness a good thing? The benefits of chronic positive affect.* Manuscript in preparation, University of California, Riverside.

MacKay, C. J. (1980). The measurement of mood and psychophysiological activity using self-report techniques. In I. Martin & P. Venables (Eds.), *Techniques in psychophysiology* (pp. 501–562). New York: Wiley.

Magnus, K., & Diener, E. (1991, May 2–4). *A longitudinal analysis of personality, life events, and subjective well-being.* Paper presented at the Sixty-third Annual Meeting of the Midwestern Psychological Association, Chicago.

Mathews, A., & MacLeod, C. (1994). Cognitive approaches to emotion and emotionaldisorders. *Annual Review of Psychology, 45*, 25–50.

McCrae, R. R., & Costa Jr., P. T. (1989). Different points of view: Self-reports and ratings in the assessment of personality. In J. P. Forgas & M. J. Innes (Eds.), *Recent advances in social psychology: An internationalperspective* (pp. 429–439). Amsterdam: Elsevier Science.

McFarland, C., Ross, M., & DeCourville, N. (1989). Women's theories of menstruation and biases in recall of menstrualsymptoms. *Journal of Personality and Social Psychology, 57*, 522–531.

Morris, W. N. (1999). The mood system. In D. Kahneman, E. Diener, & N. Schwarz (Eds.), *Well-being: The foundations of hedonic psychology* (pp. 169–189). New York: Russell Sage Foundation.

Mroczek, D. K., & Kolarz, C. M. (1998). The effect of age on positive and negative affect: A developmental perspective on happiness. *Journal of Personality and Social Psychology, 76*, 1333–1349.

Myers, D. G., & Diener, E. (1995). Who is happy? *Psychological Science, 6*, 10–19.

Neugarten, B. L., Havighurst, R. J., & Tobin, S. S. (1961). The measurement of life satisfaction. *Journal of Gerontology, 16*, 134–143.

Nozick, R. (1974). *Anarchy, State, and Utopia.* New York: Basic Books.

Oishi, S. (2000). *Culture and memory for emotional experiences: On-line vs. retrospective judgments of subjective well-being.* Unpublished doctoral dissertation, University of Illinois, Urbana-Champaign.

Oishi, S. (2002). *The function of daily vs. retrospective judgments of satisfaction in relationship longevity.* Manuscript in preparation.

Oishi, S., & Diener, E. (2001). *Culture and well-being: The cycle of action, evaluation, and decision.* Manuscript submitted for publication, University of Minnesota.

Oishi, S., Diener, E., Scollon, C. N., & Biswas-Diener, R. (2002). Cross-situational consistency of affective experiences across cultures. Manuscript submitted to *Journal of Personality and Social Psychology.*

Oishi, S., Schimmack, U., & Diener, E. (2001). Pleasures and subjective well-being. *European Journal of Personality, 15*, 153–167.

Ortony, A., & Turner, T. J. (1990). What's basic about basic emotions? *Psychological Review, 97*, 315–331.

Pinquart, M. (2001). Age differences in perceived positive affect, negative affect, and affect balance in middle and old age. *Journal of Happiness Studies, 2*, 375–405.

Robinson, M. D., & Clore, G. L. (2002). Episodic and semantic knowledge in emotional self-report: Evidence for two judgment processes. *Journal of Personality and Social Psychology, 83*, 198–215.

Ross, M. (1989). Relation of implicit theories to the construction of personal histories. *Psychological Review, 96*, 341–357.

Russell, J. A. (1980). A circumplex model of affect. *Journal of Personality and Social Psychology, 39*, 1161–1178.

Rusting, C. L. (1998). Personality, mood, and cognitive processing of emotional information: Three conceptual frameworks. *Psychological Bulletin, 124*, 165–196.

Schimmack, U., & Diener, E. (1997). Affect intensity: Separating intensity and frequency in repeatedly measured affect. *Journal of Personality and Social Psychology, 73*, 1313–1329.

Schimmack, U., Diener, E., & Oishi, S. (2002). Life satisfaction is a momentary judgment and a stable personality characteristic: The use of chronically accessible and stable sources. *Journal of Personality, 70*, 346–384.

Schwarz, N., & Clore, G. L. (1983). Mood, misattribution, and judgments of well-being: Informative and directive functions of affective states. *Personality and Social Psychology Bulletin, 18*, 574–579.

Schwarz, N., & Strack, F. (1999). Reports of subjective well-being: Judgmental processes and their methodological implications. In D. Kahneman, E. Diener, & N. Schwarz (Eds.), *Well-being: The foundations of hedonic psychology* (pp. 61–84). New York: Russell Sage Foundation.

Scollon, C. N., Diener, E., Oishi, S., & Biswas-Diener, R. (2002). *Culture, self-concept, and memory for emotions.* Manuscript in preparation.

Segerstrom, S. C. (2001). Optimism and attentional bias for negative and positive stimuli. *Personality and Social Psychology Bulletin, 27*, 1334–1343.

Seidlitz, L., & Diener, E. (1993). Memory for positive versus negative life events: Theories for the difference between happy and unhappy persons. *Journal of Personality and Social Psychology, 64*, 654–663.

Shedler, J., Mayman, M., & Manis, M. (1993). The illusion of mental health. *American Psychology, 48*, 1117–1131.

Stone, A. A. (1995). Measures of affective response. In S. Cohen, R. Kessler, & L. Gordon (Eds.), *Measuring stress: A guide for health and social scientists* (pp. 148–171). New York: Cambridge University Press.

Stone, A. A., Shiffman, S. S., & DeVries, M. W. (1999). Ecological momentary assessment. In D. Kahneman, E. Diener, & N. Schwarz (Eds.), *Well-being: The foundations of hedonic psychology* (pp. 26–39). New York: Russell Sage Foundation.

Stones, M. J., Hadjistavopoulo, T., Tuuko, H., & Kozma, A. (1995). Happiness has trait-like and state-like properties: A reply to Veenhoven. *Social Indicators Research, 36*, 129–144.

Suh, E., Diener, E., & Fujita, F. (1996). Events and subjective well-being: Only recent events matter. *Journal of Personality and Social Psychology, 70*, 1091–1102.

Suh, E., Diener, E., Oishi, S., & Triandis, H. C. (1998). The shifting basis of life satisfaction judgments across cultures: Emotions versus norms. *Journal of Personality and Social Psychology, 74*, 482–493.

Tatarkiewicz, W. (1976). Analysis of happiness. The Hague, Netherlands: Martinus Nijhoff.

Tellegen, A. (1985). Structures of mood and personality and their relevance to assessing anxiety, with an emphasis on self-report. In A. H. Tuma & J. D. Maser (Eds.), *Anxiety and the anxiety disorders* (pp. 681–706). Hillsdale, NJ: Erlbaum.

Thomas, D., & Diener, E. (1990). Memory accuracy in the recall of emotions. *Journal of Personality and Social Psychology, 59*, 291–297.

Veenhoven, R. (1994). Is happiness a trait? Tests of the theory that a better society does not make us any happier. *Social Indicators Research, 32*, 101–162.

Veenhoven, R. (1998). Two state-trait discussions on happiness. A Reply to Stones et al. *Social Indicators Research, 43*, 211–225.

Waterman, A. S. (1990). The relevance of Aristotle's conception of eudaimonia for the psychological study of happiness. *Theoretical and Philosophical Psychology, 10*, 39–44.

Watson, D., Clark, L. A., & Tellegen, A. (1988). Development and validation of brief measures of positive and negative affect: The PANAS scales. *Journal of Personality and Social Psychology, 54*, 1063–1070.

Watson, D., & Tellegen, A. (1985). Toward a consensual structure of mood. *Psychological Bulletin, 98*, 219–235.

Watson, D., & Walker, L. M. (1996). The long-term stability and predictive validity of trait measures of affect. *Journal of Personality and Social Psychology, 70*, 567–577.

Watson, D., Wiese, D., Vaidya, J., & Tellegen, A. (1999). The two general activation systems of affect: Structural findings, evolutionary considerations, and psychobiological evidence. *Journal of Personality and Social Psychology, 76*, 820–838.

Weinberger, D. A., Schwartz, G. E., & Davidson, R. A. (1979). Low-anxious, high-anxious, and repressive coping styles: Psychometric patterns and behavioral and physiological responses to stress. *Journal of Abnormal Psychology, 88*, 369–380.

Wessman, A. E., & Ricks, D. F. (1966). *Mood and personality.* New York: Holt, Rinehart, and Winston.

Wilson, W. (1967). Correlates of avowed happiness. *Psychological Bulletin, 67*, 294–306.

Wirtz, D., Kruger, J., Scollon, C. N., & Diener, E. (2003). What to do on spring break? The role of predicted, on-line and remembered experience in future choice. *Psychological Science, 14*, 520–524.

Zajonc, R. B. (1980). Feeling and thinking: Preferences need no inferences. *American Psychology, 35*, 151–175.

Zelenski, J. M., & Larsen, R. J. (2000). The distribution of basic emotions in everyday life: A state and trait perspective from experience sampling data. *Journal of Research in Personality, 34*, 178–197.

Review of the Satisfaction With Life Scale

William Pavot and Ed Diener

Abstract The Satisfaction With Life Scale (SWLS) was developed to assess satisfaction with the respondent's life as a whole. The scale does not assess satisfaction with life domains such as health or finances but allows subjects to integrate and weight these domains in whatever way they choose. Normative data are presented for the scale, which shows good convergent validity with other scales and with other types of assessments of subjective well-being. Life satisfaction as assessed by the SWLS shows a degree of temporal stability (e.g., 0.54 for 4 years), yet the SWLS has shown sufficient sensitivity to be potentially valuable to detect change in life satisfaction during the course of clinical intervention. Further, the scale shows discriminant validity from emotional well-being measures. The SWLS is recommended as a complement to scales that focus on psychopathology or emotional well-being because it assesses an individuals' conscious evaluative judgment of his or her life by using the person's own criteria.

The last decade has seen a dramatic increase in research on the construct of subjective well-being (SWB; Diener, 1984; Diener & Larsen, 1993). This research has begun to provide an important complement to one of psychology's traditional goals: the understanding of unhappiness or ill-being in the form of depression, anxiety, and unpleasant emotions. The addition of a positive orientation toward the individual's subjective experience of well-being provides an additional perspective for researchers and clinicians alike.

Research has identified two broad aspects of subjective well-being: an affective component, which is usually further divided into pleasant affect and unpleasant affect (Diener, 1990; Diener & Emmons, 1984), and a cognitive component, which is referred to as life satisfaction (Andrews & Withey, 1976). When assessed, these components of SWB are at least moderately correlated, and a number of measures of SWB include both components (Chamberlain, 1988). Several researchers, however, have found separate satisfaction and affect components (Andrews & Withey, 1976;

E. Diener (✉)
Department of Psychology, University of Illinois, Urbana–Champaign, Champaign,
Illinois 61820, USA
e-mail: ediener@uiuc.edu

E. Diener (ed.), *Assessing Well-Being: The Collected Works of Ed Diener*,
Social Indicators Research Series 39, DOI 10.1007/978-90-481-2354-4_5,
© Springer Science+Business Media B.V. 2009

Judge, 1990; Liang, 1985; Stock, Okun, & Benin, 1986). These components appear to sometimes behave differently over time and to have differing relationships with other variables (Beiser, 1974; Campbell, Converse, & Rogers, 1976; DeHaes, Pennink, & Welvaart, 1987). The affective and cognitive components of SWB are not completely independent; however, the two components are somewhat distinctive and can provide complementary information when assessed separately.

Although the affective and cognitive aspects of SWB both appear to be important, researchers have focused their attention on the measurement of affective well-being, as evidenced by the number of instruments that measure affect. For example, mood and affective well-being can be assessed by the Affectometer (Kammann & Flett, 1983), the Positive and Negative Affect Schedule (PANAS; Watson, Clark, & Tellegen, 1988), or the Memorial University of Newfoundland Scale of Happiness (MUNSCH; Kozma & Stones, 1980), among others. Scales to measure unpleasant affect (e.g., depression) are also widely used (e.g., Beck, Ward, Mendelson, Mock, & Erbaugh, 1961). Generally, the life satisfaction component of SWB has received less attention (Diener, Emmons, Larsen, & Griffin, 1985). Because life satisfaction frequently forms a separate factor and correlates with predictor variables in a unique way, it seems worthwhile to separately assess this construct.

Life satisfaction refers to a judgmental process, in which individuals assess the quality of their lives on the basis of their own unique set of criteria (Shin & Johnson, 1978). A comparison of one's perceived life circumstances with a self-imposed standard or set of standards is presumably made, and to the degree that conditions match these standards, the person reports high life satisfaction. Therefore, life satisfaction is a conscious cognitive judgment of one's life in which the criteria for judgment are up to the person.

Although there may be some agreement about the important components of "the good life," such as health and successful relationships, individuals are likely to assign different weights to these components (Diener et al., 1985). Individuals are also likely to have unique criteria for a good life as well, which in some cases might outweigh the common benchmarks in importance. Furthermore, individuals may have very different standards for "success" in each of these areas of their lives. Thus, it is necessary to assess an individuals' global judgment of his or her life rather than only his or her satisfaction with specific domains. This is the strategy adopted by the authors of the Satisfaction With Life Scale (SWLS; Diener et al., 1985). The SWLS items are global rather than specific in nature, allowing respondents to weight domains of their lives in terms of their own values, in arriving at a global judgment of life satisfaction. At the same time, it should be recognized that assessing respondents' satisfaction with common domains may also provide useful additional information (Frisch, Cornell, Villanueva, & Retzlaff, 1992).

There is evidence that satisfaction often forms a factor separate from affective indexes of well-being. If affect depends on appraisals, why do cognitive and affective measures form separate factors? First, people may ignore or deny negative emotional reactions while still recognizing the undesirable factors in their lives. Second, affective reactions are often responses to immediate factors and of short duration, whereas life satisfaction ratings can reflect a long-term perspective. Finally, a person's conscious evaluation of her or his life circumstances may reflect conscious values and goals. In contrast, affective reactions may reflect unconscious motives and the influences of bodily states to a greater extent than do life satisfaction ratings. Nevertheless, there should be a degree of convergence between life satisfaction and emotional well-being because both depend on evaluative appraisals.

The SWLS is designed to assess a person's global judgment of life satisfaction, which is theoretically predicted to depend on a comparison of life circumstances to one's standards. The brief format of the SWLS means that it can be incorporated into an assessment battery with minimal cost in time. Work on the Extended Satisfaction With Life Scale by Alfonso & Allison (1992b) has indicated that the SWLS is at the reading level of the 6th to 10th grades (depending on the scoring system used) and is thus usable with most adults. The five items of the SWLS and scoring instructions are presented in the Appendix.

Characteristics of the SWLS

Item Selection

Several authors of the original scale created 48 items to reflect life satisfaction and well-being. These items were generated on the basis of the guiding theoretical principle that life satisfaction represents a judgment by the respondent of his or her life in comparison to standards. An initial factor analysis indicated that the items formed three factors: Life Satisfaction per se, Positive Affect, and Negative Affect. Ten items had loadings on the Life Satisfaction factor of 0.60 or above. This group of 10 items was further reduced to 5, to eliminate redundancies of wording and with minimal cost in terms of alpha reliability. Further information on the original development and validation of the SWLS is provided in Diener et al. (1985), the introductory report of the SWLS.

Normative Data

Normative data for the SWLS are available for diverse populations, including older adults, prisoners, individuals under inpatient care for alcohol abuse, abused women, psychotherapy clients, elderly caregivers of demented spouses, and persons with physical disabilities, as well as college student samples. In addition, some cross-cultural data are available (e.g., Arrindell, Meeuwesen, & Huyse, 1991; Balatsky & Diener, 1993; Blais, Vallerand, Pelletier, & Briere, 1989; Shao & Diener, 1992). Table 1 gives a summary of normative data for the SWLS from several samples. As can be seen in Table 1, considerable variability in life satisfaction as reported on the SWLS has been observed between and within a number of diverse populations. The group means vary from approximately 12 for an alcoholic inpatient sample to 28 for a group of older Canadians. Thus, the range of group means spans much of the possible range of the scale (from 5 to 35).

Table 1 Normative data for the satisfaction with life scale

Sample characteristics	N	M	SD
Student samples			
American college students			
(Diener et al., 1985, Study 1)	176	23.5	6.4
American college students[a]			
(Pavot et al., 1991)	130	24.5	6.3
American college students			
(Frisch, 1991)	271	25.2	5.8
American College Students			
(Smead, 1991)	358	23.0	6.4
American College Students			
(Pavot & Diener, 1993)	244	23.7	6.4
French-Canadian college students[b]			
(Blais et al., 1989)			
Men	355	23.8	6.1
Women	472	24.8	6.2
Moscow State University students[b]			
(Balatsky & Diener, 1993)	61	18.9	4.5
Glazov University students[b]			
(Balatsky & Diener, 1993)	53	16.3	4.9
Chinese students[b]			
(Shao & Diener, 1992)	99	16.1	4.4
Disabled students			
(Chwalisz, Diener, & Gallagher, 1988)	32	20.8	8.4
Disabled students			
(Allman & Diener, 1990)	29	24.3	7.4
Korean University students			
(Suh, 1993)	413	19.77	5.84
Adult samples			
Nurses and health workers			
(Judge, 1990)	255	23.6	6.1
Older American adults[a]			
(Pavot et al., 1991)	39	24.2	6.9
Older French-Canadian adults[b]			
(Blais et al., 1989)			
Men	77	27.9	5.7
Women	2.36	26.2	6.6
Active and contemplative religious women[c]			
(McGarrahan, 1991)			
Active recent nuns	64	25.1	7.2
Active older nuns	68	23.7	8.5
Contemplative recent nuns	50	23.3	7.3
Contemplative older nuns	57	23.9	9.0
Printing trade workers[d]			
(George, 1991)	304	24.2	6.0
Military wives and nurses			
(Smead, 1991)	50	25.0	6.8
Doctoral students	50	25	6.8
(Allison, Alfonso, & Dunn, 1991)	127	24.3	6.2
Male prison inmates			
(Joy, 1990)	75	12.3	7.0

Table 1 (continued)

Veterans Affairs hospital inpatient sample[c]			
(Frisch, 1991)	52	11.8	5.6
Dutch medical out patients[b]			
(Arrindell et al., 1991)	107	23.6	7.0
Unmarried	24	21.7	6.7
Married/long relationship	69	25.2	6.7
Divorced/separated/widowed	14	19.3	6.7
Abused women[f]			
(Fisher, 1991)	70	20.7	7.4
Clinical clients, psychological private			
practitioner (Friedman, 1991)			
Intake group	27	14.4	6.7
Advanced group	16	18.3	7.1
Elderly caregivers			
(Vitaliano, Russo, Young, Becker, & Maiuro, 1991)			
Time 1	79	21.2	7.7
Time 2	79	19.7	8.1

[a] M and SD are based on multiple administrations.
[b] Scale was translated into native language of respondent.
[c] Recent nuns include women with less than 15 years in their religious order, whereas older nuns include women with 15 or more years in their religious order.
[d] Members of a printing trade association. Average age of this sample was 47.4 years. Sample was approximately 96% male.
[e] Under treatment for alcohol abuse.
[f] Women who had experienced physical, sexual, or emotional abuse, seeking help at a women's shelter. Women had obtained restraining order for protection from abuser.
Note. Frisch (1991) refers to a personal communication with M. B. Frisch on January 5, 1991; Fisher (1991) refers to a personal communication with K. Fisher on November 7, 1991; Friedman (1991) refers to a personal communication with P. Friedman on November 20, 1991. Suh (1993) refers to a personal communication with M. Suh on February 15, 1993.

Scores on the SWLS can be interpreted in terms of absolute as well as relative life satisfaction. A score of 20 represents the neutral point on the scale, the point at which the respondent is about equally satisfied and dissatisfied. For example, scores between 21 and 25 represent *slightly satisfied*, and scores between 15 and 19 represent *slightly dissatisfied* with life. Scores between 26 and 30 represent *satisfied*, and scores from 5 to 9 are indicative of being *extremely dissatisfied* with life.

In terms of the means presented in Table 1, most groups fall in the range of 23–28, or the range of *slightly satisfied* to *satisfied*. This level of satisfaction is in good agreement with the frequent finding that in Western countries a preponderance of respondents report well-being above the neutral point on a variety of measures (Andrews & Withey, 1976; Campbell, Converse, & Rogers, 1976; Veenhoven, 1984, 1991). On measures of unpleasant affect, such as the Beck Depression Inventory, most individuals in nonclinical samples score at the low end, producing a highly skewed distribution in which only a few individuals are depressed. Thus, the means on the SWLS, which fall in the *slightly satisfied* to *satisfied* range for most groups, appear to reflect the widely replicated finding that nonclinical samples are above the neutral point in SWB.

Stability and Sensitivity

Stability of measurement versus sensitivity to change is a critical issue for any assessment instrument; it becomes crucial for a measure that is intended to demonstrate temporal stability on one hand, yet maintain sensitivity to change on the other. Measures of life satisfaction must demonstrate that they are reflective of more than momentary mood states in order for researchers to make inferences about life satisfaction as a relatively stable component of subjective experience over time. To be useful in an applied setting, however, it is also essential for such an instrument to be sensitive enough to detect changes in life satisfaction, such as those occurring during psychotherapy or those due to major life events (e.g., separation or divorce, and changes in employment or financial status).

The SWLS has been examined for both reliability and sensitivity. The SWLS has shown strong internal reliability and moderate temporal stability. Diener et al. (1985) reported a coefficient alpha of 0.87 for the scale and a 2-month test-retest stability coefficient of 0.82 (Study 1). Since that time, a number of other investigators have reported both internal consistency and temporal reliability data for the scale, which are shown in Table 2.

The data of Table 2 can be used to address the issue of stability versus sensitivity. Over longer periods, the test-retest stability decreases to a level (0.54) that suggests that considerable change in the individual's life satisfaction may occur (Magnus, Diener, Fujita, & Pavot, 1993). Even when correcting for the alpha of the scale, these long-term stability coefficients suggest that only about half of the variance in life satisfaction can be accounted for by life satisfaction several years later.

Along with the decline of stability of the SWLS over longer periods, more specific evidence is available regarding the sensitivity of the SWLS. When viewed over longer periods, life events were found to be predictive of changes in life satisfaction as measured by the SWLS (Magnus et al., 1993). Changes in satisfaction were related to good and bad events in the subjects' lives during the past year. Data even more specific to the question of change over relatively shorter periods comes from the work of Friedman (P. Friedman, personal communication, November 20, 1991). He examined the life satisfaction of outpatient clients in a private practice in the eastern US. In one group (the intake group, $n = 27$), the life satisfaction of clients beginning therapy was measured. This level of satisfaction was then compared with

Table 2 Estimates of internal consistency and temporal reliability for the satisfaction with life scale

Sample	Coefficient alpha	Test–retest	Temporal interval
Alfonso and Allison (1992a)	0.89	0.83	2 weeks
Pavot et al. (1991)	0.85	0.84	1 month
Blais et al. (1989)	0.79–0.84	0.64	2 months
Diener et al. (1985)	0.87	0.82	2 months
Yardley and Rice (1991)	0.80, 0.86	0.50	10 weeks
Magnus, Diener, Fujita, and Pavot (1993)	0.87	0.54	4 years

that from an independent sample of clients (the advanced group, $n = 16$) who had been in therapy 1 to 2 months. The mean level of satisfaction as measured by the SWLS for the intake group was $14.4(SD = 6.72)$, whereas the mean satisfaction for the advanced group was $18.3(SD = 7.09)$. A t test revealed a significant difference between groups ($t = 1.77$, $p < 0.05$, one-tailed). Thus, the group that had been receiving therapy showed a significantly higher level of life satisfaction than did the group of people measured at the beginning of therapy. Friedman also administered the scale to seven clients at the beginning of outpatient therapy and again approximately 1 month into the therapy process. He found that the mean SWLS scores for these clients improved rather dramatically from $14.1(SD = 1.9)$ at Time 1 to $26.9(SD = 3.6)$ at Time 2, a significant increase, $t(6) = 4.01$, $p < 0.01$.

Vitaliano et al. (1991) also reported evidence that changing life conditions can lead to changes on the SWLS. They studied elderly caregivers who had a spouse diagnosed with primary degenerative dementia. The care recipients showed objective declines in functioning during the 15–18 month study. During this period, the caregivers showed a significant decline it life satisfaction, $t(78) = 2.14$, $p < 0.05$. It is interesting to note that only the SWLS changed significantly during this period of spousal decline, with measures of depression, anxiety, and suppressed anger not changing significantly. Furthermore, at both Times 1 and 2, the SWLS showed the strongest relation of any of the caregiver measures to the objective conditions of the patients ($rs = -0.48$ for Time 1 and -0.38 for Time 2). The change in the burden perceived by the caregiver also correlated with the change in life satisfaction ($r = -0.27$, $p < 0.05$). These data are important, because they demonstrate an instance when life satisfaction and affect appear to be diverging; therefore, they should be separately assessed. They also offer additional evidence of the discriminant validity of the SWLS.

In sum, the moderate temporal stability of the SWLS supports the idea that there is some long-term consistency of life satisfaction over time. Immediate factors, such as current mood and the situational context, are also likely to some degree to affect an individual's response to questions about life satisfaction and well-being (Yardley & Rice, 1991). Further, the stability coefficients for longer temporal periods are at a level that indicates that changes in life satisfaction do occur over time. And recent studies by Friedman (P. Friedman, personal communication, November 20, 1991), Vitaliano et al. (1991), and Diener, Sandvik, et al. (1991), have provided evidence that suggests that the SWLS can detect change over time, such as the increase of life satisfaction after a period of psychotherapy or the decrease in life satisfaction as one's spouse becomes more debilitated. From these findings, it can be concluded that life satisfaction has a long-term component (perhaps due to personality, stable life circumstances, or both), a moderate-term component (e.g., due to current life events or cognitive schemata), and a short-term state component (e.g., due to current mood and immediately salient life circumstances).

A more rigorous approach to temporal reliability would be to use multiple measures of life satisfaction in order to separate the amount of actual change in life satisfaction from the degree of error variance causing instability from one occasion to another. If a latent trait of life satisfaction can be established through multiple measures at two different points in time, one can then judge the actual change in life satisfaction and the degree of change in the SWLS, and how much of the SWLS change is due to real change versus error of measurement. This is a significant issue for future research.

Factor Structure of the SWLS

Diener et al. (1985) conducted a principal-axis factor analysis on the SWLS, from which a single factor emerged, accounting for 66% of the variance of the scale. This single-factor solution has since been replicated (Arrindell et al., 1991; Blais et al., 1989; Pavot et al., 1991), and these results are shown in Table 3. The consistent factor pattern across samples was maintained despite the fact that these samples represent translations of the SWLS into French (Blais et al., 1989) and Dutch (Arrindell et al., 1991), as well as the original English-language version (Diener et al., 1985; Pavot et al., 1991). The SWLS therefore seems to measure a single dimension. The item-total correlations and factor loadings shown in Table 3 suggest that the last item is the weakest in terms of convergence with other items. This may be because most of the items refer primarily to the present, whereas the fifth item refers primarily to the past, although this interpretation will require empirical testing.

Table 3 Item means, item factor loadings, and item-total correlations for the five items of the satisfaction with life scale

	Item number				
Sample	1	2	3	4	5
	Item means and standard deviations				
Pavot et al. (1991) ($N = 244$)					
M	4.71	4.74	5.23	4.75	4.25
SD	1.47	1.52	1.52	1.75	1.86
	Item factor loadings and item-total correlations				
Diener et al. (1985)	84/75	77/69	83/75	72/67	61/57
Blais et al. (1989)	84/51	76/54	74/71	71/60	68/57
Arrindell et al. (1991)	84/73	80/67	85/75	83/72	76/64
Pavot et al. (1991)	83/71	89/80	82/71	68/55	78/66

Note. For the factor loadings/item-total correlation section, decimal points have been omitted; numbers to the left of diagonals are component loadings, numbers to the right of diagonals are item-total correlations. Item numbers are consistent with the scale as presented in the Appendix.

Construct Validity Data

Initial validity evidence comes from groups scoring lowest on the SWLS: psychiatric patients, prisoners, students in poor and turbulent countries, and abused women. Life satisfaction as we conceptualize it currently involves a comparison with standards. So events or conditions that make the individual's circumstances better or worse will influence life satisfaction. Psychiatric patients and newly incarcerated prisoners represent groups who had suffered recent bad life events, events likely to deviate negatively from their standards. For abused women, their experience is negative in one central domain, their marriage, and their experience deviates from the ideal in our culture. For students in the countries studied, aspirations are probably higher than current conditions, a likely cause of the disquiet observed there. The data from these groups generally follow a pattern of lower satisfaction as assessed by the SWLS.

The SWLS also has been examined for its relation to an array of both self-report and external criteria in an effort to establish its validity as a measure of life satisfaction. Both Diener et al. (1985) and Pavot et al. (1991) provide considerable evidence for the convergence of the SWLS with numerous measures of subjective well-being and life satisfaction. As can be seen in Table 4, the SWLS demonstrates adequate convergence with related measures, including measures using a different methodological approach (e.g., interviewer or informant ratings) to measure life satisfaction. The modest to moderate correlations of life satisfaction using different methods compare favorably to multi-method convergence of other well-being constructs. Nevertheless, the modest size of these correlations leaves much variance unaccounted for, and points to substantial amounts of error in the measures.

The SWLS has been shown to be negatively correlated with clinical measures of distress. Blais et al. (1989) report a strong negative correlation ($r = -0.72$, $p = 0.001$) between the SWLS and the Beck Depression Inventory (Beck et al., 1961). Larsen, Diener & Emmons (1985) found a correlation of -0.31 between the SWLS and a measure of negative affect. Using a Dutch version (Arrindell & Ettema, 1986) of the Symptom Checklist-90 (SCL-90-R; Derogatis, 1977), Arrindell et al. (1991) found the SWLS to be significantly negatively correlated with all eight symptom dimensions assessed, including anxiety ($r = -0.54$), depression ($r = -0.55$), and general psychological distress ($r = -0.55$).

Table 4 Correlations of the SWLS with self-and non-self-report measures of life satisfaction and subjective well being

Sample	Andrews/ Withey Scale	Fordyce Global Scale	Interviewer ratings	Informant reports
Diener et al. (1985)	0.68	0.58	0.43	–
Larsen (1985)	0.58	0.60	–	–
Pavot et al. (1991)	–	0.82	–	0.54
Allman and Diener (1990)	0.59	0.61	–	0.58
Magnus, Diener, and Fujita (1991)	0.52	0.55	–	0.34
Frisch (1991) (VA inpatient)	0.60	0.35	0.51	–
Frisch (1991) (Student)	0.68	0.55	0.66	0.28
Pavot and Diener (1991)	–	0.45	–	0.46
Judge (1990)	–	0.55	–	0.43

Note. Frisch (1991) refers to a personal communication with M. B. Frisch on January 5, 1991.

Researchers have administered the SWLS in conjunction with measures of positive and negative affectivity. For example, Smead (1991) reported correlations of 0.44 between the SWLS and positive affect, and of −0.48 between the SWLS and negative affect, with affect measured on Watson et al.'s (1988) PANAS scales. Because the scales of the PANAS are virtually uncorrelated, the correlations of the separate subscales with the SWLS show that it does not simply measure only negative affect. George (1991) found correlations with the SWLS and the Multidimensional Personality Questionnaire (MPQ: Tellegen, 1982) of .47 for positive affectivity and −0.26 for negativity. The absolute size of these correlations, even when disattenuated for unreliability, does not support the idea that life satisfaction and affective well-being are equivalent constructs.

In terms of individual difference dimensions, the SWLS has been found to be positively correlated with extraversion and inversely correlated with neuroticism (Diener et al., 1985; Pavot & Diener, 1993), thus adding to the construct validity of the scale. Extroversion has been repeatedly found to correlated with well-being (Diener & Larsen, 1993), possibly because extroverted individuals have more sensitive reward systems. Further, neuroticism has been repeatedly found to correlate substantially with SWB (Diener & Larsen, 1993). Thus, these correlations with the SWLS support its validity.

Both marital status and health have been shown to be correlated with the SWLS (Arrindell et al., 1991). The SWLS has generally been found to be unrelated to gender and age (Arrindell et al., 1991; George, 1991; Pavot et al., 1991). Friedman (P. Friedman, personal communication, November 20, 1992) has found the SWLS to be highly correlated ($r = 0.68$) with self-esteem. Each of the above correlational patterns has been replicated with both self-report and non-self-report measures of SWB (e.g., Fujita & Diener, 1992). Thus, these correlations provide construct validity for the SWLS.

The discriminant validity of the SWLS can be approached at several levels. At the empirical level, individual difference dimensions such as affect intensity and impulsivity (Diener et al., 1985) have been found to be uncorrelated with the SWLS. Several pieces of evidence also support the discriminative power of the SWLS from measures of affective well-being.

One instance of such evidence comes from a study by Judge (1990). In a structural model. Judge allowed the covariance of the error terms of two life satisfaction measures (one being the SWLS) to be estimated separately from the hedonic measures. This produced a substantial improvement in fit, suggesting that the life satisfaction and affective measures were not adequately captured by a single latent trait. Although related, life satisfaction and affective well-being were separable.

Further, in the aforementioned study of caregivers by Vitaliano et al. (1991), the SWLS was the only scale that showed significant change when the caregiver's burden became greater. The caregivers appeared to be adapting to the change emotionally, yet they were able to recognize changes in the quality of their lives.

Thus, a number of independent sources of evidence suggest the discriminant validity of the SWLS. Nevertheless, the area of discriminant validity is in need of further exploration. For example, a confirmatory factor analysis using both self-report and informant SWLS and positive and negative affect measures would allow researchers to examine the correlation of latent satisfaction with affective SWB and to study the correlation of the SWLS with each of the three latent variables.

Response Artifacts and the SWLS

Schwarz and Clore (1983) and Schwarz and Strack (1991) have found that self-reported measures of well-being can be influenced by a number of transient factors, including the momentary mood of the respondent, the physical surroundings, and even the item that precedes the life satisfaction or well-being item on a questionnaire or survey. In a comparison of single-item versus multiple-item measures of well-being and life satisfaction (Pavot & Diener, 1991), item placement and momentary mood were found to sometimes produce a significant influence on response to single-item measures. There were no significant effects, however, for these factors found for multiple-item measures, including the SWLS.

Another frequently debated source of error is response acquiescence (Rorer, 1965). One strategy to lessen the effects of acquiescence is item reversal. The items of the SWLS are all keyed in a "positive" direction. The authors chose not to use reversed items because the degree to which acquiescence influences response may be small (Rorer, 1965), and a general acquiescence bias may not exist (Husek, 1961). Further, reverse-wording of items can confuse respondents and thereby contribute a different source of error in measurement. Nonetheless, response acquiescence is a potential problem with the SWLS, which deserves research attention.

Another potential problem for the SWLS is social desirability. Social desirability correlates with SWB scales, and it has been suggested that a large component of the variance of well-being scales is due to social desirability (Carstensen & Cone, 1983). Because of this and other similar findings, social desirability has been the subject of considerable controversy in the area of SWB research. Recent research (Diener, Sandvik, Pavot, & Gallaher, 1991) has demonstrated that when social desirability is removed from a measure of well-being, the resulting measure converges less well with peer reports of SWB. This finding suggests that social desirability may represent a substantive part of well-being and that when it is removed from such measures, valid information is lost. Botwin, Diener, & Tomarelli (1992), in a review of the social desirability literature, find no evidence that social desirability is an artifact or confound but suggest that measures of social desirability may actually include substantive personality characteristics, such as social conformity, which correlate with well-being measures. The relationship between SWB measures such as the SWLS and social desirability clearly needs to be more extensively examined with newer social desirability scales that separate the self-deception component of social desirability from the impression-management component of social desirability.

Clinical Application

The SWLS appears to have promise for use in clinical settings. It has been found that clinical and quasiclinical populations score lower on life satisfaction but also that their scores tend to increase during the course of treatment. Clearly, much more work is needed to explore which clinical populations show depressed scores on the scale and which types of problem alleviation are likely to increase scores on the scale. Evidence is reviewed in this article that indicates that life satisfaction and affective well-being are not isomorphic and that the SWLS therefore may give additional information beyond emotion or mood scales.

Cross-Cultural Use of the SWLS

The SWLS is available in several languages. Data for the French (Blais et al., 1989) and Dutch (Arrindell et al., 1991) language versions have been presented here, but versions in other languages are available, including Russian (Balatsky & Diener, 1993), Korean (Won, in progress), Hebrew (D. Shmotkin, personal communication, December 6, 1991), and Mandarin Chinese (Shao & Diener, 1992).

The existing data suggest that the SWLS has potential as a cross-cultural index of life satisfaction. Nonetheless, this issue requires substantially more exploration. It would be very helpful to have a national probability sample in which the SWLS is used so that norms for various groups such as African Americans and Latinos would be available. Further, an examination is needed in terms of the interpretation of the scale (and, indeed, the meaning of well-being) in various cultures and subcultures. For example, some of the differences between the life satisfaction of Russian and Chinese students and American student samples might be due to cultural factors rather than "real" differences in well-being and satisfaction. Although initial exploration shows the same factorial structure in different groups, a much more in-depth study would be valuable, at both the conceptual and empirical levels.

Discussion

The SWLS provides an adjunct to measures oriented toward the assessment of negative states. It assesses the positive side of the individual's experience rather than focusing on unpleasant emotions. In making a life satisfaction judgment, the SWLS emphasizes the person's own standards of evaluation. Furthermore, the respondent draws on the domains she or he finds relevant in formulating his or her judgment of global life satisfaction. Because life satisfaction judgments are at least partiallyindependent of affective measures, the SWLS is a promising instrument in terms of measuring change in subjective well-being and intervention outcomes.

Preliminary work with the SWLS reveals that life satisfaction may be a meaningful and useful psychological construct. First, the items appear to hold together in a unified factor, suggesting that there is coherence to life satisfaction. Second, life satisfaction seems to have moderate temporal stability, although it also changes in reaction to life events. In addition, life satisfaction shows some degree of autonomy from related subjective well-being constructs such as depression. Respondents seem to show moderate convergence in self-reports of life satisfaction with interviewers and informants who are asked to judge their life satisfaction. Further, informants show good levels of agreement when they judge a target person's life satisfaction using the SWLS (Pavot et al., 1991).

Along with the above strengths, the SWLS has several limitations. First, as is true of any self-report instrument, respondents can consciously distort their response to the scale if they are motivated to do so. For this reason, it is desirable to supplement the self-reported SWLS with assessments from external sources, such as informant SWLS or interviewer ratings, whenever possible. Also, the SWLS does not measure all aspects of SWB. It is a narrow-band instrument, intended to assess the cognitive rather than affective component of SWB. Although the cognitive and affective components of subjective well-being are obviously related, scores on the SWLS cannot automatically be used as direct measures of emotional well-being. Instruments with an affective focus should be included in research designs that are intended to obtain data on the broader construct of global SWB.

Several of the strengths of the SWLS in terms of allowing respondents freedom also can be seen as liabilities in terms of an unambiguous interpretation of the test score. For example, we allow the respondent to use whatever standard she or he deems to be appropriate, but this means that we do not know to what standard the person has compared the conditions of her or his life. We leave open the possibility to weight any life domains (e.g., health, marriage, hobbies) in composing an answer, but again, this means that a person may overweight domains that happen to be salient at the time of testing. Until the cognitive processes involved in arriving at a life satisfaction judgment are known and understood, we will not fully know the meaning of high life satisfaction. Thus, a crucial aspect of developing the construct validity of the SWLS will be to understand the processes involved in arriving at a life satisfaction judgment.

Several important issues remain for future research. For example, it would be useful to develop a more comprehensive data base for the SWLS, including norms for additional clinical populations. The discriminant validity of the SWLS could be investigated in greater depth, focusing on the relationship between emotional well-being and cognitive life satisfaction. Also, the relationship between global life satisfaction and other clinical and well-being constructs should be explored further, especially using a multimethod approach.

Studies in which emotion is manipulated and the influence of this on SWLS scores would be valuable. This would yield a more rigorous answer to the question of how much the SWLS is influenced by current mood. Finally, it would be interesting to explore life satisfaction in terms of different time frames of reference: the past, the present, the future, and both shorter (e.g., several weeks) and longer (the last several years) time perspectives. The stability of these various time frames could be determined, and each could be correlated with the SWLS in order to assess the time frame used by various populations. It can be noted that some of the SWLS items seem to refer to the past (e.g., "If I lived my life over, I would. . ."), whereas others appear to refer more to the present (e.g., "The conditions of my life are excellent.").

It is unknown whether an individual might score high in one time frame and low on the other. Certain items may be more susceptible to change than others because they tend to reflect a current time frame rather than a focus on the person's whole past life. Thus, the scale may mix two different meanings of life satisfaction, and an exploration of this issue is warranted.

Acknowledgments We thank Philip H. Friedman for providing clinical data on the Satisfaction with Life Scale from his ongoing research at the Foundation for Well-being, Plymouth Meeting, Pennsylvania.

Appendix: Satisfaction with Life Scale

Below are five statements with which you may agree or disagree. Using the 1–7 scale below, indicate your agreement with each item by placing the appropriate number on the line preceding that item. Please be open and honest in your responding. The 7-point scale is as follows:

1 = strongly disagree
2 = disagree
3 = slightly disagree
4 = neither agree nor disagree
5 = slightly agree
6 = agree
7 = strongly agree

_____1. In most ways my life is close to my ideal.
_____2. The conditions of my life are excellent.
_____3. I am satisfied with my life.
_____4. So far I have gotten the important things I want in life.
_____5. If I could live my life over, I would change almost nothing.

Use of the SWLS

The Satisfaction With Life Scale is in the public domain. Permission is not needed to use it.

References

Alfonso, V. C., & Allison, D. B. (1992a). *Further development of the Extended Satisfaction With Life Scale.* Manuscript submitted for publication.
Alfonso, V. C., & Allison, D. B. (1992b). *The readability of the Extended Satisfaction With Life Scale.* Manuscript submitted for publication.

Allison, D. B., Alfonso, V. C., & Dunn, G. M. (1991). The extended Satisfaction With Life Scale. *The Behavior Therapist, 5,* 15–16.

Allman, A., & Diener, E. (1990). *Measurement issues and the subjective well-being of people with disabilities.* Manuscript submitted for publication.

Andrews, F. M., & Withey, S. B. (1976). *Social indicators of well-being America's perception of life quality.* New York: Plenum Press.

Arrindell, W. A., & Ettema, J. H. M. (1986). *SCL-90: Handleiding bijeen multidimensionele psychopathologie-indicator* [SCL-90: manual for a multidimensional measure of psychopathology]. Lisse, The Netherlands: Swets Test Services.

Arrindell, W. A., Meeuwesen, L., & Huyse, F. J. (1991). The Satisfaction With Life Scale (SWLS): Psychometric properties in a non-psychiatric medical outpatients sample. *Personality and Individual Differences, 12,* 117–123.

Balatsky, G., & Diener, E. (1993). A comparison of the well-being of Soviet and American students. *Social Indicators Research, 28,* 225–243.

Beck, A. T., Ward, C. H., Mendelson, M., Mock, J., & Erbaugh, J. (1961). An inventory for measuring depression. *Archives of General Psychiatry, 4,* 561–571.

Beiser, M. (1974). Components and correlates of mental well-being. *Journal of Health and Social Behavior, 15,* 320–327.

Blais, M. R., Vallerand, R. J., Pelletier, L. G., & Briere, N. M. (1989). L'Echelle de satisfaction de vie: Validation Canadienne-Francaise du "Satisfaction With Life Scale" [French-Canadian Validation of the Satisfaction With Life Scale]. *Canadian Journal of Behavioral Science, 21,* 210–223.

Botwin, M., Diener, E., & Tomarelli, M. (1992). *On the undersirability of controlling social desirability.* Personal communication, California State University at Fresno.

Campbell, A., Converse, P. E., & Rogers, W. L. (1976). *The quality of American life.* New York: Russell Sage Foundation.

Carstenson, L. L., & Cone, J. D. (1983). Social desirability and the measurement of psychological well being in elderly persons. *Journal of Gerontology, 38,* 713–715.

Chamberlain, K. (1988). On the structure of well-being. *Social Indicators Research, 20,* 581–604.

Chwalisz, K., Diener, E., & Gallagher, D. (1988). Autonomic arousal feedback and emotional experience: Evidence from the spinal cord injured. *Journal of Personality and Social Psychology, 54,* 820–828.

DeHaes, J. C., Pennink, B. J. W., & Welvaart, K. (1987). The distinction between affect and cognition. *Social Indicators Research, 19,* 367–378.

Derogatis, L. R. (1977). *SCL-90: Administration, scoring & procedures manual-I for the r(evised) version and other instruments of the psychopathology rating scale series.* Baltimore, MD: Clinical Psychometrics Research Unit, Johns Hopkins University School of Medicine.

Diener, E. (1984). Subjective well-being. *Psychological Bulletin, 95,* 542–575.

Diener, E. (1990). *Issues in defining and measuring subjective well-being.* Manuscript submitted for publication.

Diener, E., & Emmons, R. A. (1984). The independence of positive and negative affect. *Journal of Personality and Social Psychology, 47,* 1105–1117.

Diener, E., Emmons, R. A., Larsen, R. J., & Griffin, S. (1985). The Satisfaction With Life Scale. *Journal of Personality Assessment, 49,* 71–75.

Diener, E., & Larsen, R. J. (1993). The subjective experience of emotional well-being. In M. Lewis & J. M. Haviland (Eds), *Handbook of emotions* (pp. 405–415) New York: Guilford Press.

Diener, E., Magnus, K., & Fujita, F. (1991). *A longitudinal examination of life events and subjective well-being.* Unpublished Manuscript, University of Illinois.

Diener, E., Sandvik, E., Pavot, W., & Gallaher, D. (1991). Response artifacts in the measurement of subjective well-being. *Social Indicators Research, 24,* 36–56.

Fordyce, M. W. (1977). *The happiness measures: A sixty-second index of emotional well-being and mental health.* Unpublished manuscript, Edison Community College, Ft. Myers, FL.

Frisch, M. B., Cornell, J., Villanueva, M., & Retzlaff, P. (1992). Clinical validation of the Quality of Life Inventory: A measure of life satisfaction for use in treatment planning and outcome assessment. *Psychological Assessment, 4*, 92–101.

Fujita, F. & Diener, E. (1992). *Social comparison and domain satisfactions.* Research in progress.

George, J. M. (1991). Time structure and purpose as a mediator of work-life linkages. *Journal of Applied Psychology, 21*, 296–314.

Husek, T. R. (1961). Acquiescence as a response set and as a personality characteristic. *Educational and Psychological Measurement, 21*, 295–307.

Joy, R. H. (1990). *Path analytic investigation of stress-symptom relationships: Physical and psychological symptom models.* Unpublished doctoral dissertation, University of Illinois at Urbana-Champaign.

Judge, T. (1990). *Job satisfaction as a reflection of disposition: Investigating the relationship and its effects on employee adaptive behaviors.* Unpublished doctoral dissertation, University of Illinois.

Kammann, R., & Flett, R. (1983). Affectometer 2: A scale to measure current level of general happiness. *Australian Journal of Psychology, 35*, 257–265.

Kozma, A., & Stones, M. J. (1980). The measurement of happiness: Development of the Memorial University of Newfoundland Scale of Happiness (MUNSCH). *Journal of Gerontology, 35*, 906–912.

Larsen, R. J., Diener, E., & Emmons, R. A. (1985). An evaluation of subjective well-being measures. *Social Indicators Research, 17*, 1–18.

Liang, J. (1985). A structural integration of the Affect Balance Scale and the Life Satisfaction Index A. *Journal of Gerontology, 40*, 552–561.

Magnus, K., Diener, E., Fujita, F., & Pavot, W. (1993). Extraversion and neuroticism as predictors of objective life events: A longitudinal analysis. *Journal of Personality and Social Psychology, 65*, 1046–1053.

McGarrahan, J. F. (1991). *Family of origin, antecedents of religious vocation, community experience, and life satisfaction of active and contemplative religious women.* Unpublished doctoral dissertation, Temple University.

Pavot, W., & Diener, E. (1993). The affective and cognitive context of self-reported measures of subjective well-being. *Social Indicators Research, 28*, 1–20.

Pavot, W., Diener, E., Colvin, C. R., & Sandvik, E. (1991). Further validation of the Satisfaction With Life Scale: Evidence for the cross-method convergence of well-being measures. *Journal of Personality Assessment, 57*, 149–161.

Rorer, L. G. (1965). The great response-style myth. *Psychological Bulletin, 63*, 129–156.

Schwarz, N., & Clore, G. L. (1983). Mood, misattribution, and judgments of well-being: Informative and directive functions of affective states. *Journal of Personality and Social Psychology, 45*, 513–523.

Schwarz, N., & Strack, F. (1991). Evaluating one's life: A judgment model of subjective well-being. In F. Strack, M. Argyle, & N. Schwarz (Eds.), *Subjective well-being: An interdisciplinary perspective* (pp. 27–47). Oxford, England: Pergamon Press.

Shao, L., & Diener, E. (1992). *Multilanguage comparability of life satisfaction and happiness measures in mainland Chinese and American Students.* Unpublished master's thesis, University of Illinois.

Shin, D. C., & Johnson, D. M. (1978). Avowed happiness as an overall assessment of the quality of life. *Social Indicators Research, 5*, 475–492.

Smead, V. S. (1991). *Measuring well-being is not easy.* Paper presented at the Annual Convention of the American Association of Applied and Preventive Psychology.

Stock, W. A., Okun, M. A., & Benin, M. (1986). Structure of subjective well-being among the elderly. *Psychology and Aging, 1*, 91–102.

Tellegen, A. (1982). *Brief manual of the Differential Personality Questionnaires.* Minneapolis: University of Minnesota Press.

Veenhoven, R. (1984). *Conditions of happiness.* Hingham, MA: Kluwer Boston Academic Publishers.

Veenhoven, R. (1991). Questions on happiness: Classical topics, modern answers, blind spots. In F. Strack, M. Argyle, & N. Schwarz (Eds.), *Subjective well-being: An interdisciplinary perspective* (pp. 7–26). Oxford, England: Pergamon Press.

Vitaliano, P. P., Russo, J., Young, H. M., Becker, J., & Maiuro, R. D. (1991). The screen for caregiver burden. *The Gerontologist, 31,* 76–83.

Watson, D., Clark, L. A., & Tellegen, A. (1988). Development and validation of brief measures of positive and negative affect: The PANAS scales. *Journal of Personality and Social Psychology, 54,* 1063–1070.

Won, H. (in progress). Unpublished doctoral dissertation, University of Oregon.

Yardley, J. K., & Rice, R. W. (1991). The relationship between mood and subjective well-being. *Social Indicators Research, 24,* 101–111.

Subjective Well-Being: The Convergence and Stability of Self-Report and Non-Self-Report Measures

Ed Sandvik, Ed Diener, and Larry Seidlitz

Abstract The validity of self-report measures of subjective well-being (SWB) was examined and compared with non-self-report measures using a sample of 136 college students studied over the course of a semester. A principal axis factor analysis of self- and non-self-report SWB measures revealed a single unitary construct underlying the measures. Conventional single-item and multi-item self-report measures correlated highly with alternative measures, with theoretical correlates of SWB, and with a principal axis factor underlying five non-self-report measures of well-being. Comparisons of family versus friend informant reports demonstrated the considerable cross-situational consistency and temporal stability of SWB. Evidence of the discriminant validity of the measures was provided by low correlations of the various SWB measures with constructs theoretically unrelated to well-being. It was concluded that conventional self-report instruments validly measure the SWB construct, and that alternative, non-self-report measures are useful for providing a comprehensive theoretical account of happiness and life satisfaction.

The present article provides evidence concerning the construct validity of various self-report and non-self-report measures of subjective well-being (SWB). The analyses serve several major purposes: (a) to assess the convergence of conventional single- and multi-item self-report measures of SWB with each other and with alternative measures of the construct, (b) to provide evidence of the unitary nature of the well-being construct, (c) to assess the convergence of conventional and alternative SWB measures with a number of theoretical correlates of well-being, (d) to assess the consistency of individual differences in SWB over time and across situations, and (e) to provide evidence of the discriminant validity of conventional and alternative well-being measures. These analyses are necessary to clarify what traditional well-being scales measure as well as to elucidate the nature of individual differences in SWB.

E. Diener (✉)
Department of Psychology, University of Illinois, Urbana-Champaign, Champaign, IL 61820, USA
e-mail: ediener@uiuc.edu

E. Diener (ed.), *Assessing Well-Being: The Collected Works of Ed Diener,*
Social Indicators Research Series 39, DOI 10.1007/978-90-481-2354-4_6,
© Springer Science+Business Media B.V. 2009

In recent years interest in SWB has increased both in the frequency with which well-being is assessed in research and survey projects, and in the diversity of research interests which have found it to be a useful construct. These include sociology (Phillips, 1967), geriatric research (McNeil, Stones, & Kozma, 1986), clinical psychology (Cameron, Titus, J. Kostin, & M. Kostin, 1973), personality trait (Diener, 1984), and cognitive affect (Schwarz & Strack, 1991). Although few concepts have more intuitive reality and relevance to life than personal happiness, it is a construct which presents unique challenges to its assessment.

The single most common form of well-being assessment has been the collection of self-reports. A variety of such well-being measures have commonly been used, such as the Delighted-Terrible (D-T) Scale (Andrews and Withey, 1976) and the Fordyce Happiness Measure (1977). These two scales are comprised of single-item, face-valid inquiries into personal well-being: "How do you feel about how happy you are?" (response possibilities ranging from "delighted" to "terrible"), and "In general, how happy or unhappy do you usually feel?" (response possibilities ranging from "extremely happy" to "neutral" to "extremely unhappy"). Regardless of the simple face-validity of such inquiries, there are reasons for not automatically accepting responses to them as valid.

There has always existed considerable skepticism in the social sciences concerning the validity and interpretation of self-report data in general (e.g., Nisbett & Wilson, 1977), and there are reasons for more rather than less skepticism in the case of reports of personal well-being. It is possible that society imposes strong norms concerning the social desirability of happiness that are less of a problem for other constructs such as extraversion. To claim to be happy may be the ultimate assertion of success in our society, and to admit unhappiness could be the single greatest summary of failure in life that an individual could concede. The potential for social desirability artifacts provides good grounds for initial skepticism in the interpretation of self-reports of well-being. Another possibility for artifactual interpretation of self-reports, the influence of current mood, has been addressed elsewhere (Diener, Sandvik, Pavot, & Gallagher, 1991).

Demonstrations that self-reports of well-being are not simply interpretable in various artifactual terms, although important, do not establish the construct validity of such measures. If SWB research findings are to be interpretable, it is also necessary to determine the extent to which well-being shows itself to be a unitary construct which converges across a variety of measures. Because no one type of SWB measure by itself can be considered the touchstone of the well-being construct, the nomological network in which well-being exists must be elaborated in terms of the construct's converging and discriminating relations with affiliated constructs (Cronbach & Meehl, 1955).

Most previous research on construct validity in well-being assessment has focused on the relation of self-reports of well-being to other self-reports of well-being or related self-reports of personality traits. For example, in his recent review of his Happiness Measure, Fordyce (1988) reports on the correlations between his well-being measure and a host of similar measures, such as the D-T Scale (Andrews and Withey, 1976), the Affectometer 2 (Kammann & Flett, 1983), as well as measures such as the Beck Depression Inventory (Beck, 1978), the Mood Survey (Underwood & Froming, 1980), the Institute for Personality and Ability Testing (IPAT) Depression Scale (Krug & Laughlin, 1970), and omnibus inventories such as the Minnesota Multiphasic Personality Inventory (Hathaway & McKinley, 1951), the Personality Research Form (Jackson, 1967), and the California Personality Inventory (Gough, 1957). Similarly, in their classic study, Andrews and Withey (1976) report on the intercorrelations of a host of self-report scales of well-being and personality. They find a high concordance among many different phrasings of self-report well-being scales, and based on such comparisons, provide estimates on the true well-being variance accounted for in measures such as their D-T happiness measure. Although such information is important, the cautious researcher may hesitate to incorporate happiness measures in his or her research or to interpret findings without greater evidence that scores on self-report happiness scales correspond with something other than similar self-reports. Cogent arguments have been voiced against naive interpretations of self-reports as such (Nisbett & Ross, 1980; Nisbett & Wilson, 1977). Although such concerns have been considered in abstract (Dulany, 1968; Ericsson & Simon, 1980), it is clearly desirable for well-being researchers to demonstrate convergence between the commonly used, traditional one-time self-report well-being measures and other diverse sources of information which would not be subject to the same limitations or biases as traditional self-report inventories.

In their recent review, Hogan & Nicholson (1988) note that, although the idea of construct validity is familiar, it has not been practiced as thoroughly as it has been preached. The result, they claim, has been a rehash of what they term "1960s-vintage criticisms" in assessment. The concern for construct validity arose out of a need to develop scientifically rigorous justification and procedures for dealing with the measurement of inferred states, and a skepticism about a naive interpretation of self-reports.

Unfortunately, there are unique difficulties involved in attempting to collect diverse forms of evidence in the case of subjective well-being. Andrews and Withey (1976) stated the situation as follows:

> Evaluating measures of people's feelings about their lives presents major problems because there seem to be no clear and directly observable phenomena that can serve as criteria. People's behavior and the conditions under which they live, while related to their perceptions of well-being, are influenced by many factors in addition to their feelings and hence are not appropriate criterion variables. It is the feelings themselves that we seek to measure. Although very real and important to the people who hold them, they are internal and inherently unobservable phenomena. (p. 215)

Thus, special care must be used in selecting objective indices of SWB, and caution must be exercised in their interpretation.

Several studies, however, have attempted to go beyond self-report information on well-being. One such attempt was by Andrews and Withey (1976). In addition to collecting self-report information, they gathered reports from two or three individuals who knew the subject. They found low correlations between these ratings by knowledgeable others and the D-T Scale and concluded that future collection of such information is unlikely to be useful. Recent methodological reviews have suggested, however, that because informed others usually see individuals only in a limited number of settings, a greater number of reports than that collected by Andrews and Withey is necessary to show convergence (Moskowitz, 1986). Other studies gathering peer reports have in fact had greater success. Carroll (1952), for example, reported a 0.39 correlation between self- and other reports of well-being. Similarly, Hartmann (1934) reported a 0.34 correlation between self-reports and those of four associates, and Goldings (1954) reported a 0.38 correlation between self-reports and those of five experimenters who knew the subject moderately well.

Although each of the studies mentioned above assessed the convergence of a self-report measure of well-being with a non-self-report measure, none have attempted a broad study of the relation between commonly used traditional self-report measures of SWB and a broad spectrum of non-self-report measures. We have examined standard single-item and multiple-item self-reports, as well as various alternative strategies, including informant reports, a forced-choice measure which controls for social desirability, a memory sampling measure, expert ratings, and a longitudinal study of daily mood over 42 days. The convergence among these diverse well-being measures should provide important information on the construct of SWB, on how traditional well-being scales should be interpreted, and on how much is gained by using non-self-report strategies in addition to traditional self-report measures.

Although well-being is inherently internal and experiential, there are reasons to believe that methods other than self-report might be valid indicators of this experience. Furthermore, it does not seem that simple self-report should be automatically afforded privileged status in the assessment of private experience. For example, experts should be able to estimate participants' SWB based on information provided in a written interview. Although based on self-report, the written interview can be much more detailed, ideographic, and complex than the traditional self-report of well-being. Such an interview can include a subject's hopes and concerns, goals and interests, and pleasures and pains. It is harder for respondents to avoid unpleasant aspects of their lives when formulating their responses because information about these domains is directly requested. The expert rater then judges this complex material and converts it into a numeric response. Thus, the method avoids problems associated with traditional self-report measures such as differences between subjects in the strategies used to retrieve and integrate relevant information, and differences in numerically scaling their level of happiness.

A measure of daily moods over an extended period is another alternative that avoids other problems associated with traditional self-reports of SWB. The advantage to a daily score is that subjects' memories are likely to be much more accurate for a single day than for a prolonged period. Furthermore, although subjects might be loathe to admit that they are very unhappy, they would be much more likely to admit that they had a bad day. Therefore, the daily score is likely to give a good indication of subjects' average moods.

The reports of informants are likely to summarize emotional information expressed by subjects over time—information conveyed in both verbal and nonverbal channels. Because some nonverbal channels (e.g., vocal parameters) are less controllable than self-reports (DePaulo & Rosenthal, 1979), knowledgeable others may gain an accurate idea of a subject's emotional life. The reports of informants have a strength which is complementary to self-report: Respondents are less likely to be able to hide their true feelings from knowledgeable others.

A memory measure of SWB is based on the idea that important emotional experiences will be encoded in subjects' memories. Indeed, a primary source of self-reports of well-being must be the recall of such remembered material. A number of studies have shown that happy persons recall more positive versus negative life events than unhappy persons (e.g., Diener, Sandvik, Pavot, & Gallagher, 1991; Pavot, Diener, Colvin, & Sandvik, 1991). Seidlitz and Diener (1993) demonstrated that happy individuals can recall more positive events and fewer negative events because they initially encode the events in this manner. Differences between happy and unhappy persons in the encoding of life events may be due to both differences in the incidence of positive versus negative objective events and to differences in the interpretation of events. Other research has indicated that mood, both at the time of encoding (Bower, Gilligan, & Monteiro, 1981) and retrieval (Clark & Teasdale, 1985; Forgas, Bower, & Krantz, 1984), has effects on the valence of information recalled (for a review, see Blaney, 1986). Thus, there are empirical and theoretical reasons to believe that counts of memories for positive and negative events will tap SWB. The idea that a simple count of such memories will be a valid index is based on the finding that happy persons frequently experience positive feelings and infrequently experience negative feelings (Diener, Sandvik, & Pavot, 1991), and therefore should have more positive events available for easy recall. Thus, memory for happy versus unhappy events is likely to tap SWB, and will be complementary to self-report in that it is less susceptible to response artifacts such as differences in using numbers to rate SWB or social desirability.

Finally, a forced-choice measure was specifically designed to control social desirability. In assessing the frequency with which various positive versus negative emotions are experienced, this measure requires subjects to choose between emotions and personality traits that have been balanced for the social desirability of the items. Scores on this measure are based on the positive and negative emotion terms chosen by subjects over trait adjectives having approximately equal social desirability. Thus, the measure complements traditional self-report measures in that it taps the SWB construct uncontaminated by social desirability.

Therefore, in this study a number of nontraditional measures of SWB which appear to have promise as alternative ways to assess subjects' private experiences were employed. Although some of these alternative measures rely on self-report to some degree, they all guard against at least some important threat to traditional self-report measures, and thus as a group represent an index of SWB which is relatively free from traditional self-report biases.

We compared the construct validity of various well-being measures by examining their correlations with measures of various constructs theoretically related to SWB such as extraversion, neuroticism, optimism, and symptoms of ill-being. Extraversion and neuroticism have been found to be related to well-being in a number of studies (e.g., Costa & McCrae, 1980; Emmons & Diener, 1985), but the exact reasons for these relations are not yet firmly established (Pavot, Diener, & Fujita,

1990). Emmons and Diener (1986) found that the extraversion-SWB relation resulted from a relation of the sociability component of extraversion with positive affect, and speculated that the reinforcement and satisfaction of needs provided by others lead to an increase in positive affect. Emmons and Diener (1986) also found that neuroticism was related to negative but not positive affect, and that impulsivity may have contributed in small degree to the neuroticism–negative affect relation.

Optimism has been theoretically and empirically related to SWB in previous studies through its association with successful coping with stress and physical ill-being. Scheier, Weintraub, and Carver (1986) found that optimists were more likely than pessimists to use problem-focused coping strategies, seek social support, and emphasize positive aspects of stressful situations. Carver and Gaines (1987) found that optimism moderated the tendency toward depression after a stressful life change, the birth of a child. In a study with coronary bypass surgery patients, Scheier, Matthews, and Owens (1989) found optimism to be associated with problem-focused coping, faster recovery, and higher quality of life 6 months after surgery. Thus, optimism was expected to be associated with SWB because of its association with successful coping strategies.

Symptoms of illness are predicted to correlate inversely with well-being because of causal paths in both directions. Evidence from a number of studies suggests that illness makes people less happy (Okun, Stock, Haring, & Witter, 1984); however, other studies suggest that the relation between self-reported health and SWB results primarily from unhappy people perceiving more symptoms of illness (Costa, McCrae, & Norris, 1981; Okun & George, 1984). Similarly, a high grade point average might correlate with well-being both because it is a valued resource, and also because depressed individuals may function less well academically.

For empirical and theoretical reasons, both family income and divorce or death of parents are expected to be associated with SWB. E. Diener, Sandvik, Seidlitz, and M. Diener (1992) have shown income to be associated with SWB in both a cross-country study and a longitudinal study within the United States. Their evidence suggested that income is a resource that not only satisfies basic needs but also contributes to SWB after basic needs have been met. Divorce and death within a family are among the most stressful life events and have been shown to be associated with lower SWB (Diener, 1984).

To test the discriminant validity of SWB instruments, we have also examined the correlations of the various measures with several constructs which are a priori theoretically independent of SWB: stimulus screening (Mehrabian, 1976), intelligence (Otis, 1939), and affect intensity (Larsen, 1984). Larsen's (1984) Affect Intensity Measure, for a variety of theoretical reasons, was predicted not to correlate substantially with measures of well-being. First, this measure assesses the intensity of *both* a person's pleasant and unpleasant emotions, and thus should not be correlated with happiness. Second, Diener, Sandvik, et al. (1991) have empirically demonstrated that happiness is more related to emotional frequency than to its intensity. Larsen and Diener (1987) review evidence showing that individual differences in emotional intensity are unrelated to individual differences in happiness. Finally, Diener, Colvin, Pavot, and Allman (1991) have shown that intense positive emotions can entail costs. Thus, based on theoretical reasons as well as past empirical work, affect intensity was predicted to exhibit low, discriminant correlations with measures of SWB.

Stimulus screening is the individual difference characteristic of the automatic screening out of irrelevant stimuli, and of the habituation to distracting, irrelevant stimuli. The characteristic is closely related to arousability, such that screeners impose a structure on complex situational stimuli, resulting in lower arousal. Unlike extraversion, however, this concept does not emphasize sociability, which is associated with well-being. Thus, screeners have lower arousal and less distraction due to irrelevant stimuli than nonscreeners, but there is no theoretical relation between these characteristics and frequencies of positive and negative affect or cognitive judgments of overall life satisfaction, on which SWB is based.

The third discriminant variable, intelligence, consistently has been found to be unrelated to SWB in past studies (Diener, 1984). It has been conjectured that the rewards of being intelligent are offset by higher expectations and by an ability to understand problems and counterfactual alternatives more clearly. Thus, based on previous research using a variety of measures of mental ability and well-being, intelligence was hypothesized to be unrelated to SWB.

Method

Participants

Participants included 136 University of Illinois students enrolled in a course that involved extended participation in research in SWB during the fall of 1986. Before any statistical analyses were performed, the number of participants was reduced to 130, 46 men and 84 women, due either to suspect or largely incomplete data by 6 respondents. The number of participants included in particular analyses varied due to a number of cases with partially missing data.

Happiness Measures

Standard self-report. Participants completed a number of conventional and non-conventional SWB measures during the semester. Conventional measures included the Fordyce Happiness Measure (Fordyce, 1977), the D-T Scale (Andrews and Withey, 1976), the Bradburn Affect Balance Scale (1969), and the Affectometer 2 (Kammann & Flett, 1983).

Alternative Measures

An alternative SWB measure included a written interview that participants were given to complete at home during the first week. The written interview contained open-ended questions pertaining to the participants' happiness and satisfaction with life. The detailed five-page, 19-item questionnaire included diverse questions on topics such as subjects' typical moods, suicidal ideation, and the happiest and unhappiest times in their life. Examples of items include the following: "Describe your life right now; the good points and bad." "When, how intensely, and how often do you feel excited and enthusiastic about your life?" "Describe your average moods, your ups and downs, your pleasant and unpleasant feelings and when these occur." These questionnaires were later given global ratings by the senior investigator (Diener) and two research assistants for evidence of SWB on a 7-point scale on which 0 represented "very depressed in general" and 6 represented "elated most of the time." All ratings were made blind to the identity of subjects.

Subjects also completed daily affect reports on 42 occasions over a period of 6 weeks during the latter part of the semester, after the traditional self-report measures had been taken. Participants were asked to recall their daily mood each evening by rating the degree to which they experienced each of four positive emotions and four negative emotions on a 0–6 scale ranging from "not at all" to "extremely much." The ratings of the negative adjectives were reverse-scored and added to the ratings of the positive adjectives to yield a total daily affect score. The average score for each subject for the 42 days was then computed.

As a non-self-report measure of happiness, a minimum of seven informants rated each participant's happiness using the Fordyce scale. Informants included at least three family members and at least three friends of the subject. Comparisons of reports from family members with those of friends would provide information concerning the situational consistency of subjective well-being. These informant reports were confidential and sent directly to the experimenters.

Participants were given a 3-min, timed test to recall as many positive life events as they could that had occurred during their lifetimes, and a separate 3-min test to recall as many negative life events as they could. Participants also were given separate 2-min, timed tests to recall as many positive and negative life events as they could that had occurred during the past year. Subjects generally recall different types of events under the different instruction sets, with a tendency for major life events to be recalled under the lifetime set, and minor hassles and uplifts to be recalled under the past year set. Because the life and year memory tasks are included in the same testing period, subjects assume that nonredundant information is being requested and thus list different events. The 2- and 3-min tests were combined and an event memory index of SWB was derived by subtracting the total number of negative events recalled from the total number of positive events recalled.

To obtain a social desirability–free assessment of SWB, a measure was constructed based on Edwards's forced-choice approach. Participants were asked to make a choice between 54 pairs of affect versus personality trait adjectives that were previously matched for social desirability by raters (across the entire list, not item by item). Subjects were asked to choose the one alternative for each pair that was most self-descriptive. Examples of item pairs were "happy-kind" and "unhappy-dishonest." The number of times participants chose the mood adjective of the pair was summed to yield separate positive and negative affect scores. An overall forced-choice affect balance well-being score was computed by subtracting the negative affect score from the total number of negative affect adjectives, and adding this reversed negative affect score to the positive affect score. This score represented subjects' affect balance, uninfluenced by need for approval or social desirability. When considered on an item-by-item basis, words were paired such that always answering in the socially desirable direction would yield a score of only one higher than would be obtained if a subject answered randomly. Because the range of the scale was 54 points and the standard deviation of scores was 10, social desirability could have only a trivial effect on scores. Thus the scores were likely to be highly saturated by affect information uncontaminated by social desirability.

Theoretical Correlates and Noncorrelates of Well-Being

Measures of a number of theoretical correlates of SWB were also collected during the semester to examine the construct validity of the various measures. These included the Brief Symptom Inventory (BSI; Derogatis, 1975), the Life Orientation Test (LOT; Scheier & Carver, 1985), and the extraversion and neuroticism scales of the NEO Personality Inventory (NEO-PI; Costa & McCrae, 1985). The positive affect subscale of the NEO-PI extraversion scale was omitted so that correlations with the SWB measures would not be artifactually inflated.

Other SWB correlates included self-reported grade point average, a trouble index (composed of the sum of unit weighting of below-median self-reported parental income, parental divorce, and death of father or mother), and a daily ill-feeling index (composed from the sum of two standardized items included on a questionnaire completed daily over a period of 42 days—the items inquired how many aspirin or other pain relievers had been taken and whether the participant had felt under the weather that day).

Several personality measures of constructs theoretically independent of SWB were also completed. These included the Affect Intensity Measure (AIM; Larsen, 1984), the Otis Quick Scoring Mental Abilities Test (Otis, 1939), and the Stimulus Screening Measure (Mehrabian, 1976).

Results

The means, standard deviations, and reliabilities of the various measures are presented in Table 1. The numbers of participants completing the measures varied because of partially missing data for several of the participants. The reliabilities of the well-being instruments were obtained using several methods. Although most reliabilities shown in Table 1 are alphas, in some cases traditional alpha coefficients were unavailable. The coefficient for the single-item Fordyce is based on the 2-week test-retest, whereas the reliability for the D-T Scale was provided by an estimate from Andrews and Withey (1976). The alpha for the written interview uses three raters as items, and the alpha for the informant reports uses seven informants as

Table 1 Means, standard deviations, and reliabilities of measures

Measures	N	Mean	SD	Reliability[a]
Standard self-report measures				
Fordyce	126	7.32	1.16	0.72[b]
D-T Scale	128	2.76	1.20	0.70[c]
Affectometer 2	128	111.60	23.27	0.96
Bradburn	128	6.48	1.81	0.53
Alternative measures				
Written interview	119	3.56	0.92	0.68
Daily affect	129	31.15	4.70	0.88
Informant reports	126	7.44	0.89	0.72
Event memory	126	3.98	6.44	0.69
Forced-choice	130	82.67	9.73	0.89
Theoretical correlates				
Trouble index	130	0.46	0.70	
Daily ill-feeling index	129	0.00	1.76	
Grade point average (5-point scale)	127	4.07	0.61	
Brief Symptom Inventory	120	11.00	3.62	
Optimism (LOT)[d]	126	19.46	5.27	
NEO extraversion	117	98.70	13.37	
NEO neuroticism	117	91.02	23.39	
Discriminant variables				
Stimulus Screening	128	174.27	67.71	
Otis	127	64.55	7.13	
Affect Intensity Measure	112	152.29	20.32	

[a] Reliabilities are alpha coefficients unless otherwise noted. Alphas for the written interview and informant reports are based on agreement between raters or informants, instead of items.
[b] Two-week test-retest reliability.
[c] Provided as estimate for D-T Scale (Andrews and Withey, 1976).
[d] Life Orientation Test.

items. The alpha for the event memory uses the two tests (past year and lifetime) as items. In addition to the alphas shown in the table, the daily affect measure's test-retest reliability (first 21 daily reports vs. second 21 reports) may be of interest—it was 0.94. All remaining reliability coefficients shown in the table are traditional alphas.

Intercorrelations of SWB Instruments

The intercorrelations of the various SWB measures are presented in Table 2. The conventional scales are listed first, followed by the alternative SWB measures. The intercorrelations show satisfactory convergent validity for all of the measures. Of the alternative measures, the written interview, daily affect reports, and informant reports correlated most highly with the conventional measures, most ranging between 0.50 and 0.70. The event memory measure correlated moderately with most of the measures, generally in the 0.30 to 0.50 range, its indirect methodology probably contributing to the lower correlations. The forced-choice measure also correlated in the 0.30 to 0.50 range with the other SWB measures.

Table 2 Intercorrelations of subjective well-being measures

	1	2	3	4	5	6	7	8	9
1. Fordyce	–								
2. D-T Scale	0.62	–							
3. Affectometer 2	0.57	0.72	–						
4. Bradburn	0.46	0.54	0.69	–					
5. Written interview	0.68	0.71	0.76	0.60	–				
6. Daily affect	0.54	0.66	0.70	0.56	0.59	–			
7. Informant reports	0.58	0.58	0.54	0.34	0.60	0.52	–		
8. Event memory	0.33	0.41	0.41	0.20	0.47	0.45	0.34	–	
9. Forced-choice	0.27	0.50	0.50	0.35	0.47	0.37	0.36	0.18	–

Note. $N = 110$ to 128. For $r > 0.17$, $p < 0.05$. For $r > 0.22$, $p < 0.01$.

Principal Axis Factor Analyses

Table 3 shows the factor loadings of the SWB measures on the first factor obtained in an exploratory principal axis factor analysis of the self-report instruments and the five alternative measures. The purpose of the analysis was to explore the number of factors needed to adequately describe the data. The first factor extracted had an eigenvalue of 4.82 and accounted for 53.6% of the variance. It was the only factor with an eigenvalue above one, and the scree plot distinctly indicated a single factor. Both the self-report and non-self-report measures loaded highly on the first factor, indicating convergence on a single underlying construct. Although the various measures have acceptably high levels of reliability, an estimate of what the factor loadings would be if there were no measurement error was obtained by disattenuating the correlation matrix for unreliability using a standard formula (Ghiselli, Campbell, & Zedeck, 1981), and then factoring the disattenuated matrix. As seen in the right-hand column, the disattenuated loadings are quite high. The first factor underlying the disattenuated correlation matrix accounted for 61.1% of the variance.

Because the first factor analysis included a preponderance of self-report measures, we performed a second exploratory factor analysis including only the five alternative measures to determine if a single factor would emerge. The first factor in the principal axis factor analysis had an eigenvalue of 2.31 and explained 46.2%

Table 3 Factor loadings of subjective well-being measures

Measure	Factor loading	Disattenuated loading
Fordyce	0.74	0.78
D-T Scale	0.85	0.92
Affectometer 2	0.89	0.85
Bradburn	0.66	0.81
Written interview	0.85	0.92
Daily affect	0.77	0.79
Informant reports	0.68	0.74
Event memory	0.53	0.58
Forced-choice	0.52	0.57

Table 4 Factor loadings of alternative well-being measures

Measure	Factor loading	Disattenuated loading
Written interview	0.84	1.00
Daily affect	0.73	0.79
Informant reports	0.71	0.82
Event memory	0.55	0.64
Forced-choice	0.51	0.56

of the variance in the measures. It was the only factor with an eigenvalue above one, and again the scree plot of eigenvalues clearly suggested a one-factor solution. Table 4 shows the loadings of the five alternative measures on the first factor. As indicated in the table, the factor analysis shows strong convergence of the nonconventional measures. The factor loadings average 0.67, and the loadings based on the correlation matrix disattenuated for unreliability average 0.76. The single factor based on the correlation matrix of disattenuated measures accounted for 60.2% of the variance. Given the extremely different methodologies used in the alternative measures, this finding is very encouraging in terms of pointing to a unified underlying construct of SWB.

Neither factor analysis indicates that variance due simply to the self-report method is a major component of the SWB measures. Several of the highest-loading variables are self-report. It should be noted, however, that the one measure which is most clearly not a self-report assessment, informant reports, loads highly in both factor analyses, and that the self-report forced-choice method fares more poorly. If one compares the average correlation between the four conventional self-report measures with each other (0.60) to the average correlation of these measures with the informant reports (0.46), an estimate of 15% of the variance in self-report measures due to the self-report methodology would be obtained (0.60^2 minus 0.46^2).

Correlations of SWB Measures with Theoretical Correlates

Table 5 shows the correlations of the traditional self-report and alternative SWB measures with the theoretically related variables and with the principal axis factor underlying the five alternative measures. The conventional measures again are listed first, followed by the alternative measures. The conventional self-report measures compared favorably to the nonconventional measures in predicting several of the theoretical correlates, including the trouble index, optimism, extraversion, and neuroticism. Even the single-item measures performed at a level comparable to the more elaborate alternative measures. Nevertheless, it is encouraging that the nonconventional measures often correlated significantly with the theoretical correlates, indicating that the correlation of these variables is not simply due to self-report artifacts.

The correlations of the self-report measures with the SWB factor underlying the alternative measures were very respectable. Indeed, the average correlation of

Table 5 Correlations of subjective well-being measures with theoretical correlates

Measures	TI	DIFI	GPA	BSI	LOT	EXT	NEUR	FAC
Fordyce	−0.36	−0.01	0.16	−0.22	−0.59	0.40	−0.41	0.71
D-T Scale	−0.18	−0.14	0.14	−0.12	−0.59	0.30	−0.57	0.79
Affectometer 2	−0.11	−0.21	0.17	−0.17	−0.72	0.49	−0.73	0.82
Bradburn	−0.06	−0.22	0.04	−0.06	−0.50	0.36	−0.57	0.61
Written interview	−0.15	−0.21	0.20	−0.20	−0.67	0.42	−0.60	–
Daily affect	−0.21	−0.23	0.21	−0.17	−0.50	0.46	−0.55	–
Informant reports	−0.27	−0.07	0.29	−0.14	−0.51	0.38	−0.34	–
Event memory	−0.16	−0.33	0.25	−0.21	−0.36	0.22	−0.29	–
Forced-choice	−0.06	−0.25	0.02	−0.09	−0.38	0.13	−0.39	–

Note. $N = 99$ to 128. For $r > 0.17$, $p < 0.05$. For $r > 0.22$, $p < 0.01$. TI = trouble index, composed of the sum of unit weightings of parental death, parental divorce, and below-median parental income (less than $43,000); DIFI = daily ill-feeling index, composed of two standardized items: daily self-reports of feeling under the weather (yes or no) and number of aspirin taken; GPA = grade point average; BSI = Brief Symptom Inventory; LOT = Life Orientation Test; EXT = NEO extraversion, excluding positive affect subscale; NEUR = NEO neuroticism; FAC = principal axis factor underlying the five alternative subjective well-being measures.

the self-report measures with the non-self-report factor (0.73) slightly outstripped the average loading of the alternative measures (0.67) from which the factor was derived. These high correlations are especially encouraging because the common factor underlying the alternative method measures reflects the SWB construct untainted by many of the problems associated with self-report methodology.

Although it is encouraging that the SWB measures correlate with the theoretically related variables, their correlations with the LOT and NEO-PI neuroticism scales are as high as the intercorrelations among the well-being scales themselves. An analysis of the neuroticism items of the NEO-PI indicates that they essentially measure negative affect. Indeed, Watson and Clark (1984) suggest that neuroticism is the propensity to experience negative affect. In confirmatory factor-analytic work, Fujita, Diener, and Pavot (1993) find that neuroticism and negative affect are indistinguishable. Similarly, generalized expectancies about the future as measured by the LOT might be based on feelings of positive or negative affect. Thus, several personality constructs may have a strong affective underpinning and not be discriminable from the construct of SWB. Further work is needed in order to fully assess the discriminant validity of neuroticism and optimism from SWB—work with large samples and with multiple measures of each construct.

Comparisons Among Self-Report Instruments

The correlations of the four self-report instruments with the alternative SWB measures and with the theoretically related constructs were compared to determine which self-report instruments had greater convergent validity. Direct comparisons of the self-report instruments may be of interest to survey researchers and others who, because of practical constraints, are forced to choose between available conventional instruments. Four types of comparisons were made: (a) between the two single-item

Table 6 Z scores for differences in correlations for pairs of alternative subjective well-being measures

	D-T Scale vs. Fordyce	Affectometer vs. Bradburn	Affectometer vs. D-T	Affectometer vs. Fordyce
Fordyce	–	ns	ns	–
D-T Scale	–	3.40	–	ns
Affectometer 2	2.59	–	–	–
Bradburn	ns	–	3.02	3.60
Written interview	ns	2.96	ns	ns
Daily affect	2.03	2.76	ns	2.70
Informant reports	ns	3.17	ns	ns
Event memory	ns	3.12	ns	ns
Forced-choice	3.25	2.52	ns	3.13
Trouble index	−2.43	ns	ns	−3.28
Daily ill-feeling	ns	ns	ns	2.52
Grade point average	ns	ns	ns	ns
Brief Symptom Inventory	ns	ns	ns	ns
Optimism (LOT)[a]	ns	3.97	2.66	2.66
NEO extraversion	ns	1.96	3.01	ns
NEO neuroticism	2.29	2.90	3.04	4.53

[a] LOT = Life Orientation Test.
Note. Positive value indicates the first instrument of the pair had the higher correlation with the measure.

measures, (b) between the two multi-item measures, (c) between the multi-item Affectometer 2 and the Fordyce measure, and (d) between the Affectometer 2 and the single-item D-T Scale.

Table 6 shows the Z scores for the differences in correlations between the two instruments in each comparison with the various well-being measures and related constructs listed in the left column. For example, the first entry, 2.59, represents the Z score for the difference between (a) the correlation of the D-T Scale with the Affectometer 2, and (b) the correlation of the Fordyce measure with the Affectometer 2. The positive value of the Z score indicates that the first instrument of the pair listed in the heading, the D-T Scale, had the higher correlation with the Affectometer 2. In comparisons between the D-T Scale and the Fordyce measure, the D-T Scale also correlated more highly with two alternative well-being measures and with neuroticism, whereas the Fordyce measure better-predicted the trouble index. The Affectometer 2 was substantially superior to the Bradburn Affect Balance Scale in correlations with the other well-being instruments and with several related variables, not surprising given the relatively low reliability of the Bradburn scale. Shortcomings of the Bradburn scale have been discussed elsewhere (Diener, 1984). The D-T Scale's correlations were generally comparable to those of the Affectometer 2, but it had lower correlations with the Bradburn scale and several of the theoretically related variables. The Fordyce measure compared less favorably to the Affectometer 2; it had lower correlations with the Bradburn, daily affect, and forced-choice measures, as well as with several of the theoretical correlates.

Cross-Situational Consistency

To examine more systematically the long-term cross-situational consistency of SWB, we separately analyzed the informant reports completed by family members and those completed by friends. Family members observed the student participants in very different situations from those in which the informant friends encountered them. The participants, mostly juniors and seniors, had lived away from home for several years. Family members primarily interacted with the participants several years before in a home setting. In contrast, friends primarily saw the participants in a large university setting, living in an apartment with other students, at parties, etc. Thus, convergence of these two sets of informant reports would provide evidence of the long-term cross-situational consistency of SWB.

Table 7 shows the separate intercorrelations of the two sets of informant reports with self-report measures, the alternative well-being measures, and the theoretically related variables. As shown in Table 7, the two sets of informant reports correlated 0.44 with each other, and correlated highly and similarly with the alternative well-being measures. They also correlated similarly and at a moderate level with several variables theoretically related to well-being. The nonsignificant correlations of the informant reports with the daily ill-feeling index and the BSI probably resulted because the minor health problems assessed by these measures were frequently unobservable. Overall, the results support the cross-situational consistency of SWB.

If one disattenuates the correlation between friends and family for the reliability of these measures (0.85 and 0.74), one obtains an estimated correlation of 0.70. The coefficient of determination based on this number suggests that about half of the

Table 7 Informant reports separated by family versus friends

	Family reports	Friends' reports
Friends' reports	0.44	
Fordyce (Self)	0.48	0.50
D T Scale	0.52	0.49
Affectometer 2	0.46	0.46
Bradburn	0.34	0.26
Written interview	0.54	0.52
Daily affect	0.50	0.42
Event memory	0.37	0.27
Forced-choice	0.34	0.28
Trouble index	−0.30	−0.18
Daily ill-feeling index	−0.13	−0.04
Grade point average	0.33	0.23
Brief Symptom Inventory	−0.11	−0.12
Optimism (LOT)[a]	−0.40	−0.47
NEO extraversion	0.31	0.33
NEO neuroticism	−0.33	−0.27

[a] LOT = Life Orientation Test.

Note. $N = 113$ to 126. For $r > 0.17$, $p < 0.05$. For $r > 0.23$, $p < 0.01$.

variance in SWB can be attributed to long-term and cross-situational factors such as personality and stable environmental conditions. The average intercorrelation of individual friends with each other was 0.49, of family members with each other was 0.65, and of family with friends, 0.32. This pattern suggests some stability across life periods, but greater levels of stability of SWB within a life period because there is greater agreement within groups than between groups. It could be, however, that the greater agreement within groups arises because there is more discussion of the individual within the rated groups than between them. Thus, the greater consensus within groups might be a function of discussion rather than behavioral consistency per se.

Discriminant Validity

Although the previous results show a unitary construct underlying the various SWB measures and consistency across situations, the discriminant validity of the well-being measures remains to be demonstrated. If the various scales and measures correlated substantially with constructs which were theoretically independent of SWB, the precise nature of the underlying construct would be in doubt. Table 8 presents the correlations of the various SWB measures with several constructs theoretically distinct from well-being: stimulus screening (Mehrabian, 1976), intelligence (Otis, 1939), and affect intensity (Larsen, 1984). Only 2 of the 27 correlations reached significance: the correlation of the daily affect with the Otis Quick Scoring Mental Abilities Test, and the correlation of the Affectometer 2 with the Stimulus Screening Measure. There were no particular SWB measures that showed substantially higher or lower correlations with the discriminant constructs than the other measures.

Table 8 Discriminant validity

	Stimulus Screening Measure	Intelligence[a]	Affect Intensity Measure
Fordyce	0.17	−0.06	0.11
D-T Scale	0.10	0.07	0.02
Affectometer 2	0.19*	0.02	0.01
Bradburn	0.17	0.05	0.03
Written interview	0.16	0.12	0.02
Daily affect	0.15	−0.22*	0.09
Informant reports	−0.03	−0.03	0.18
Event memory	0.15	0.02	0.04
Forced-choice	0.12	0.14	−0.15

[a] Measured by the Otis Quick Scoring Mental Abilities Test.
* $p < 0.05$.
Note. $N = 104$ to 128.

Discussion

The results are encouraging for the use of self-reports in the assessment of well-being. For instance, it could be concluded that standard self-report well-being scales are adequate for many or most research purposes. The traditional self-report measures of SWB demonstrated high convergent validity by their agreement with alternative SWB measures and their relations with theoretically related constructs. In this respect they appear as or more valid and useful than most personality measures in use today. The results thus indicate a unitary core of experience for well-being, which self-reports reflect to a great extent. This core of experience has some temporal and situational stability. Thus, researchers using standard well-being scales can generally expect they are obtaining meaningful, interpretable information from these scales under ordinary conditions.

Situational influences, however, should still be considered. The correlations obtained between our diverse measures and standard self-report scales are high, but certainly not perfect. There is room in these relations for situational effects and momentary mood to have significant influences on the outcome of individual studies. Schwarz and his colleagues (Schwarz & Clore, 1983; Schwarz & Strack, 1991; Schwarz, Strack, Muller, & Chassein, 1988) have demonstrated that situational effects such as the weather or question ordering can influence self-reports of well-being. Momentary effects and simple error may also account for a part of this variance. Such effects may be minimized by increasing reliability through use of multi-item measures and by repeated measurements. Other problems associated with self-reports of SWB, such as repression or denial of negative emotions, and cultural differences in emotional experience and labeling, are more difficult to correct (Diener, 1994).

Several practical implications can be drawn from the present findings. First, the results imply several recommendations concerning the self-report instruments. The Affectometer 2 was shown to be a superior instrument to Bradburn's Affect Balance Scale. In other work (Diener, Emmons, Larsen, & Griffin, 1985; Pavot & Diener, 1993; Pavot et al., 1991), we have demonstrated that the Satisfaction with Life Scale is also a reliable and valid SWB instrument. The multi-item Affectometer 2 showed greater reliability and validity than the single-item measures, and thus its use is preferable when practical considerations permit. Nevertheless, the two single-item measures loaded highly on the factor underlying the various well-being measures and showed respectable convergent and discriminant validity. Thus, their use in survey research, when practical considerations preclude more elaborate measures, is defensible. Although both single-item measures demonstrated significant convergent and discriminant validity, comparisons between the two scales suggested the D-T Scale to be slightly preferable.

Second, although self-report well-being scales may be adequate for many purposes, they do not tell the whole story or necessarily contain all the information a given researcher might want or need. When possible, a broader base of measures is desirable to investigate the experiential, communicative, behavioral, and physiological components of well-being, and their interconnections. For example, if groups differed in informant report versus self-report assessments, this would point to interesting hypotheses about the processes underlying the two types of assessment. Various assessment strategies are also useful for generating research hypotheses concerning the internal and external determinants of well-being. It may be, for example, that self-reports are adequate when comparing persons within a homogenous culture, but that additional measures are desirable when comparing persons' SWB across different cultures. In addition, alternative measurement methods such as informant reports and event memory seem desirable when time permits because they help rule out various artifactual explanations of results.

Finally, what do the results indicate about the stability of SWB? The answer seems to be that there are both long-term consistencies in average mood and a fair amount of fluctuation in short-term moods (Diener & Larsen, 1984). The present study clearly indicates that there are long-term consistencies in average mood, and that a variety of self-report and non-self-report methods can tap into this long-term average. Thus, SWB or happiness is a scientifically defensible area of study for personologists.

References

Andrews, F. M., & Withey, S. B. (1976). *Social indicators of well-being: America's perception of life quality*. New York Plenum Press.

Beck, A. (1978). *Beck depression inventory*. Philadelphia: Center for Cognitive Therapy.

Blaney, P. H. (1986). Affect and memory: A review. *Psychological Bulletin, 99*, 229–246.

Bower, G. H., Gilligan, S. G., & Monteiro, K. P. (1981). Selectivity of learning caused by affective states. *Journal of Experimental Psychology: General, 110*, 451–473.

Bradburn, N. M. (1969). *The structure of psychological well-being*. Chicago: Aldine.

Cameron, P., Titus, D. G., Kostin, J., & Kostin, M. (1973). The life satisfaction of nonnormal persons. *Journal of Consulting and Clinical Psychology, 41*, 207–214.

Carroll, J. B. (1952). Ratings on traits measured by a factored personality inventory. *Journal of Abnormal Social Psychology, 47*, 626–632.

Carver, C. S., & Gaines, J. G. (1987). Optimism, pessimism, and postpartum depression. *Cognitive Therapy and Research, 11*, 449–462.

Clark, D. M., & Teasdale, J. D. (1985). Constraints on the effects of mood on memory. *Journal of Personality and Social Psychology, 48*, 1595–1608.

Costa, P. T., Jr., & McCrae, R. R. (1980). Influence of extraversion and neuroticism on subjective well-being: Happy and unhappy people. *Journal of Personality and Social Psychology, 38*, 668–678.

Costa, P. T., Jr., & McCrae, R. R. (1985). *The NEO Personality Inventory manual*. Odessa, FL: Psychological Assessment Resources.

Costa, P. T., Jr., McCrae, R. R., & Norris, A. H. (1981). Personal adjustment to aging: Longitudinal prediction from neuroticism and extraversion. *Journal of Gerontology, 36*, 78–85.

Cronbach, L. J., & Meehl, P. E. (1955). Construct validity in psychological tests. *Psychological Bulletin, 52*, 281–302.

DePaulo, B. M., & Rosenthal, R. (1979). Ambivalence, discrepancy, and deception in nonverbal communication. In R. Rosenthal (Ed.), *Skill in nonverbal communication* (pp. 204–248). Cambridge, MA: Oelgeschlager, Gunn, & Hain.

Derogatis, L. R. (1975). *Brief symptom inventory*. Baltimore: Clinical Psychometric Research.

Diener, E. (1984). Subjective well-being. *Psychological Bulletin, 95,* 542–575.

Diener, E. (1994). Assessing subjective well-being: Progress and opportunities. *Social Indicators Research, 31,* 103–157. (2005 reprinted in *Citation classics from Social Indicators Reserch*)

Diener, E., Colvin, C. R., Pavot, W., & Allman, A. (1991). The psychic costs of intense positive affect. *Journal of Personality and Social Psychology, 61,* 492–503.

Diener, E., Emmons, R. A., Larsen, R. J., & Griffin, S. (1985). The Satisfaction with Life Scale. *Journal of Personality Assessment, 49,* 71–75.

Diener, E., & Larsen, R. J. (1984). Temporal stability and cross-situational consistency of affective, behavioral, and cognitive responses. *Journal of Personality and Social Psychology, 47,* 871–883.

Diener, E., Sandvik, E., & Pavot, W. (1991). Happiness is the frequency, not the intensity, of positive versus negative affect. In F. Strack, M. Argyle, & N. Schwarz, (Eds.), *Subjective well-being: An interdisciplinary perspective* (pp. 119–139). London: Pergamon.

Diener, E., Sandvik, E., Pavot, W., & Gallagher, D. (1991). Response artifacts in the measurement of subjective well-being. *Social Indicators Research, 24,* 35–56.

Diener, E., Sandvik, E., Seidlitz, L., & Diener, M. (1992). The relationship between income and subjective well-being: Relative or absolute? *Social Indicators Research, 28,* 253–281.

Dulany, D. E. (1968). Awareness, rules, and propositional control: A confrontation with S-R behaviorism. In T. Dixon & D. Horton (Eds.), *Verbal behavior and general behavior theory* (pp. 340–387). Englewood Cliffs, NJ: Prentice-Hall.

Emmons, R. A., & Diener, E. (1985). Personality correlates of subjective well-being. *Personality and Social Psychology Bulletin, 11,* 89–97.

Emmons, R. A., & Diener, E. (1986). Influence of impulsivity and sociability on subjective well-being. *Journal of Personality and Social Psychology, 50,* 1211–1215.

Ericsson, K. A., & Simon, H. A. (1980). Verbal reports as data. *Psychological Review, 87,* 215–251.

Fordyce, M. W. (1977). *The happiness measures: A sixty-second index of emotional well-being and mental health.* Unpublished manuscript, Edison Community College, Ft. Myers, FL.

Fordyce, M. W. (1988). A review of research on the Happiness Measures: A sixty-second index of happiness and mental health. *Social Indicators Research, 20,* 355–381.

Forgas, J. P., Bower, G. H., & Krantz, S. E. (1984). The influence of mood on perception of social interactions. *Journal of Experimental Social Psychology, 20,* 497–513.

Fujita, F., Diener, E., & Pavot, W. (1993). *An investigation of the relations between extraversion, neuroticism, positive affect, and negative affect.* Manuscript submitted for publication.

Ghiselli, E. E., Campbell, J. P., & Zedeck, S. (1981). *Measurement theory for the behavioral sciences.* San Francisco: Freeman.

Goldings, H. J. (1954). On the avowal and projection of happiness. *Journal of Personality, 23,* 30–47.

Gough, H. (1957). *California personality inventory.* Palo Alto, CA: Consulting Psychologists Press.

Hartmann, G. W. (1934). Personality traits associated with variations in happiness. *Journal of Abnormal and Social Psychology, 29,* 202–212.

Hathaway, S. R., & McKinley, J. C. (1951). *Minnesota multiphasic personality inventory.* New York: Psychological Corporation.

Hogan, R., & Nicholson, R. A. (1988). The meaning of personality test scores. *American Psychologist, 43,* 621–626.

Jackson, D. (1967). *Personality research form.* Port Huron, MI: Research Psychologists Press.

Kammann, R., & Flett, R. (1983). *Sourcebook for measuring well-being with Affectometer 2.* Dunedin, New Zealand: Why Not? Foundation.

Krug, S., & Laughlin, J. (1970). *IPAT depression checklist.* Champaign, IL: Institute for Personality and Ability Testing.

Larsen, R. J. (1984). Theory and measurement of affect intensity as an individual difference characteristic. *Dissertation Abstracts International, 85,* 2297B. (University Microfilms No. 84-22112).

Larsen, R. J., & Diener, E. (1987). Affect intensity as an individual difference variable: A review. *Journal of Research in Personality, 21*, 1–39.

McNeil, J. K., Stones, M. J., & Kozma, A. (1986). Subjective well-being in later life: Issues concerning measurement and prediction. *Social Indicators Research, 18*, 35–70.

Mehrabian, A. (1976). *Manual for the questionnaire measure of Stimulus Screening and Arousability*. University of California, Los Angeles.

Moskowitz, D. S. (1986). Comparison of self-reports, reports by knowledgeable informants, and behavioral observation data. *Journal of Personality, 54*, 294–317.

Nisbett, R. E., & Ross, L. (1980). *Human inference: Strategies and shortcomings of social judgment*. Englewood Cliffs, NJ: Prentice-Hall.

Nisbett, R. E., & Wilson, T. D. (1977). Telling more than we can know: Verbal reports on mental processes. *Psychological Review, 84*, 231–259.

Okun, M. A., & George, L. K. (1984). Physician- and self-ratings of health, neuroticism and subjective well-being among men and women. *Personality and Individual Differences, 5*, 533–539.

Okun, M. A., Stock, W. A., Haring, M. J., & Writter, R. A. (1984). Health and subjective well-being: A meta-analysis. *Journal of Aging and Human Development, 19*, 111–132.

Otis, A. S. (1939). *Otis Quick Scoring Mental Abilities Test*. New York: Harcourt, Brace & World.

Pavot, W., & Diener, E. (1993). Review of the satisfaction with life scale. *Psychological Assessment, 5*, 164–172.

Pavot, W., Diener, E., Colvin, C. R., & Sandvik, E. (1991). Further validation of the Satisfaction with Life Scale: Evidence for the cross-method convergence of well-being measures. *Journal of Personality Assessment, 57*, 149–161.

Pavot, W., Diener, E., & Fujita, F. (1990). Extraversion and well-being. *Personality and Individual Differences, 11*, 1299–1306.

Phillips, D. L. (1967). Social participation and happiness. *American Journal of Sociology, 72*, 479–488.

Scheier, M. F., & Carver, C. S. (1985). Optimism, coping, and health: Assessment and implications of generalized outcome expectancies. *Health Psychology, 4*, 219–247.

Scheier, M. F., Matthews, K. A., & Owens, J. F. (1989). Dispositional optimism and recovery from coronary artery bypass surgery: The beneficial effects on physical and psychological well-being. *Journal of Personality and Social Psychology, 57*, 1024–1040.

Scheier, M. F., Weintraub, J. K., & Carver, C. S. (1986). Coping with stress: Divergent strategies of optimists and pessimists. *Journal of Personality and Social Psychology, 51*, 1257–1264.

Schwarz, N., & Clore, G. L. (1983). Mood, misattribution, and judgments of well-being: Informative and directive functions of affective states. *Journal of Personality and Social Psychology, 45*, 513–523.

Schwarz, N., & Strack, F. (1991). Evaluating one's life: A judgment model of subjective well-being. In F. Strack, M. Argyle, & N. Schwarz (Eds.), *Subjective well-being: An interdisciplinary perspective* (pp. 27–48). London: Pergamon.

Schwarz, N., Strack, F., Muller, G., & Chassein, B. (1988). The range of response alternatives may determine the meaning of the question: Further evidence on informative functions of response alternatives. *Social Cognition, 6*, 107–117.

Seidlitz, L., & Diener, E. (1993). Memory for positive versus negative life events: Theories for the differences between happy and unhappy persons. *Journal of Personality and Social Psychology, 64*, 654–664.

Underwood, B., & Froming, W. (1980). The mood survey: A personality measure of happy and sad moods. *Journal of Personality Assessment, 44*, 404–414.

Watson, D., & Clark, L. A. (1984). Negative affectivity: The disposition to experience aversive emotional states. *Psychological Bulletin, 96*, 465–490.

Measuring Positive Emotions

Richard E. Lucas, Ed Diener, and Randy J. Larsen

Abstract When researchers want to assess positive feelings, they need to understand the various definitions and models of emotion. The current chapter describes the theories and various measures that derive from them, and reviews the strenghts and weaknesses of different measures of positive emotions. In addition, nonself-report measures of positive feelings are reviewed.

The diverse chapters in this handbook illustrate that the field of positive psychology encompasses areas of research that extend beyond the psychology of positive subjective experience. Positive psychologists value characteristics such as creativity, wisdom, and empathy, even if these characteristics do not always lead to feelings of happiness. Yet the field would be incomplete if it failed to incorporate individuals' subjective experiences. It would be hard to argue that an individual had a positive, fulfilling life if he or she did not have the sense that life was rewarding. One central feature of the subjectively rewarding life is the experience of pleasant emotions. Judgments of happiness and life satisfaction are consistently and moderately to strongly correlated with the frequency with which one experiences pleasant emotions such as joy, contentment, excitement, affection, and energy (Diener & Lucas, 2000). These emotions often indicate that one's life is going well.

Yet the role of positive emotions extends beyond a simple signal that one's life is on the right track. Positive emotions also may serve specific functions and may play a role in helping individuals achieve positive outcomes. Research suggests that positive emotions cause people to become more creative (e.g., Estrada, Isen, & Young, 1994; Isen, Daubman, & Nowicki, 1987) and more affiliative (e.g., Cunningham, 1988; Isen, 1987). Happy people even make more money than unhappy people (Diener, Nickerson, Lucas, & Sandvik, 2002). Furthermore, individual differences in the tendency to experience positive emotions have implications for personality traits: Some researchers claim that positive emotionality forms the core of the extraversion personality dimension (Lucas, Diener, Grob, Suh, & Shao, 2000; Tellegen, 1985; Watson & Clark, 1997). Therefore, positive emotions must assume

R.E. Lucas (✉)
Department of Psychology, Michigan State University, East Lansing, MI 48824, USA
e-mail: lucasri@msu.edu

E. Diener (ed.), *Assessing Well-Being: The Collected Works of Ed Diener,*
Social Indicators Research Series 39, DOI 10.1007/978-90-481-2354-4_7,
© Springer Science+Business Media B.V. 2009

a central role, both as an outcome variable and an input variable, in a comprehensive positive psychology.

To understand positive emotions, it is essential that our measures of positive emotions are adequate. However, it is not enough simply to examine the reliability and validity of our emotion scales. Emotions are complex phenomena with a broad array of components that range from purely subjective feelings to action tendencies, and from observable behaviors to specific physiological changes. Often, these various components are only modestly related, and by measuring only one or two of these components, researchers may miss part of the picture. In this chapter, we will discuss some of the issues surrounding the measurement of positive emotions. This will enable psychologists to understand, evaluate, and select positive emotionl measures.

Definition and Models of Positive Emotions

What is an *emotion*? Unfortunately, there is no single, widely agreed on answer to this question (see, e.g., Frijda, 1999; Kleinginna & Kleinginna, 1981; Larsen & Fredrickson, 1999; Ortony and Turner, 1990). Instead, most theorists define emotions in terms of multiple components, each of which is included in some, but not all definitions of the construct. Frijda (1999), for example, argued that emotions are made up of the following components: (a) affect, or the experience of pleasure or pain; (b) appraisal of an object or event as good or bad; (c) action readiness, or the readiness for changes in behavior toward the environment; (d) autonomic arousal; and (e) cognitive activity changes. Yet some researchers have included certain non-valenced feeling states in their lists of basic emotions even though these states do not meet these criteria. For example, Ortony and Turner (1990) pointed out that surprise, interest, and desire often are included in lists of basic emotions, even though these feelings are not clearly affectively valenced. Surprise, interest, and desire can all be pleasant, unpleasant, or completely neutral. Similarly, Fredrickson (1998) noted that many positive emotions do not have easily identifiable action tendencies. Therefore, the components that Frijda listed can be seen as a description of possible components rather than a definition of emotions.

It may seem that some of these definitional issues are made moot by this chapter's focus on positive emotions. One may argue that a positive emotion by definition must be affectively valenced. Unfortunately, there also are disagreements about what is positive about positive emotions. For some, positive emotions are simply those that have a pleasant valence (e.g., Larsen & Diener, 1992). For others, however, positive emotions result from a behavioral activation system that motivates approach behavior. According to this approach, positive emotions are not simply pleasant. Instead, they are positive if they lead to approach behavior. Affectively neutral feelings like interest would be considered positive emotions, whereas pleasantly valenced feelings like contentment and relaxation would not. These definitional issues become measurement issues when psychologists have specific hypotheses about the nature of the positive emotions they are investigating. If psychologists are interested in approach behavior and activity in approach systems, they may want to assess emotions such as interest or engagement; whereas if they are interested solely in pleasantness, they may want to ensure that their measures include such emotions as contentment and relaxation. In our experience, however, different types of positive emotion scales often behave similarly (e.g., Lucas & Fujita, 2000), and the use of these different emotion scales may not make much practical difference as long as a broad range of positive emotions are sampled.

Structural Models of Positive Emotions

Emotion researchers often try to develop models that can organize the large number of emotions that exist into a smaller list of basic emotions or emotional dimensions. There are a number of alternative approaches to accomplishing this goal. Some researchers, for example, argue for the existence of a small number of basic emotions. Among the various advocates of the basic emotions approach, there is some disagreement about what constitutes a basic emotion and which emotions satisfy these requirements (Ekman, 1992a, 1992b; Izard, 1992; Ortony and Turner, 1990; Panksepp, 1992; Turner & Ortony, 1992). Fortunately, only a few distinct positive emotions have been proposed to be basic. In Ortony and Turner's (1990) review, most theorists only included a single general pleasantness emotion (e.g., joy, happiness, elation, or pleasure). More specific emotions such as courage, hope, love, and wonder (along with the questionably positive emotions of interest, surprise, and desire) were included as basic emotions less frequently. If basic emotions do exist, basic positive emotions seem to be fewer in number than basic negative emotions.

An alternative to the basic emotion approach is the dimensional approach to understanding the associations among different emotions (e.g., Russell, 1980; Watson & Tellegen, 1985). According to the dimensional approach, the covariance among distinct emotions can be reduced to a small number of important dimensions through factor analysis. Some researchers suggest that three dimensions are necessary to account for the covariance (e.g., Schimmack & Grob, 2000), but there is somewhat greater consensus that two dimensions satisfactorily account for the variability in emotion terms (e.g., Russell, 1980; Watson & Tellegen, 1985). In some of the two-factor approaches, emotion terms are described as having a circumplex structure: The emotions are thought to be equally spaced in a circle around a point formed from the intersection of the two independent emotion dimensions (for a review of circumplex approaches see Larsen & Diener, 1992; for recent evidence on the circumplex structure, see Watson, Wiese, Vaidya, & Tellegen, 1999).

Among the two-dimensional models of emotion, there are alternative approaches to understanding the specific dimensions that emerge. Specifically, within any factorial representation of mood terms, the factors can be rotated differently, and the dimensions that emerge will have different interpretations. Russell and his colleagues (Russell, 1980; Russell & Feldman Barrett, 1999), for example, argued that the factor space can be described well by independent pleasantness and arousal dimensions. Watson, Tellegen, and their colleagues (Watson & Tellegen, 1985; Watson et al., 1999), on the other hand, argued that these dimensions should be rotated

45 degrees to create independent positive affect or positive activation and negative affect or negative activation dimensions. Positive affect is a combination of high pleasantness and high arousal and includes such emotions as interested, engaged, and active; negative affect is a combination of high unpleasantness and high arousal and includes such emotions as nervous, distressed, and afraid (for a similar view see Thayer, 1978). These researchers argue that these rotated dimensions are aligned with the major clusters of emotions, and that they represent fundamental emotional systems.

It also is possible that the structure of affect and emotions may be hierarchical. Watson (2000) argued that although positive and negative affect formed two higher level factors in a hierarchy, a larger number of correlated lower order factors were needed to fully describe emotion structure. In his model, positive affect can be broken down into three distinct facets: joviality, self-assuredness, and attention. Similarly, in a theoretical analysis of positive emotions, Fredrickson (1998) argued that there were at least four distinct types of positive emotions: joy, interest, contentment, and love. Diener, Smith, and Fujita (1995) took a more systematic, empirical approach and selected emotion terms from a variety of research traditions (including cognitive approaches to emotion, biological/evolutionary approaches, and empirical approaches). Their analyses suggested that two distinct types of positive emotion were necessary to account for the variability: joy and love. All three groups of researchers (Diener et al., 1995; Fredrickson, 1998; Watson & Clark, 1992) noted, however, that positive emotions are often strongly correlated and relatively undifferentiated.

One other debate concerns whether positive emotions and negative emotions represent opposite poles of a single dimension or whether they are in fact independent dimensions. In other words, there is a question about whether one could experience positive emotions at the same time as negative emotions, or whether the presence of one indicates the absence of the other. A number of studies have investigated this issue (e.g., Diener & Emmons, 1984; Diener & Iran-Nejad, 1986; Feldman Barrett & Russell, 1998; Green, Salovey, & Truax, 1999), yet we do not believe that any resolution has been proposed that can satisfy all sides of the debate. The independence of positive and negative emotions probably depends on the time frame during which emotions are measured (e.g., Diener & Emmons, 1984), the response scale that is used, and whether multiple methods are used to measure the constructs (Green, Goldman, & Salovey, 1993). We recommend that researchers and clinicians explicitly measure positive emotions and not take the absence of negative emotions as evidence for the existence of the positive. At least in certain cases, the two are independent; and in fact, positive and negative emotions may result from different brain systems (Cacioppo, Gardner, & Berntson, 1999).

One final structural issue concerns the time frame in which positive emotions are measured. Emotions can be short-lasting responses to specific events and objects or long-lasting responses that may not be associated with anything specific. In general, the term "emotion" refers only to the former (Frijda, 1999), whereas the term "mood" refers to the latter (Morris, 1999). However, the terms have sometimes been used interchangeably, and when we talk about positive emotions in the current chapter, we refer to both emotions and moods. Both researchers and practitioners should be aware, however, that the structure and processes of emotions may differ when they are assessed during a single moment versus over long periods of time. Psychologists must decide which types of emotional reactions are of interest when they choose specific response scales and measures.

Summary and Implications of Emotion Models

Each of the approaches to understanding the nature of emotional experience has resulted in a slightly different model of positive emotions. Our discussion of these issues has necessarily been brief, and readers are advised to consult the sources cited previously if they believe that these issues will affect their assessment of positive emotions. We must point out, however, that there are a number of similarities among the different models, and for most psychologists, the major debates in the field will have few practical implications for the assessment of positive emotions. At most, there are a small number of highly correlated basic positive emotions or positive emotional dimensions. There are many short emotion questionnaires available (which we review subsequently), and most provide a broad sampling of these emotions. If one is unsure whether to measure activated positive emotions versus unactivated positive emotions, he or she could reliably assess both with only a few extra items. If the two types of positive emotions exhibited different correlations, researchers could keep them separate in their analyses; if they exhibited similar correlations, researchers could combine them to form a single measure. Of course, psychologists who are interested in the dynamics of a specific positive emotion (e.g., love, joy, contentment) should make sure that they use reliable, multiple item scales.

Methods of Assessment

Emotions are complex phenomena that comprise multiple components ranging from the purely subjective to the purely physiological. No single method of emotion assessment can possibly capture the entirety of emotional phenomena, and a complete understanding of emotion phenomena can only be gained through multiple-method investigations. Therefore, psychologists interested in positive emotions always should use multiple methods when possible. In this section, we review the different methods that have been used, and we discuss the promises and problems of using these methods for the assessment of positive emotions.

Self-Reports of Positive Emotions

Self-report emotion scales generally require respondents to indicate how frequently or intensely they are experiencing or have experienced positive emotions. The specific format of the scales can vary along a number of dimensions, and these differences can profoundly affect the measurement properties of the scale.

Number of items. The simplest way to assess positive emotions is to ask how a respondent feels using a single, broad positive emotion. For example, he or she could be asked, "How pleasant are you feeling in general" or "How happy do you feel in general?" Alternatively, if a psychologist was interested in a specific positive emotion such as excitement, he or she could ask, "How excited do you feel right now?" Scales such as these have some amount of validity and have the advantage of brevity. Unfortunately, they might suffer from low reliability.

Multiple-item scales offer the advantage of greater reliability and, in many cases, greater breadth of coverage. Multiple aspects of a single basic emotion can be assessed (e.g., contentment, happiness, joy, and elation all reflect various intensities of a single basic emotion), or multiple basic emotions can be included so that a broad range of positive emotions is sampled.

Although emotion scales can run as long as 132 items [e.g., Zuckerman and Lubin's (1985). Multiple Affect Adjective Checklist-Revised (MAACL-R)], most scales are much shorter. Because the various positive emotions are highly correlated, even scales as short as four of five items often exhibit very strong reliability (see, e.g., Diener et al., 1995; Watson and Clark, 1994).

Response scale. A variety of response scales have been used to measure positive emotions. Many instruments use a simple checklist approach in which participants are presented with a list of emotions and are asked to check which ones they are experiencing or have experienced during some discrete period of time (e.g., Zuckerman and Lubin, 1985). A variation of this approach asks participants to indicate, using a yes-no response scale, whether they agree with various statements that describe their emotional states (e.g., Bradburn and Caplovitz, 1965). In both cases, checks or "yes" responses are summed for an overall positive emotion score. Checklists may be more likely than other response scales to be influenced by certain response sets, and some researchers caution against their use (e.g., Green et al., 1993).

An alternative to the checklist is the Likert response scale. Again, participants are presented with a list of emotion terms or statements describing their emotional states. They are then asked to indicate how strongly they feel the emotion, how frequently they have felt the emotion in the past or how much they agree with the statement using a numbered Likert scale.

The number of points on the scales varies (generally, from five to nine points), and the specific anchors change depending on the focus of the measure. Some scales assess the strength with which a respondent has experienced an emotion, and these scales often use labels that range from "not at all or slight," "a little," "moderately," "quite a bit," to "very much" (e.g., Watson, Clark, and Tellegen, 1988). Other scales assess the frequency with which a respondent has experienced an emotion, and these scales may use anchors that refer to specific percentages of time (e.g., "0% of the time," "10% of the time," etc.) or general frequency descriptors (e.g., "never," "about half the time," "always"; Diener et al., 1995). Frequency and intensity are separable components of emotional experience and they may reflect different processes (Schimmack & Diener, 1997).

Diener, Sandvik, and Pavot (1991), for example, argued that overall happiness reflects the frequency, but not the intensity, of positive versus negative affect over time. Because these components are separable, we recommend using response scales that refer to the frequency or intensity of emotion (or both measured separately) and to avoid response scales that ambiguously measure both (e.g., "not much" or "a lot").

A variation of the Likert response scale is the visual analog scale. This approach uses a visual representation of the response options on the Likert scale. For example, participants may be presented with a series of faces that range from frowning to neutral to smiling. They can then circle the face that best reflected their own feeling state. Similarly, participants may be presented with a line separating two opposing adjectives, or a thermometer indicating intensity of an emotion. Participants can indicate how they feel by making a mark somewhere on the visual analog. Visual analog scales are a useful alternative to traditional emotion measures when participants are likely to have difficulty understanding the words on a scale. For example, research with young children or with participants who speak different languages would benefit from the use of visual analog scales.

Time frame. Perhaps the most important feature to consider when deciding how to assess emotion is the time frame of the instructions. As noted previously, most theorists distinguish between the short-lived reactions to specific stimuli (emotions) and the long-lasting feelings that tend to be unrelated to specific objects and events (moods). Furthermore, long-term individual differences in emotions and moods may reflect one's underlying personality dispositions. The processes that underlie moods, emotions, and temperament may differ and may be differentially related to other phenomena. Therefore, it is essential for researchers and clinicians to decide which aspect of emotional experience they wish to study and to select appropriate measures.

Many emotion questionnaires have different instructions for measuring different types of emotional experiences. For example, Watson et al. (1988) noted that their Positive And Negative Affect Schedule (PANAS) scale can be administered with instructions that ask participants to indicate how they feel "right now," "today," "in the last week," "in the last month," or "in the last few months." The shorter the time frame, the more likely one is to capture emotional responses; the longer the time frame, the more likely one is to capture mood or personality differences in emotionality. The instructions for most emotion questionnaires can be altered to assess various aspects of emotional experience.

On-line versus retrospective reports. The issue of time frame should alert researchers to a related problem in emotion assessment: The dynamic nature of emotional experience. Emotions vary considerably over time. We may feel angry if we are cut off in traffic, and this event may significantly affect our mood for the rest of the day. Yet the intensity and subjective experience of anger would change dramatically in the hours following the event. Asking participants to retrospectively evaluate their emotions requires participants to remember their feelings and to accurately aggregate across this dynamic experience, a task that may be very difficult (Fredrickson & Kahneman, 1993). Often researchers who wish to capture the temporal dimension of emotional experience use on-line measures of emotion and mood (e.g., Kahneman, 1999). For example, researchers can ask participants to carry palm-top computers programmed to assess positive emotions at random times throughout the day. A low-cost alternative to this procedure can be undertaken using inexpensive watches that have alarms to remind participants to complete paper-and-pencil emotion questionnaires (though compliance cannot be assessed with paper-and-pencil inventories). Alternatively, psychologists who are interested in shorter emotional experiences can use a variety of new techniques to assess changes in emotion over time in the laboratory. For example, sliding meters and rotating dials can be used to assess emotional experience over time. Participants can change the dials and meters as their emotions change.

By assessing emotions over time, psychologists can examine a number of features of emotional experience. Multiple emotion reports can be decomposed into distinct components. For example, separate frequency and intensity scores can be calculated; and emotional reactivity can be examined by calculating variability in emotions or peak levels of emotional experience. Similarly, different sampling strategies can be used to emphasize emotions versus mood. An event sampling strategy, where participants are asked to complete a report any time a significant emotional even takes place, is likely to capture emotional reactions to specific events. A random-sampling strategy, where participants are signaled randomly throughout the day, may capture context-free mood to a greater extent. The use of different strategies allows different aspects of emotional experience to be investigated. Furthermore, participants often have difficulty remembering and accurately aggregating across multiple affective experiences when they are asked how much positive emotion they have experienced over long periods of time (Robinson & Clore, 2000). On-line experience can be compared to retrospective judgments of positive emotions to assess how well participants can remember and report the emotions they experienced. On-line emotion assessment is becoming an increasingly important part of a comprehensive study of positive emotional experience.

Specific positive emotion measures. Table 1 presents a list of 12 widely used self-report positive emotion scales. Most are embedded within larger emotion questionnaires that assess a broad range of emotional experiences. Some were designed specifically to measure individual differences in emotionality [e.g., Tellegen and Waller's (1994) Multidimensional Personality Questionnaire], whereas most can be used to measure individual differences or momentary experience of emotion depending on the specific instructions and response scales. As noted previously, theories about the structure of positive emotions differ, and the measures described in Table 1 reflect these differences. Some measures focus on basic positive emotions or lower level facets of positive emotional experience; whereas others focus on broad pleasantness or activated positive emotion dimensions. Most lower order scales can be combined to form a single higher order positive emotion scale. Because most positive emotions are highly intercorrelated (especially at an individual difference level; see Zelenski & Larsen, 2000), all of the scales listed in Table 1 exhibit strong internal consistency and strong evidence of validity (with the possible exception of the Affect Balance scale; see Larsen, Diener, & Emmons, 1985). Also included is a measure of cognitive well-being, the Satisfaction With Life scale (Diener, Emmons, Larsen, and Griffin, 1985). Measures of cognitive well-being are

Table 1 Summary of positive emotion measures

Measure items	Authors	Subscales	Items	Positive emotions subscales
Activation-deactivation Adjective checklist	Thayer (1967)	2	28	Energetic arousal
Affect balance scale	Bradburn and Caplovitz (1965)	2	10	Positive emotions
Affect grid	Russell, Weiss, and Mendelsohn (1989)	2	1	Pleasantness
Differential emotion scale	Izard, Dougherty, Bloxom, and Kotsch (1974)	10	30	Surprise, interest, enjoyment
Intensity and time affect scale	Diener, Smith, and Fujita (1995)	6	24	Love, joy
Mood adjective checklist	Nowlis and Green (1957)	12	190	Surgency, elation, social affection, vigor
Multiple affect adjective checklist	Zuckerman and Lubin (1985)	5	132	Positive affect
Multidimensional personality questionnaire	Tellegen and Waller (1994)	11	300	Positive emotionality
Positive and negative affect schedule	Watson, Clark, and Tellegen (1988)	2	20	Activated positive affect
Positive and negative affect schedule (expanded)	Watson and Clark (1994)	11	55	Joviality, self-assurance, attentiveness
Profile of mood states	McNair, Lorr, and Droppleman (1971)	6	72	Vigor
Satisfaction with life scale	Diener, Emmons, Larsen, and Griffin (1985)	1	5	Life satisfaction

moderately correlated with the experience of positive emotions (Lucas, Diener, & Suh, 1996). Appendix 1 and 2 show examples of standard positive emotion and life satisfaction scales.

Summary. Self-report methods of assessment are probably the easiest and most efficient way to assess positive emotions. These methods are reliable and valid, and they map closely on to the layperson's understanding of what a positive emotion actually is. Furthermore, by changing the specific items, response scales, time frames, or the specific method of assessment, self-report scales are quite flexible. Separate intensity, frequency, reactivity, and variability scores (as well as other components) can be easily computed from various emotion measures.

These separable components allow for a rich understanding of emotional experience. Yet self-reports do not provide the only insight into emotional processes, and they are certainly not infallible. Participants may be unable or unwilling to report on their true emotional experiences. Their responses may be influenced by social desirability, extreme responding, or other response styles and response sets. Furthermore, there may be aspects of emotional experience that are simply not available to subjective awareness. Therefore, self-report emotion scales should be supplemented with non-self-report measures when possible.

Non-Self-Report Methods

Most non-self-report measures of positive emotions are based on the assumption that an emotional experience comprises multiple components. For example, emotion theorists argue that emotions have an expressive component that can be recognized by others. Therefore, informant reports of emotional experience can provide a useful alternative to self-reports. Similarly, most emotion theorists argue that there are physiological correlates of emotional experience. By assessing physiological processes, researchers may be able to tap aspects of emotions that cannot be recognized by the person who is experiencing the emotion. In this section, we review the various non-self-report measures of positive emotions that have been proposed.

Observer reports. One simple and easily administered alternative to self-reports is the observer report. Most self-report positive emotion measures can be easily altered to create reliable and valid observer measures of emotion. By asking friends and family members to rate how frequently or intensely a target participant has experienced an emotion, researchers can get additional information about emotional experience. Informants likely have different response sets, response styles, and memory biases, and the combination of self- and informant-reports of emotion may provide more valid measures of positive emotions (Diener et al., 1995).

Although it may seem difficult for informants to judge the private and subjective emotional feelings experienced by a target, research shows that informants and targets generally agree fairly well about a target's emotional experiences. For example, Diener et al. (1995) found that self-reports of positive emotions correlated over 0.50 with informant reports of positive emotions.

An alternative to the known-informant approach is the expert-rater approach. Using this technique, informants who do not know the target can be trained to interpret specific signs of emotional experience (e.g., Gottman, 1993). Alternatively, untrained judges can simply be asked to judge a person's emotion after observing the target in an emotion-provoking situation. The former approach involves extensive training of raters but provides more valid and reliable emotion reports than the latter.

Facial measures. In addition to training raters to judge emotional experience holistically, it is possible to train raters to look for specific signs of emotions in the facial expressions that targets exhibit. For example, the Facial Action Coding System (FACS; Ekman & Friesen, 1975, 1978) allows raters to make judgments about emotions based on specific muscle movements in the face. Substantial training is required, and facial coding of temporal sequences can be very time-consuming. Nonetheless, reliable and valid measures of individual differences in positive emotions can be obtained from static pictures such as yearbook photos (e.g., Harker & Keltner, 2001). Furthermore, the measurement of facial expressions can be automated using electromyographical techniques (Cacioppo, Berntson, Larsen, Paehlmann, & Ito, 2000; Cacioppo & Tassinary, 1990). These techniques measure muscle contractions in the face and compare these muscle contractions to known changes that occur when emotions are expressed.

Electromyography has the added advantage of being able to capture muscle changes that may be too small to be noticed by the naked eye. We should note that although facial measures of positive emotions offer a promising alternative to self-reports, it is unlikely that differentiated measures of positive emotions can be obtained from facial measures (Fredrickson, 1998). Instead, these techniques can probably only reliably measure general pleasantness.

Physiological measures. Other psychophysiological measures have been used to measure emotion, but again, these tend to distinguish general happiness from negative emotions or to distinguish among various negative emotions. For example, Cacioppo et al. (2000) presented a meta-analysis of the literature examining the physiological correlates of different emotional experiences. The studies they reviewed measured such variables as heart rate, heart rate acceleration, blood pressure, bodily temperature, finger temperature, respiration amplitude, skin conductance, and many others. Several of these variables were able to distinguish positive from negative emotions, but they had limited success in discriminating among discrete emotions.

Other researchers have noted that certain brain regions tend to be involved in the experience and expression of distinct types of emotions and that the measurement of activity in these regions may provide a useful measure of emotional activity (either on an individual difference or momentary state level). For example Davidson (1992) reviewed evidence that the left anterior region of the brain may be responsible for positive emotions, whereas the right anterior region may be involved in the expression of negative emotions. Electroencephalogram (EEG) measures as well as PET scans and functional MRI can index this differential activity to assess positive emotional experience. Again, however, discrete emotions are unlikely to be captured by this psychophysiological approach.

Emotion-sensitive tasks. Because emotions affect cognitive processing and action tendencies, researchers can sometimes take advantage of these effects to measure emotions themselves. Seidlitz and Diener (1993), for example, simply asked people to recall as many happy experiences from their lives as they could in a short amount of time. The number of recalled experiences was positively correlated with happiness reports. Thus, recall of positive events can be used as an indicator of elevated mood. Other studies have used other cognitive tasks such as word-completion and word-recognition tasks. Happy participants are quicker than participants in neutral states to identify positive words as words, and happy participants are more likely than unhappy participants to complete word stems to form positive words. When researchers are concerned about social desirability or other issues that may make respondents answer in untruthful ways, cognitive tasks such as these may help identify how happy the respondent really is. Rusting (1998) reviewed evidence that these cognitive tasks are sensitive to both individual differences in positive emotions as well as positive emotional states.

Summary. Because emotions are known to involve more than just subjective experience, non-self-report measures are essential to our understanding of emotions and emotional processes. There is much work that is needed, however, before the various non-self-report measures can be incorporated into standard assessment batteries. Although there are a number of facial and physiological indicators that have been shown to be associated with self-reports of emotion, these indicators also are associated with other nonemotional processes. Therefore, they often are only weakly correlated with the subjective experience of emotion. Nonphysiological measures such as informant reports, behavioral tasks, and cognitive measures can easily be incorporated into research programs. However, they are often only weakly to moderately correlated with self-reports. Therefore, although we encourage multiple-method investigations, researchers should not expect strong convergence across these diverse methods.

Future Developments in the Measurement of Positive Emotions

There are four main challenges regarding the measurement of positive emotions. First, a number of the debates regarding the definition and structure of positive emotions will need to be settled. Studies are beginning to take advantage of multiple methods of assessment and modern analytical techniques such as structural equation modeling and hierarchical linear modeling to address the structure of emotions between persons and within persons over time. These sophisticated measurement approaches will help us understand the nature of emotional experience and the processes that underlie emotions themselves.

Second, psychologists must develop a better understanding of the ways that the various components of positive emotions converge. Most emotion theorists believe that emotions have multiple components including subjective experience, cognitive changes, action tendencies, and physiological changes. Yet measures of the various components are only modestly intercorrelated. Future research must determine when the components converge and why.

Third, research on the measurement of positive emotions will benefit from a closer examination of the structure of discrete positive emotions. Although many theorists argue that there are distinct basic positive emotions or at least discriminable positive emotion facets, the specific positive emotions that are identified vary across different models. Furthermore, most research shows that these different positive emotions are strongly intercorrelated. Future research must determine whether there are distinct, discriminable, basic positive emotions, and what features (appraisal patterns, physiological changes, action tendencies, etc.) can distinguish among them. Fredrickson (1998) suggested that to accomplish this goal, researchers may need to shift their strategy from the methods and theories that have been used to study negative emotions. Fredrickson argued that positive emotions are fundamentally different from negative emotions, and theories of positive emotions may need to focus on different characteristics to distinguish among and explain the various ways of feeling positive.

Fourth, clinicians and other practitioners must determine what implications these theoretical debates have for practical issues associated with the experience of positive emotions. For example, although distinct positive emotions may be strongly intercorrelated, they may exhibit differential relations with other psychological problems or clinical treatments. Understanding these relationships can help researchers and practitioners alike understand the mechanisms underlying the experience of positive emotions.

Conclusion

Positive psychologists can confidently assess positive emotions using a variety of well-validated measurement techniques. The simplest and most flexible are self-reports of emotions; and self-reports probably provide the best insight into the experience of emotion within individuals over time. In general, any reasonably diverse collection of positive emotion adjectives will capture the positive emotion dimension with a fair amount of reliability and validity. However, these self-reports must be complemented with a broad array of non-self-report measures including informant reports, facial coding, and psychophysiological measures before a complete understanding of emotional experience can be attained.

Appendix 1: Intensity and Time Affect Survey (ITAS)

Instructions: [During the past month/During the past week/During the past day/Right now], how [frequently/intensely] [did you experience/are you experiencing] each of the following emotions?

1	2	3	4	5	6	7
Never			About half the time			Always

1. Affection
2. Joy
3. Fear
4. Anger
5. Shame
6. Sadness
7. Love
8. Happiness
9. Worry
10. Irritation
11. Guilt
12. Loneliness
13. Caring
14. Contentment
15. Anxiety

16. Disgust
17. Regret
18. Unhappiness
19. Fondness
20. Pride
21. Nervous
22. Rage
23. Embarrassment
24. Depression

Note. Items 1, 7, 13, and 19 make up the "love" subscale; items 2, 8, 14, and 20 make up the "joy" subscale. The love and joy subscales can be combined to form an overall positive emotions scale. Different response options can be used to measure affect over different lengths of time. Frequency and intensity instructions can be used to measure different components of affective experience.

Appendix 2: The Satisfaction With Life Scale

Instructions: Please use one of the following numbers from 1 to 7 to indicate how much you agree or disagree with the following statements.

7 Strongly agree
6 Agree
5 Slightly agree
4 Neither agree nor disagree
3 Slightly disagree
2 Disagree
1 Strongly disagree

1. ____ In most ways my life is close to my ideal.
2. ____ The conditions of my life are excellent.
3. ____ I am satisfied with my life.
4. ____ So far I have gotten the important things I want in my life.
5. ____ If I could live my life over, I would change almost nothing.

Note. Scores for all items are summed to calculate a total score.

References

Bradburn, N. M., & Caplovitz, D. (1965). *Reports on happiness*. Chicago: Aldine.
Cacioppo, J. T., Berntson, G. G., Larsen, J. T., Paehlmann, K. M., & Ito, T. A. (2000). The psychophysiology of emotion. In M. Lewis & J. M. Haviland-Janes (Eds.), *Handbook of emotions* (2nd ed., pp. 173–191). New York: Guilford Press.
Cacioppo, J. T., Gardner, W. L., & Berntson, G. G. (1999). The affect system has parallel and integrative processing components: Form follows function. *Journal of Personality and Social Psychology, 76,* 839–855.
Cacioppo, J. T., & Tassinary, L. G. (1990). Inferring psychological significance from physiological signals. *American Psychologist, 45,* 16–28.
Cunningham, M. R. (1988). Does happiness mean friendliness? Induced mood and heterosexual self-disclosure. *Personality and Social Psychological Bulletin, 14,* 283–297.

Davidson, R. J. (1992). Anterior cerebral asymmetry and the nature of emotion. *Brain and Cognition, 20,* 125–151.

Diener, E., & Emmons, R. A. (1984). The independence of positive and negative affect. *Journal of Personality and Social Psychology, 47,* 1105–1117.

Diener, E., Emmons, R. A., Larsen, R. J., & Griffin, S. (1985). The Satisfaction With Life scale. *Journal of Personality Assessment, 49,* 71–75.

Diener, E., & Iran-Nejad, A. (1986). The relationship in experience between various types of affect. *Journal of Personality and Social Psychology, 50,* 1031–1038.

Diener, E., & Lucas, R. E. (2000). Subjective emotional well-being. In M. Lewis & J. M. Haviland-Jones (Eds.), *Handbook of emotions* (2nd ed., pp. 325–337). New York: Guilford Press.

Diener, E., Nickerson, C., Lucas, R. E., & Sandvik, E. (2002). Dispositional affect and job outcomes. *Social Indicators Research, 59,* 229–259.

Diener, E., Sandvik, E., & Pavot, W. (1991). Happiness is the frequency, not the intensity, of positive versus negative affect. In F. Strack, M. Argyle, & N. Schwarz (Eds.), *Subjective well-being: An interdisciplinary perspective. International series in experimental social psychology* (pp. 119–139). Oxford: Pergamon Press.

Diener, E., Smith, H., & Fujita, F. (1995). The personality structure of affect. *Journal of Personality and Social Psychology, 50,* 130–141.

Ekman, P. (1992a). An argument for basic emotions. *Cognition and Emotion, 6,* 169–200.

Ekman, P. (1992b). Are there basic emotions? *Psychological Review, 99,* 550–553.

Ekman, P., & Friesen, W. (1975). *Unmasking the face.* Englewood Cliffs, NJ: Prentice Hall.

Ekman, P., & Friesen, W. (1978). *Facial action coding system.* Palo Alto, CA: Consulting Psychologists Press.

Estrada, C. A., Isen, A. M., & Young, M. J. (1994). Positive affect improves creative problem solving and influences reported source of practice satisfaction in physicians. *Motivation and Emotion, 18,* 285–299.

Feldman Barrett, L., & Russell, J. A. (1998). Independence and bipolarity in the structure of affect. *Journal of Personality and Social Psychology, 74,* 967–984.

Fredrickson, B. L. (1998). What good are positive emotions? *Review of General Psychology, 2,* 300–319.

Fredrickson, B. L., & Kahneman, D. (1993). Duration neglect in retrospective evaluations of affective episodes. *Journal of Personality and Social Psychology, 65,* 45–55.

Frijda, N. H. (1999). Emotions and hedonic experience. In D. Kahneman, E. Diener, & N. Schwarz (Eds.), *Well-being: The foundations of hedonic psychology* (pp. 190–210). New York: Russell Sage Foundation.

Gottman, J. M. (1993). Studying emotion in social interaction. In M. Lewis & J. M. Haviland (Eds.), *Handbook of emotions* (pp. 475–487). New York: Guilford Press.

Green, D. P., Goldman, S. L., & Salovey, P. (1993). Measurement error masks bipolarity in affect ratings. *Journal of Personality and Social Psychology, 64,* 1029–1041.

Green, D. P., Salovey, P., & Truax, K. M. (1999). Static, dynamic, and causative bipolarity of affect. *Journal of Personality and Social Psychology, 76,* 856–867.

Harker, L., & Keltner, D. (2001). Expressions of positive emotion in women's college yearbook pictures and their relationship to personality and life outcomes across adulthood. *Journal of Personality and Social Psychology, 80,* 112–124.

Isen, A. M. (1987). Positive affect, cognitive processes, and social behavior. In L. Berkowitz (Ed.), *Advances in experimental social psychology* (Vol. 20, pp. 203–253). San Diego, CA: Academic Press.

Isen, A. M., Daubman, K. A., & Nowicki, G. P. (1987). Positive affect facilitates creative problem solving. *Journal of Personality and Social Psychology, 52,* 1122–1131.

Izard, C. E. (1992). Basic emotions, relations among emotions, and emotion–cognition relations. *Psychological Review, 99,* 561–565.

Izard, C. E., Dougherty, F. E., Bloxom, B. M., & Kotsch, W. E. (1974). *The differential emotions scale: A method of measuring the subjective experience of discrete emotions.* Unpublished manuscript, Vanderbilt. University, Nashville, TN.

Kahneman, D. (1999). Objective happiness. In D. Kahneman, E. Diener, & N. Schwarz (Eds.), *Well-being: The foundations of hedonic psychology* (pp. 3–25). New York: Russell Sage Foundation.

Kleinginna, P. R., & Kleinginna, A. M. (1981). A categorized list of emotion definitions, with suggestions for a consensual definition. *Motivation and Emotion, 5*, 345–379.

Larsen, R. J., & Diener, E. (1992). Promises and problems with the circumplex model of emotion. In M. S. Clark (Ed.), *Review of personality and social psychology: Emotion* (Vol. 13, pp. 25–59). Newbury Park, CA: Sage.

Larsen, R. J., Diener, E., & Emmons, R. A. (1985). An evaluation of subjective well-being measures. *Social Indicators Research, 17*, 1–17.

Larsen, R. J., & Fredrickson, B. L. (1999). Measurement issues in emotion research. In D. Kahneman, E. Diener, & N. Schwarz (Eds.), *Well-being: The foundations of hedonic psychology* (pp. 40–60). New York: Russell Sage Foundation.

Lucas, R. E., Diener, E., Grob, A., Suh, E. M., & Shao, L. (2000). Cross-cultural evidence for the fundamental features of extraversion. *Journal of Personality and Social Psychology, 79*, 452–468.

Lucas, R. E., Diener, E., & Suh, E. M. (1996). Discriminant validity of subjective well-being measures. *Journal of Personality and Social Psychology, 71*, 616–628.

Lucas, R. E., & Fujita, F. (2000). Factors influencing the relation between extraversion and pleasant affect. *Journal of Personality and Social Psychology, 79*, 1039–1056.

McNair, D. M., Lorr, M., & Droppleman, L. F. (1971). *Manual: Profile of mood states.* San Diego, CA: Educational and Industrial Testing Service.

Morris, W. N. (1999). The mood system. In D. Kahneman, E. Diener, & N. Schwarz (Eds.), *Well-being: The foundations of hedonic psychology* (pp. 169–189). New York: Russell Sage Foundation.

Nowlis, V., & Green, R. (1957). *The experimental analysis of mood.* Technical report, contract no. Nonr-668 (12). Washington, DC: Office of Naval Research.

Ortony, A., & Turner, T. J. (1990). What's basic about basic emotions? *Psychological Review, 97*, 315–331.

Panksepp, J. (1992). A critical role for "affective neuroscience" in resolving what is basic about basic emotions. *Psychological Review, 99*, 554–560.

Robinson, M., & Clore, G. L. (2000). *Belief and feeling: Evidence for an accessibility model of emotional self-report.* Manuscript submitted for publication, University of Illinois at Urbana-Champaign.

Russell, J. A. (1980). A circumplex model of affect. *Journal of Personality and Social Psychology, 39*, 1161–1178.

Russell, J. A., & Feldman Barrett, L. (1999). Core affect, prototypical emotional episodes and other things called emotion: Dissecting the elephant. *Journal of Personality and Social Psychology, 76*, 805–819.

Russell, J. A., Weiss, A., & Mendelsohn, G. A. (1989). The Affect Grid: A single-item scale of pleasure and arousal. *Journal of Personality and Social Psychology, 57*, 493–502.

Rusting, C. L. (1998). Personality, mood, and cognitive processing of emotional information: Three conceptual frameworks. *Psychological Bulletin, 124*, 165–196.

Schimmack, U., & Diener, E. (1997). Affect intensity: Separating intensity and frequency in repeatedly measured affect. *Journal of Personality and Social Psychology, 73*, 1313–1329.

Schimmack, U., & Grob, A. (2000). Dimensional models of core affect: A quantitative comparison by means of structural equation modeling. *European Journal of Personality, 14*, 325–345.

Seidlitz, L., & Diener, E. (1993). Memory for positive versus negative life events: Theories for the difference between happy and unhappy persons. *Journal of Personality and Social Psychology, 64*, 654–663.

Tellegen, A. (1985). Structures of mood and personality and their relevance to assessing anxiety, with an emphasis on self-report. In A. H. Tuma & J. D. Maser (Eds.), *Anxiety and the anxiety disorders* (pp. 681–706). Hillsdale, NJ: Erlbaum.

Tellegen, A., & Waller, N. (1994). Exploring personality through test construction: Development of the Multidimensional Personality Questionnaire. In S. R. Briggs & J. M. Cheek (Eds.), *Personality measures: Development and evaluation* (Vol. 1, pp. 133–161). Greenwich, CT: JAI Press.

Thayer, R. E. (1967). Measurement of activation through self-report. *Psychological Reports, 20*, 663–678.

Thayer, R. E. (1978). Toward a psychological theory of multidimensional activation (arousal). *Motivation and Emotion, 2*, 1–34.

Turner, T. J., & Ortony, A. (1992). Basic emotions: Can conflicting criteria converge? *Psychological Review, 99*, 566–571.

Watson, D. (2000). *Mood and temperament*. New York: Guilford Press.

Watson, D., & Clark, L. A. (1992). On traits and temperament: General and specific factors of emotional experience and their relation to the five-factor model. *Journal of Personality, 60*, 441–476.

Watson, D., & Clark, L. A. (1994). *The PANAS-X: Manual for the Positive and Negative Affect Schedule Expanded Form*. Unpublished manuscript, University of Iowa, Iowa City.

Watson, D., & Clark, L. A. (1997). Extraversion and its positive emotional core. In R. Hogan. J. Johnson, & S. Briggs (Eds.), *Handbook of personality psychology* (pp. 767–793). San Diego, CA: Academic Press.

Watson, D., Clark, L. A., & Tellegen, (1988). Development and validation of brief measures of positive and negative affect: The PANAS scales. *Journal of Personality and Social Psychology, 54*, 1063–1070.

Watson, D., & Tellegen, A. (1985). Toward a consensual structure of mood. *Psychological Bulletin, 98*, 219–235.

Watson, D., Wiese, D., Vaidya, J., & Tellegen, A. (1999). The two general activation systems of affect. Structural findings, evolutionary considerations, and psychobiological evidence. *Journal of Personality and Social Psychology, 76*, 820–838.

Zelenski, J. M., & Larsen, R. J. (2000). The distribution of basic emotions in everyday life: A state and trait perspective from experience sampling data. *Journal of Research in Personality, 34*, 178–197.

Zuckerman, M., & Lubin, B. (1985). *Manual for the MAACL-R: The multiple affect adjective check list revised*. San Diego, CA: Educational and Industrial Testing Service.

Experience Sampling: Promises and Pitfalls, Strengths and Weaknesses

Christie Napa Scollon, Chu Kim-Prieto, and Ed Diener

Abstract The experience-sampling (ESM) technique is a method in which record-ing of feelings and activities is done on-line at the moment, either at randomly selected moments or at predetermined times. This method has the advantage of being able to not only assess people's general feelings, but to link feelings with situations, times of day, and other circumstances. Thus, ESM provides a powerful way of moving beyond simple questions about who is "happy" and who is not, to more intricate questions about when and why people experience positive and negative feelings. Compared to retrospective reports of feelings, ESM is less influ-enced by memory biases. ESM also allows researchers to analyze the patterning and relationships of feelings as they unfold over time. Despite the strengths and promise of this method, there are also limitations. For example, the heavy demand placed on research participants means that the sample might be biased toward highly con-scientious individuals, and repeatedly reporting one's moods might itself influence feelings. How to analyze ESM data is discussed, including the issue of how to aggre-gate momentary feelings into global measures of the average subjective well-being of individuals.

Since its inception in the late 1970s, experience sampling methodology (ESM) has enjoyed an explosion of popularity in psychological research. A literature search for ESM and related terms, such as ecological momentary assessment, on PsychINFO yielded 343 articles and dissertations, most of which have been undertaken in the past dozen years. Much of its popularity can be attributed to its ability to delve beyond single-time self-report measurement to answer complex questions about lives, such as the role of situations in individual functioning, as well as its ability to provide solutions to nagging methodological problems, such as memory biases.

Investigators have long recognized the need for an assessment tool that is more true to life experiences than laboratory assessments, global questionnaires, or ob-server ratings. Brunswik (1949) and Cattell (1957) addressed the importance of understanding how various psychological variables manifest themselves in different situations in order to understand the full constellation of behaviors and conditions

C.N. Scollon (✉)
University of Illinois, Urbana-Champaign, Champaign, IL 61820, USA
e-mail: scollon@s.psych.uiuc.edu

E. Diener (ed.), *Assessing Well-Being: The Collected Works of Ed Diener*,
Social Indicators Research Series 39, DOI 10.1007/978-90-481-2354-4_8,
© Springer Science+Business Media B.V. 2009

that elicit them. Later, the call for studies of on-line experience was again taken up by Fiske (1971), who wrote that the assessment of on-line experiences should be one of the essential tools in assessing personality. More recently, Funder (2001) brought attention to the necessity of studying personality in a wide variety of settings, and the utility of ESM in meeting that need.

What is ESM? A Brief History

ESM refers to a method of data collection in which participants respond to repeated assessments at moments over the course of time while functioning within their natural settings. Although no single person or research program can be credited with inventing ESM per se, the precursor to today's ESM can be seen as early as Flügel's (1925) 30-day study of mood. However, the methodology that most resembles its current form is usually credited to Csikszentmihalyi, Larson, and Prescott (1977) investigation of adolescents in their natural environments or Brandstaetter's (1983) study of mood across situations. ESM was also used extensively by Diener and his colleagues in the early 1980s for measuring mood across situations (e.g., Diener & Larsen, 1984; Diener & Emmons, 1985). What distinguishes these current forms from their earlier precursors is the introduction of random signaling and attempts to study intrapsychic phenomena.

The use of random sampling of behaviors used in the past by industrial researchers and behavior therapists (e.g., Ayllon & Haughton, 1964; Case Institute of Technology, 1958) were usually observer reports, and hence limited to the study of overt behaviors in institutional settings. The use of self-reports allowed for the sampling of a greater range of situations and investigation of more intra-psychic phenomena; however, participants were often required to keep track of the sampling times themselves, by either keeping a schedule of the times when one would be required to record one's behavior, or else setting alarm watches for the next assessment period (e.g., Barnes, 1956; Brandstaetter, 1983; Diener & Larsen, 1984; Heiland & Richardson, 1957; Hinricks, 1964; Case Institute of Technology, 1958). The disadvantage to this approach is that participants might anticipate alarms (although Diener and Larsen noted that most participants said they usually forgot about the alarms after they programmed the watch).

Fortunately for today's ESM researcher, technological advances have made many former problems moot. The tools of ESM have evolved to allow greater ease of data collection for the researchers as well as the participant. At its nascence, participants carried pagers or alarm watches, along with a stack of paper on which they recorded their responses when signaled. While the paging devices were usually small enough to be carried around comfortably, investigators still had to call the paging device. Other researchers telephoned the participants at home at random times. This approach, too, had its limitations; the participants could only be studied at certain times and while at home (see Stone, Kessler, & Haythornwaite, 1991 for a discussion of the advantages). Alternatives included pre-programmed alarm devices (Hormuth, 1986) that were relatively large.

Today, hand-held computers (a.k.a. personal digital assistants (PDAs) or palmtop computers) can be pre-programmed to signal participants at random moments. Participants can respond directly on the computer, negating the need to carry around a separate stack of response sheets. Besides the time-saving advantage and the convenience for the participant, the decrease in the cost of electronic goods makes hand-held computers cost-effective as well. The palmtop computers allow data to be directly transferred to statistical software packages or other programs for immediate analysis, and with no data entry, mistakes are minimized or eliminated altogether. Furthermore, participants cannot as easily fake their responses as with the paper-pencil measures (see below).

Types of Experience Sampling

Under the broad umbrella of experience sampling methods, three distinct types of experience sampling exist (Reis & Gable, 2000; Wheeler & Reis, 1991). Interval-contingent sampling refers to the type of data collection in which participants complete self-reports after a designated interval for a pre-set amount of time (e.g., hourly reports, Nowlis & Cohen, 1968; daily reports, Wessman & Ricks, 1966). Event-contingent sampling occurs when participants complete self-reports when a pre-designated event occurs (e.g., reporting after every social interaction, Cote & Moskowitz, 1998). Last, signal-contingent sampling requires participants to complete their self-reports when prompted by a randomly-timed signal. This last form of sampling is what is typically labeled ESM. For the most part, the present paper focuses on signal-contingent sampling. Signal-contingent sampling is advantageous in that it allows for the sampling of a representative schedule of times, and avoids any expectancy effects that may come from having prior knowledge of the sampling period (Alliger & Williams, 1993).

Besides the three broad categories that distinguish between the timing and method of gathering data, other researchers distinguish ESM from three other methods based on the type of data generated. First, thought-sampling, developed independently by Hurlburt (1997) and Klinger (1978–1979), differs from ESM in that it focuses on recordings of inner thoughts and mostly dispenses with external events. Hurlburt (1997) also distinguishes descriptive-experience sampling from ESM, in that the former is used only for gathering qualitative data. Second, Stone and his colleagues distinguish ESM from ecological momentary assessment (EMA). In EMA, measurement is concerned with not just the participant's momentary subjective experience, but also with the elements of the environment related to momentary experience (Stone, Shiffman, & DeVries, 1999). It should be noted that many researchers do not make sharp distinctions between ESM and other random-sampling methods (Hurlburt, 1997; Reis & Gable, 2000).

Promises and Strengths

From the brief outline of ESM's historical roots and description, it is easy to see why ESM and its predecessors have enjoyed researchers' enduring interest. Even decades earlier, when technology made experience sampling difficult, time-consuming, and costly, researchers recognized the need for the type of data made possible through ESM. Five major strengths of experience sampling are discussed in detail below. First, ESM allows researchers to better understand the contingencies of behavior. Second, ESM takes psychology out of the laboratory and into real-life situations, thus increasing its ecological validity. Third, ESM allows for the investigation of within-person processes. Fourth, researchers can avoid some of the pitfalls associated with traditional self-reports, such as memory biases and the use of global heuristics. Fifth, ESM answers the call for the greater use of multiple methods to study psychological phenomena.

Contingencies Can Be Noted

Mischel (1968) highlighted the problem of understanding individual behavior across situations in his criticism of personality research, and suggested a need for "direct experience sampling" in order to understand the covariation in stimulus conditions and responses of human behavior. In fact, one of the strongest benefits of ESM is that it allows for the investigation of complex questions about the contingencies of behaviors. For example, research exploring the link between extraversion and happiness tracked whether extraverts' greater levels of positive emotion were due to greater time spent in social activities (e.g., Diener, Larsen, & Emmons, 1984; Pavot, Diener, & Fujita, 1990). But also, ESM has been used to investigate the effects of momentary pleasant affect on social activity (Lucas, 2000). As Lucas (2000) demonstrated, ESM is better suited to this task than global reports because current levels of pleasant affect can predict future social activity, even after controlling for previous levels of social activity.

Through the use of ESM, other researchers have shown the intricacies of the interaction between persons and situations. Brandstatter (1983), for example, found that the types of situations and the social interactions encountered in daily lives were correlated with the personality of the individuals, and that the subsequent emotions were dependent on both situational and personality variables (see also Diener et al., 1984 for an example of situational selection using time-contingent sampling). Others have shown situation interactions with gender (Larson, Richards, & Perry-Jenkins, 1994) and culture (Oishi, Diener, Scollon, & Biswas-Diener, 2004), as well as personality variables (Flory, Raeikkoenen, Matthews, & Owens, 2000). Indeed, these types of studies allow for a better understanding of the mutual role of the individual and the situation that gives rise to various psychological phenomena.

Ecological Validity

In addition to allowing the researcher to investigate the various situational contingencies of a psychological phenomenon, ESM also permits greater generalizability of the research findings. That is, psychologists can ecologically validate their theoretical concepts and empirical findings in real-life settings. For example, experience sampling studies have identified diurnal and weekly patterns of moods. That is, people tend to experience greater pleasant affect later in the day, versus in the morning, and on the weekends, versus on weekdays, (e.g., Egloff, Tausch, Kohlmann, & Krohne, 1995; Larsen & Kasimatis, 1990; Lucas, 2000). In another illustrative example, Lucas (2000) found that individuals who scored high on global measures of extraversion did not engage in more social behaviors on a moment-to-moment basis than individuals who scored low on the global measures. This finding demonstrates the usefulness of ESM in informing our theories; in this case, ESM data challenged the traditional and implicit beliefs about what it means to be extraverted.

Investigating Within-Person Processes

While psychologists over the years have emphasized the need for idiographic research (e.g., Lamiell, 1997; McAdams, 1995; Pelham, 1993), nomothetic investigations have largely formed the mainstay of research. However, with ESM, researchers are not limited to between-person investigations. This is important because within-person analyses can reveal interesting patterns that may be masked at mean levels. For example, researchers are often interested in what emotions occur together. However, this question can be framed at two different levels of analysis, and can sometimes lead to different conclusions depending on the level of analysis. Correlations computed at the within-person level represent state conceptions of emotions, while between-person correlations computed from aggregated moment data reflect trait conceptions of emotion (see Zelenski & Larsen, 2000, pp. 180–181, for a detailed explanation). In other words, at the within-person level, we are primarily interested in what states go together at a given moment (e.g., Can a person feel both happy and guilty simultaneously?). On the other hand, at the between-person level, we can examine the "long-term structure" of affect (Diener & Emmons, 1985). For example, does knowing a person's mean level of happiness tell us anything about that person's mean level of guilt? Because the two levels are logically independent, positive and negative emotions can be negatively correlated at one level and yet independent or positively correlated at another level (e.g., Diener & Emmons, 1985).

Two studies illustrate the importance of distinguishing between the distinct levels of analysis. Zelenski & Larsen (2000) found that like-valenced emotions were only weakly correlated at the within-person or state level. On the other hand, like-valenced emotions were more strongly correlated at the between-person or trait level (see also Schimmack, 2003). Similarly, Scollon et al. (2002) found cross-cultural similarities in within-person correlations of pleasant and unpleasant affect, but cross-cultural differences in between-person correlations.

Yet another valuable aspect of ESM is its sensitivity to differences within individuals that emerge over time or across situations, in terms of the variability or intensity of behavior and feelings. For instance, in spite of cultural differences in mean levels of pleasant and unpleasant emotion, Oishi and colleagues (2004) found that across cultures, being with friends increased pleasant mood and decreased negative mood. But the benefit of being with others was qualified by culture and gender such that people in some cultures, as well as men, received a greater boost from being with friends.

At an idiographic level, ESM has helped understand the role of resources in personal goal strivings and subjective well-being (e.g., Diener & Fujita, 1995; Emmons, 1986; Zirkel & Cantor, 1990). Case studies also have been conducted using ESM, such as delle Fave and Massimini's (1992) charting of an agoraphobic patient's treatment progress and her experiences and moods during the nine week sampling period.

Reduction in Memory Bias

The problem of memory biases has been noted for years, but researchers were not always able to distill the biases from the self-reports themselves, or understand the processes that underlie the biases in self-reports. For example, problems of global self-reports include biases in retrospective recall (Cutler, Larsen, & Bruce, 1996; Redelmeier & Kahneman, 1996; Ross, 1989), autobiographical memory (Han, Leichtman, & Wang, 1998; Henry, Moffitt, Caspi, Langley, & Silva, 1994; Wang, 2001), and the use of heuristics in response patterns (Robinson & Clore, 2002; Schwarz, 1994, 1999; Tversky & Kahneman, 1973).

In response to problems with global self-reports, researchers use ESM to separate on-line experiences from recall and global biases. This is possible because in ESM, not much room for recall bias exists between the signal and the response because of the shortness of the timelag between the signal and the response. Discrepancies between on-line and global self-report measures have been demonstrated in a variety of research areas, such as coping and emotion. For example, Ptacek, Smith, Espe, and Raffety (1994) found that on-line reports of the usage of coping strategies correlated 0.58 with retrospective reports. Also, Stone and his colleagues (1998) found that in global reports, cognitive coping was underreported while behavioral coping was over-reported.

On the other hand, several studies have demonstrated convergent validity between aggregated experience sampling data and global or retrospective reports (Diener, Smith, & Fujita, 1995; Feldman Barrett, 1997). One reason for the mixed findings is that there are multiple ways of conceptualizing accuracy (see Thomas & Diener, 1990). For instance, it would be misleading to say that participants were inaccurate because they were not 100% accurate. In fact, the study by Ptacek et al. (1994) demonstrates both accuracy and inaccuracy. After all, a correlation of 0.58 between on-line and recalled reports, while not perfect, still indicates a good deal of overlap between participants' memories and reality.

One alternative is to examine the rank ordering of individuals or groups on both on-line and retrospective measures to determine if the measures converge. For example, Scollon et al. (2002) found that global, on-line, and retrospective measures of emotion converged in that the rank ordering of different groups was preserved across the various measures. Again, retrospective measures were not entirely unrelated to actual experience. However, retrospective measures overlapped considerably with individuals' self-beliefs, and this was consistent across various cultures. Nevertheless, greater cultural differences emerged with some of the recall measures than with the on-line measures (albeit those displayed differences as well).

To further complicate matters, researchers can ask participants to recall the past in a variety of ways. For example, people are very inaccurate in estimating absolute frequencies (e.g., In the past hour, how many minutes did you feel happy?), but are very good at remembering which type of emotion is experienced relatively more frequently than others (e.g., happy more than sad; Schimmack, 2003). Similarly, Scollon et al. (2002) showed that the recall of frequency was often colored by the intensity of on-line experiences presumably because intense emotions are more salient in memory.

Multiple Methods Assessment

ESM is most useful when applied in conjunction with other methods, for instance, traditional global reports. Since Campbell and Fiske's (1959) landmark paper explicating the need to assess multiple traits through multiple methods, psychologists have been acutely aware of the need for multi-method approaches. Mischel (1968) repeated this call in his caution against common method variance, and in recent years Bank, Dishion, Skinner, and Patterson (1990) echoed similar warnings of what they called the problem of "glop" associated with common method variance. By allowing the researcher to study the differential effects of on-line versus other measures, ESM enables the researcher to adopt a multi-method strategy.

The study by Diener et al. (1995) provides a good example of the multimethod approach. In applying a multitrait-multimethod (MTMM) analysis to global self-reports, informant reports, and daily reports of emotion, Diener and his colleagues found that the different measures displayed substantial convergent validity. Like-valenced emotions were highly correlated even when measured with different methods, demonstrating that individuals who tended to experience one emotion (e.g., joy) also experienced similar emotions (e.g., love). Additionally, using structural equation modeling to identify the structure of affect, they found that despite the coherence among like-valenced emotions revealed in the MTMM, a model with only pleasant and unpleasant affect did not fit as well a model with specific emotions influencing pleasant and unpleasant affect. Thus, the authors cautioned against using the specific emotion terms interchangeably because the discrete emotions were still necessary for describing individual differences in emotion.

Clearly, there are accuracies and inaccuracies in retrospective measures. Nevertheless, global recall measures can compliment ESM data because they avoid some of the pitfalls of ESM that are reviewed later. One major advantage of global reports is that they often cover a much longer time frame than can be covered in an experience sampling study, and this makes them better trait-indicators than aggregates over one week. Recently, global reports have been shown to be especially useful in predicting behavioral choices. For example, Wirtz, Kruger, Scollon, and Diener (2003) investigated the differential roles of on-line experiences, retrospective recall, and expectation for determining future behavior. In their study, vacationing students completed self-reports measuring expectations of pleasure, on-line reports of pleasure, and retrospective recall of pleasure. Results indicated that only recalled affect, not on-line experience or expections, directly and strongly predicted the desire to take a similar vacation in the future. Similarly, the strongest predictor of enduring romantic relationships was not partners' daily reports during times spent together, but rather their retrospective reports of their experiences together (Oishi, 2002). These studies suggest that it is absolutely essential to measure both aspects of experience.

Pitfalls and Weaknesses

Clearly, the main strength of experience sampling lies in its ability to provide fine-grained, detailed pictures of human experience. However, investigators should be a ware of potential pitfalls before investing both the time and money in an intensive ESM study. The bulk of problems associated with experience sampling studies can be divided into participant issues, situation issues, and measurement and data analytic issues. These are discussed in detail in the next section.

Who are We Studying? Participant Issues

Self-Selection Bias and Attrition

Self-selection bias and attrition are potential problems for all studies, but the intensive nature of the data-gathering strategy creates special difficulties for the ESM researcher. A typical study lasts 1–2 weeks, during which participants respond to 2–12 signals per day (see Reis & Gable, 2000). This is an onerous task for most people. Imagine oneself as a participant. (Or better yet, investigators should try carrying the palmtop device around just as a participant would.) The alarms disrupt one's activities, conversations, and work, and may not only annoy one self but surrounding others as well, such as in church, classrooms, or meetings. Furthermore, even with short forms that only take 1 min to complete, a participant answers 1,000 or more questions over the course of an entire study, totaling well over an hour.

Who volunteers for such intrusive studies and who completes them? Who provides the most data? The difficult nature of these tasks might lead certain types of individuals to be over- or underrepresented in ESM studies. Some individuals will refuse to participate outright. The less motivated participants may drop out after a few days of being interrupted during their daily activities. The remaining participants may show greater motivation, conscientiousness, agreeableness, or other characteristics that may not make them a representative sample. After all, participants who forget the palmtop at home half of the time are likely to differ from participants who remember to take the palmtop with them everywhere and everyday; unfortunately, there will be a preponderance of data on the latter.

Motivation

Indeed research shows that motivation plays a significant role in determining whether a participant will successfully complete an ESM study. Wilson, Hopkins, deVries, and Copeland (1992) found that poor volition and concentration made it difficult for depressed older people to complete experience sampling studies. Chronic illness also hindered participation (Wilson et al., 1992), although with high motivation, subjects were remarkably perseverant despite difficulties. The degree of motivation needed to complete an ESM study may also vary by groups. Because the signals are interruptive, those who have more time (e.g., unemployed people or college students) might require less motivation than those with little free time (e.g., Young harried professionals with children).

Other Sample Limitations

ESM may not be suitable for studying some people or groups. For example, Csikszentmihalyi & Larson (1987) found that blue collar workers in the 1980s found the task too unusual and were less compliant than clerical workers—although we suspect this gap has narrowed and will continue to do so due to the spread of technology. The elderly and children may be uncomfortable with the task, although Csikszentmihalyi & Larson (1987) report that their youngest participant was 10 and their oldest participant was 85 (although in that study they did not use palmtop computers). Beidel, Neal, and Lederer (1991) noted that children in grades 3–6 could successfully complete ESM studies. Additionally, ESM has been used to study the naturally occurring moods of schizophrenics, showing that it is a viable method that can be used with special populations.

Beyond technological familiarity, however, people must be able to hear and respond to the signals. The elderly and people who spend a lot of time in loud, crowded settings (e.g., bartenders) might be excluded from experience sampling studies. Of course, these problems can be circumvented if researchers use devices that send vibrating signals or devices with a high volume setting. Similarly, Wilson et al. (1992) found that elderly participants had trouble reading digital displays. Even if a signal can be heard, the nature of some jobs makes it more difficult to participate (e.g., truck drivers). In fact, it would be dangerous for some people to try to complete reports during their work (e.g., air traffic controllers).

Possible Solutions and Recommendations

Naturally, one source of motivation for participants is money, and monetary incentives have been shown to significantly improve compliance (Lynn, 2001). However, incentives for completion might not be appropriate for some participants, such as anxious or perfectionistic subjects who are already apprehensive and concerned about completing the study. Also, caution must be exercised in deciding how much compensation to provide—a point to which we will return later. Interestingly, in one study reported by Stone et al. (1991), the monetary incentive of $250 resulted in overall poor quality of data (e.g., missing data, evidence of faking, etc.) because the high desirability of the reward attracted participants who were not intrinsically motivated to participate. In other words, when determining the appropriate amount of compensation, more may not be better.

A possibly more effective way of ensuring participant cooperation is to gain participant trust, or establish what Csikszentmihalyi & Larson (1987) called a "viable research alliance" (p. 529). In other words, participants need to understand the importance of the study (without necessarily knowing the hypothesis), and they need to be thoroughly trained on the procedures and on the usage of the equipment. Furthermore, researchers should convey to participants the importance of continuing with the study even if they forget to carry the palmtop for one or two days (Stone et al., 1991).

Limiting the Number of Variables in the Design

By reducing the burdensome nature of the task, researchers are likely to narrow the gap between those who participate and those who do not or cannot. One way to do this is to signal participants less frequently and select as few items as possible per occasion. A general rule of thumb is: the more signals per day, the shorter the form should be. Unfortunately, the small number of questions one can ask in ESM studies is in itself a limitation of the methodology. On the other hand, multiple items are not necessary for establishing reliability because reliability can be computed from the aggregate of the single items over time (Csikszentmihalyi & Larson, 1987).

Cautious Generalizations

The most compliant participants for experience sampling studies will be conscientious, agreeable, non-depressed, young people who are not too busy—essentially, college students. Thus, researchers need to consider what effects, if any, these subject characteristics may have on the results of the study and the ability to generalize to broad populations. Although generalization issues are endemic to any psychological research based on college samples, because ESM attempts to link basic psychological processes to situations in the daily lives and experiences of the participants, dangers are even greater. That is, the types of situations—classroom learning, living in dorms, meals in cafeterias—encountered by college students are necessarily different from the types of situations that working adults encounter in their daily lives. On the other hand, most of these situations are social and/or involve the pursuit of one's daily goal. In this sense, perhaps college students are not so different from the larger population. However, the generalizability of findings is one that must be explored.

When are We Studying People? Situation Issues

Quality of Data

Even if a variety of participants volunteer, the quality of data is another problem that is exacerbated by the nature of ESM. Stone et al. (1991) wrote that declining quality of data reporting is estimated to occur after 2–4 weeks of data collection. With wrist watches or beepers and paper-pencil reports, participants can easily fake their responses by completing all their forms in one sitting. This problem can be alleviated by requiring participants to turn in their completed forms on a daily basis. Palmtop computers further reduce the problem of faked responses by recording the exact date and time of each report, making it painfully obvious if a participant completes all forms in one sitting, and allowing researchers to compute the time lag between the signal and response.

Unfortunately, even with the newer technology, people might simply use the same responses across time. Brandstaetter (1983) argued that participants' responses would become more accurate over time through increased self-awareness. However, it is not clear how accuracy and habitual responding can be separated. Individuals may not use the full range of responses over time (as indicated by decreased variability or increased stability in ratings), but this could be indicative of either habitual, repeated responding or greater self-awareness and accuracy (Hormuth, 1986). Stone and colleagues (1991) detail weighting procedures that can help correct for habitual responding, and Reis & Gable (2000) suggest pilot-testing and refining procedures to minimize the problem.

Select Situations

Random sampling from a person's everyday life invites a host of problems not associated with random sampling from a set of stimuli or variables, because ultimately it is the participant who decides whether to respond to an experience sampling signal. There may be some instances in which one is less likely to respond to a signal, or in which it is impossible to do so. Response rates tend to decreases slightly in the evenings (Alliger & Williams, 1993), in the home (Pawlik & Buse, 1982 as cited in Hormuth, 1986), and in places where the signaling device could not be carried, such as swimming pools (Hormuth, 1986) or where the signal could be disruptive (e.g., church). Of course, the ecological strength of the ESM depends on the degree to which a full range of participants' activities and situations are sampled. This requires that subjects respond to signals and complete forms, even when it is inconvenient and they do not feel like doing so. Again this underscores the need to provide participants with explicit instructions and to help them understand the importance of sampling all situations, not simply select ones.

The fact that some situations (e.g., swimming, being in church, operating machinery, driving) will not get sampled is a difficult problem. Although response rates increase if participants are allowed to respond to the signal afterwards, this practice raises its own concerns. Similarly, rare situations or emotions might not be sampled, such as being the victim of crime or intense fear. Even events that might seem frequent, for instance studying among students, might be recorded relatively infrequently in on-line reports (see Wong & Csikszentmihalyi, 1991). For infrequent events, Wheeler & Reis (1991) and Reis & Gable (2000) recommend event-contingent sampling because "the rarer the event in question, the less useful the signal-contingent method—there is not much chance that the signal and the event will coincide" (Wheeler & Reis, 1991, p. 347). Hormuth (1986) argues that while situation selectivity is a potential problem for ESM studies, other methods are even more vulnerable to threats of ecological validity.

Time Lag Between Signal and Response

The quality of ESM data is best if participants respond to signals immediately. The trade-off here is that more responses will be gained if participants are allowed to respond to signals at a more convenient, later time. However, with greater time lag, memory biases and the use of heuristics can contaminate reports, and thus defeat the purpose of experience sampling. Thus, when participants are allowed to make delayed responses, researchers typically restrict responses to no more than 30 min after the signal (e.g., Cerin, Szabo, & Williams, 2001; Diener & Larsen, 1984; 20 min in Csikszentmihalyi & Larson, 1987; Stone et al., 1998). Fortunately, much of the data on this issue are encouraging. Hormuth (1986) reported that half of his participants responded immediately to the signal, 70% within 3 min, and 80% within 5 min. Similar figures are reported in Csikszentmihalyi and Larson's (1984) study of adolescents: 64% immediately responded when signaled, and 87% responded within 10 min.

Admittedly, the 20 min- or the 30 min-response window is an arbitrary cut-off, although it provides some uniformity as to when to use the data. Future researchers should consider whether differences in the data exist between timely and tardy responses, in terms of types of participants, time periods, events, moods, or other variables of concern. We suspect more industrious participants will respond on time or closer to the time of the signal. Similar to compliance in timeliness is compliance in response. Future research should aim to identify the factors that increase or decrease response rates. For example, what are the differences in the subject characteristics of those who might respond to 80% of the signals versus those who respond to only 40%? Are some people more willing to respond to signals when they are in a happy mood than when they are feeling irritated? Research showing that positive moods result in increasing helpfulness (Isen, 1970; Isen & Levin, 1972) suggests that this may be a possibility, but it has yet to be tested.

Reactivity

Psychologists must contend with their own version of Heisenberg's Uncertainty Principle – in this case reactivity or the potential for any phenomenon under study to change as a result of measurement or reporting (Wheeler & Reis, 1991). Although reactivity is a problem for many researchers interested in human behavior, it is especially problematic for ESM studies because the repeated assessments may lead people to pay unusual attention to their internal states and own behavior. For example, completing mood measures 7 times a day might alert someone to insights such as, "I am the kind of person who is sad a lot," or "I am happy when I am with my friends." Reflections of the latter sort, in particular, may lead to behavioral changes such as spending more time with one's friends which in turn may change the person's moods. With non-random sampling techniques (i.e., event-contingent or interval-contingent sampling), people might look for events or anticipate behaviors or situations (Hormuth, 1986). In fact, self-monitoring was believed to be so strongly associated with experience sampling that behaviorists used this method as a tool for behavior modification (Wheeler & Reis, 1991). Schimmack (personal, communication, 2002) recalls one incident in which a participant was advised by his therapist not to participate in an experience sampling study for fear that the constant self-awareness would trigger a relapse. Similarly, alcoholics who participated in an ESM study said that reporting on drinking made them more aware of their drinking, although greater awareness did not lead to behavioral changes (Litt, Cooney, & Morse, 1998).

In a provocative study on premenstrual symptoms, Ruble (1977) manipulated participants' beliefs about their menstrual cycle and showed its effects on attending to bodily symptoms. Some women were led to believe they were premenstrual while others were led to believe they were not, when in fact all of them were tested 6 days before the onset of their next menses. The women who thought they were premenstrual reported greater pain, water retention, change in eating habits, and sexual arousal than women who were led to believe they were mid-cycle. Ruble's (1977) findings suggested that beliefs about premenstrual status alerted the women to look for symptoms that they normally might not have noticed. Arguably, because participants in Ruble's study were asked to report their symptoms for the "last day or two," the observed differences in symptoms between the groups may have been due to implicit theories of menstruation (see also Mc-Farland, Ross, & DeCourville, 1989; Ross, 1989), rather than any differences in attention.

Few studies have directly examined the reactivity effects of experience sampling. Cruise, Broderick, Porter, Kaell, and Stone (1996) had chronic arthritis sufferers complete pain dairies several times a day and observed that pain levels and affect ratings remained constant over time, suggesting no reactivity effects. Cerin et al. (2001) randomly assigned participants in a week-long study to either (a) an ESM condition, (b) a repeated measures condition that sampled emotions four times, roughly once every three days, or (c) a retrospective assessment condition that asked participants to recall their emotions on four previous days. The authors compared ratings on four days using (a) the average of the day's ratings for the ESM participants, (b) the day's rating made by the repeated measures group, and (c) the recalled ratings made by the retrospective group. Results revealed higher estimates of feeling energetic, enjoyment, and worry, and lower estimates of feeling anger and irritation, in retrospective reports than in on-line or daily reports. Arguably, these results are inconclusive because group differences may have been driven by memory reconstruction rather than reactivity per se. The pattern of emotions for the retrospective group appeared to conform to implicit beliefs of how a person should feel before competition.

Besides priming participants to pay attention to certain states, the intrusive nature of the ESM experiment may actually *make* participants more irritated. This would certainly have ethical as well as methodological implications. Fortunately, Cerin and colleagues (2001) did not find that use of the ESM increased negative mood due to its intrusiveness. In fact, ESM measures of cognitive intrusion were lower than repeated or retrospective measures.

Even if experience sampling does not have an effect on participants' current moods, some evidence suggests that repeated assessments might influence the recall of emotions. For instance, Thomas & Diener (1990) found that daily and momentary reports correlated higher with retrospective estimates of emotion than with prospective estimates. Similarly, Schimmack (2003) found that absolute estimates of emotions after a daily diary study were more accurate than those before the study. On the other hand, if experience sampling influences accuracy of recall, then we would expect greater accuracy with more repeated assessments. However, Thomas & Diener (1990) found that momentary reporting did not have a greater effect on retrospective accuracy than daily reporting.

In short, we currently know surprisingly little about the effects of ESM on a person's subjective experience. Clearly, more studies are needed. Until reactivity is better understood, researchers cannot be certain that ESM is indeed tapping a phenomenon as it exists, or as it has been transformed by measurement. Future research on reactivity can lead to improvements in testing procedures to minimize reactivity. For example, if researchers find that responding to the same question five times a day results in greater self-monitoring of behavior and alterations in the variable in question, but responding to the same question twice a day does not, this information can guide the design of future research. Because such information is not available, the number of sampling occasions each day typically represents a compromise between maximizing the number of data points while minimizing participant drop-out.

Future research should also explore whether reactivity differs across groups and across variables. Many ESM studies of emotion have, thus far, been conducted in Western cultures where the norm is to think about one's own emotional states (cf. Ji, Schwarz, & Nisbett, 2000). Cultures that are less emotion-focused may experience greater reactivity to the constant reporting of emotions. Even within cultures, however, differential reactivity may even occur among people of different classes or educational levels (e.g., Csikszentmihalyi & Larson, 1987), or may vary according to what is being measured. For example, attention to anxiety or worry may trigger cognitions or ruminations that may lead to greater anxiety and worry (e.g., Mathews & MacLeod, 1994; Nolen-Hoeksema, 1993).

The Limits of Self-Report

Although the on-line reporting of emotions eliminates retrospective bias to some extent, it is still subject to some of the same problems as any self-report measure (see Schwarz, 1999). Social desirability, cognitive biases, and cultural norms might influence responses even at the momentary level of reporting. For example, if there is a cultural norm that feeling negative emotions is undesirable, there may be reluctance to reporting feelings such as sadness. Similarly, highly defensive people may "filter" their responses, and even the most honest person might find it difficult to report on some states, such as unconscious motives or feelings (Shedler, Mayman, & Manis, 1993).

Experience sampling also relies on the use of numerical scales that, although useful among college participants, might be inappropriate or awkward for some people. In fact, Wilson and colleagues (1992) found that Likert scales were too confusing for elderly depressed participants, whereas visual scales were better understood.

Perhaps the best remedy to these problems is to take a multi-method approach and supplement ESM with other non-self-report measures. Promising possibilities include informant reports, on-line physiological measures (e.g., ambulatory measures, Fahrenberg & Myrtek, 2001), or on-line ambient recording, a new methodology developed by Mehl, Pennebaker, Crow, Dabbs, and Price (2001) that captures random 30-s recordings of a participant's surrounding sounds. However, no other method besides self-reports is able to capture the hedonic tone of people's emotional experiences, an aspect of emotion phenomena that is arguably most relevant to subjective well-being research.

The Issue of Scaling

Schwarz (1999) demonstrated that the time frame of the question can influence participants' responses. For example, when asked to recall how often they felt angry in the past year, participants' estimates were lower in frequency but higher in intensity than when they recalled how often they felt angry in the past week (Winkielman, Knäuper, & Schwartz, 1998). Presumably as the time frame increases, participants discount low levels of anger and retrieve instances of more salient, intense anger. But with repeated assessments every few hours or so, what frame of reference do respondents use? Some researchers instruct participants to respond according to how they were feeling at the moment, while others instruct participants to recall their experiences since the last report. In any case, the time of reference is much shorter than with global reports. The threshold for what is considered an angry state, for example, might be lower when one considers the past few hours as opposed to the past week. Additionally, participants might rate their present state in reference to their previous states (e.g., Compared to my other reports, how happy am I right now?). Thus, the meaning of momentary reports might change compared to between-subject responses. These are empirical questions that, unfortunately, have not received much attention thus far.

Data Issues: Now What?

Once the data are successfully collected, the ESM researcher is often left staring at 10,000–50,000 data points, wondering how to proceed. After all, as Larson & Delespaul (1992) note, "ESM data have a complexity which defies textbook analysis" (p. 58). With the ability to capture more of the complexities of life comes the complexities of data analysis, and ESM researchers face the challenge of choosing a statistical strategy that addresses the unique nature of the data.

Aggregation Issues

One way to handle the massive amount of data that experience sampling studies generate is to aggregate momentary data, for example, computing a mean intensity rating of happiness for each participant over the entire week. This procedure has the main advantage of being straightforward and manageable. Furthermore, aggregation increases reliability and gives higher correlations (Epstein, 1980). But does the meaning of one's construct change as variables are aggregated over time? Diener & Larsen (1984) found that personal consistency and stable patterns emerged when responses were aggregated over several occasions, whereas for single moments, there was little consistency for most variables. Thus, the two levels of analysis are independent of one another, and aggregate level data cannot be used to make assertions about what occurs at the momentary level (Snijders & Bosker, 1999). Ultimately, the nature of one's research questions should specify the level of inquiry (see Larson & Delespaul, 1992), and one's theories will determine which level is most appropriate.

A second concern is that response sets might get amplified through aggregation. For example, factor analysis at the within-person level, which controls for response styles, reveals more negative correlations between positive and negative affect than between-person correlations. However, positive and negative affect are more independent (e.g., Diener & Emmons, 1985) or positively related (e.g., Diener, Larsen, Levine, & Emmons, 1985; Larsen & Diener, 1987; Schimmack & Diener, 1997) when aggregated states are used. This difference in correlations between momentary data and aggregated data may be partly an effect of response style, such as number use, which might cancel the inverse relation between different types of emotion. Although Schimmack and his colleagues (Schimmack, 2003; Schimmack, Bockenholt, & Reisenzein, 2002) have documented the operation of response sets on aggregated data, their results show that the effect is negligible and unlikely to bias correlations in a strong way. Nevertheless, the problem of aggregation is central to subjective well-being research because of the increasing reliance on aggregate experience sampling data as measures of trait affect.

Challenges in Analyzing Data

ESM data can be analyzed at the event, subject, and group level (Larson & Delespaul, 1992). At the event level, it is typical to count frequencies of certain events. However, the researcher must take care that first, the event is common enough that the frequency count is meaningful, and second, that a few individuals who experience a given event frequently do not skew mean levels. For example, at a cursory glance, the researcher may find that attending church service may be associated with heightened feelings of joy and gratitude. However, a closer look may show that most of the participants did not respond to the signal while actually attending the service because of its disruptive nature. The few participants who did respond might therefore have a greater influence on the overall results. While some of these issues may be solved by conducting a subject-level analysis supplement to the event-level analysis, events that do not recur several times a day, such as church attendance, may be too rare for such analysis to be meaningful.

If the target variable can be recorded with requisite frequency, then the researcher can simply consider differences in the within-person variability in the frequency of the target event or behavior (Larson & Delespaul, 1992). Furthermore, the researcher can make use of multi-level modeling, such as hierarchical linear modeling (HLM), that allow the simultaneous estimation of within- and between-person effects, and the interactions between the within and the between variables (Reis & Gable, 2000). Multilevel modeling is particularly useful in analyzing ESM data because it allows the researcher to take full advantage of the fact that multiple data points were gathered from a single individual. Furthermore, multilevel analyses tend to handle missing data well (Snijders & Bosker, 1999); thus, the missed signals by the respondents pose a smaller problem for the researcher.

Another challenge in the analysis of ESM data is the existence of time dependencies in the data. That is, not only are the data nonindependent within individuals, various patterns that may be present in the data may be time-dependent as well (Reis & Gable, 2000; West & Hepworth, 1991). As mentioned earlier, various factors can influence mood, such as time of day (Rusting & Larsen, 1998), day of week (Egloff et al., 1995; Larsen & Kasimatis, 1990), or mood from the previous day or moment (Larsen, 1987). Researchers should be careful to control for such factors when modeling their data. Additionally, time series analysis may help clarify the time-dependencies in the data. For example, spectral analysis is one way in which the frequency of change over time can be analyzed, as opposed to simple examination of within-person standard deviations. In other words, fluctuation in the responses can be understood idiographically, but also can be used as an index through which between-person comparisons can be made (see Larsen, 1987, for more in-depth explanation and example of this analytic technique).

Because spectral analysis assumes a curvilinear relation, one needs to first make sure that the data support such a relationship. For example, Larsen & Kasimatis (1990) report that daily fluctuations in mood follow a 7-day cycle, such that the pattern assumes the shape of a sine curve. That is, a curvilinear relation between the day of the week and mood exists, such that the daily hedonic level increases from a low-point on Monday to a high-point on Saturday, then drops again to the Monday low. In contrast, a linear relationship would assume that a straight line would best capture the relationship between the days of the week and hedonic levels. That is, hedonic level would either continue to increase, decrease, or remain the same over the number of days.

While new analytic methods allow researchers to better understand the various nested relationships within the data, the robustness of these new methods remains largely untested (Reis & Gable, 2000). Furthermore, assumptions that underlie the analytic strategy must also be considered before these methods can be used. For example, while hierarchical linear models assume a linear relationship, spectral analytic models assume a curvilinear relationship. Unless these assumptions are met, such analyses may be inappropriate or misleading. New statistical techniques are needed that take into account the time dependencies in ESM data, and which are compatible with the uneven time periods between assessments.

Special Ethical Issues

As mentioned earlier, participants must be provided with just compensation for their cooperation in the burdensome tasks of an experience sampling study. But as Tennen, Suls, and Affleck (1991) note, "At what point does incentive shade into coercion?" (p. 320). For this reason, IRB committees may frown upon too much compensation for participation, leaving ESM researchers with the challenge of providing fair, yet non-coercive, incentives.

Also, through the use of ESM, are researchers intruding into people's private lives? Compared to other forms of behavioral assessment or experiments, the privacy of individuals is considerably protected in experience sampling studies. First and foremost, the participant retains a great deal of control over experience sampling information – for instance, when to respond to signals, and what to report. Of course, from the researcher's perspective, this is a limitation. For example, as Csikszentmihalyi & Larson (1987) pointed out, if employers used ESM to assess worker productivity, or if ESM were used to investigate sensitive, perhaps even illegal activities, then the veracity of such reports would be questionable. But still, from the participants' perspective, privacy would be preserved. However, technological advances may force researchers to reexamine the boundaries of privacy and science in the future, for example if global positioning satellite devices were to be implanted in palmtop computers.

Future Direction

Researchers looking for a panacea in ESM will be sorely disappointed. Like all other methods and measures, it has both strengths and weaknesses. Clearly, future research should turn towards testing reactivity, clarifying the meaning of scales, and validating data analytic procedures such as aggregation and modeling techniques.

Until these issues are resolved, experience sampling measures, although highly valuable and informative, should not be accepted as the "gold-standard" of measures.

Nevertheless, ESM remains a powerful tool that can aid researchers in tackling new questions as well as investigating current questions in greater depth. Our lengthy discussion of the pitfalls associated with ESM should not discourage the potential and current ESM user. We have highlighted some areas of concern so that these concerns can be resolved and addressed. By drawing attention to these deficits, we hope to stimulate research that will address some of these concerns and bolster ESM's usage in psychological research.

Conclusions

In spite of ESM's relatively short history, it is enjoying increasing popularity among researchers in various fields. The growing afford-ability of the tools used in ESM, such as palmtop computers, should make ESM even more attractive to many researchers. Of course, ESM entails greater commitment in terms of time and monetary resources than a single time questionnaire, but it is likely to produce greater payoffs, in terms of deeper understanding and more detail. Plus, when the researcher is aware of the pitfalls and takes precautions to avoid potential hazards, ESM can be a boon to research. Ultimately, the nature of one's research questions should guide the decision of whether to use experience sampling.

When paired with other methods of assessment, ESM may be particularly beneficial to the study of happiness. First, given the definition of subjective well-being (SWB: a combination of pleasant affect, low unpleasant affect, and satisfaction with life, see Diener, 1984), ESM is most useful in assessing the affective components of SWB, particularly because these components are vulnerable to distortions in memory (Kahneman, 1999). Experience sampling of the cognitive component, however, may not be necessary because this component shows high consistency (see Conner, Feldman Barrett, Bliss-Moreau, Lebo, & Kaschub, 2003; Diener & Larsen, 1984). On the other hand, momentary satisfaction judgments might still prove useful in understanding the different ways in which people incorporate satisfaction with specific domains or satisfaction on specific occasions with global life satisfaction (Diener, Lucas, Oishi, & Suh, 2002). Second, experience sampling can enable SWB research to move beyond the understanding of the demographics of happiness towards identifying the specific mechanisms and causal influences of SWB (Diener & Biswas-Diener, 2000).

The potential pitfalls outlined above underscore the need to pilot test materials before embarking on long studies with actual participants. Oneself and one's research group make excellent trial participants, and we recommend that researchers carry the signaling device for the expected duration of the study, or for at least several days, prior to actual data collection. This allows the researcher to experience first-hand the various difficulties that a participant may encounter and make necessary adjustments to the research plan instead of subjecting participants to impossible tasks. This experience also allows the researcher to better train participants, and with better training, greater compliance will follow. Compliance is especially important in ESM studies because the ecological strength of ESM is dependent on this compliance. But if the participant is compliant only under certain circumstances, such as when he or she is bored and has nothing else to do, or when he or she is in a good mood, then the assumption of ecological validity is weakened.

In sum, while ESM provides the researcher with a helpful tool with which one can further one's research goals, like any other tool, its utility can only be measured by the care with which the researcher plans and conducts the research, analyzes the findings, and interprets the results. ESM is one of the more effective tools in a growing repertory of means from which the researcher can delve into important psychological questions.

References

Alliger, G. M., & K. J. Williams. (1993). Using signal-contingent experience sampling methodology to study work in the field: A discussion and illustration examining task perceptions and mood. *Personnel Psychology, 46,* 525–549.

Ayllon, T., & E. Haughton. (1964). Modification of symptomatic verbal behavior of mental patients. *Behavioral Research Therapy, 2,* 87–98.

Bank, L., Dishion, T. J., Skinner, M., & Patterson, G. R. (1990). Method variance in structural equation modeling: Living with "glop". In G. R. Patterson (Ed.), *Depression and Aggression in family interaction: Advances in family research* (pp. 247–279). Lawrence Erlbaum Hillsdale, NJ: Associates Inc.

Barnes, R. M. (1956). *Work sampling.* New York: Wiley.

Beidel, D. C., Neal, A. M., & Lederer, A. S. (1991). The feasibility and validity of a daily diary for the assessment of anxiety in children. *Behavior Therapy, 22,* 505–517.

Brandstaetter, H. (1983). Emotional responses to other persons in everyday life situations. *Journal of Personality and Social Psychology, 45,* 871–883.

Brunswik, E. (1949). *Systematic and representative design of psychological experiments.* Berkeley, CA: University of California Press.

Campbell, D. T., & Fiske, D. W. (1959). Convergent and discriminant validation by the multitrait-multimethod matrix. *Psychological Bulletin, 56,* 81–105.

Case Institute of Technology. (1958). An operations research study of the scientific acitivy of chemists. Cleveland, Ohio: Operations Research Group.

Cattell, R. B. (1957). *Personality and motivation: Structure and measurement.* New York: World Book.

Cerin, E., Szabo, A., & Williams, C. (2001). Is the experience sampling method (ESM) appropriate for studying pre-competitive emotions? *Psychology of Sport and Exercise, 2,* 27–45.

Conner, T., Feldman Barrett, L., Bliss-Moreau, E., Lebo, K., & Kaschub, C. (2003). A practical guide to experience-sampling procedures. *Journal of Happiness Studies, 4,* 53–78.

Cote, S., & Moskowitz, D. S. (1998). On the dynamic covariation between interpersonal behavior and affect: Prediction from neuroticism, extroversion, and agreeableness. *Journal of Personality and Social Psychology, 75,* 1032–1046.

Cruise, C. E., Broderick, J., Porter, L., Kaell, A., & Stone, A. A. (1996). Reactive effects of diary self-assessment in chronic pain patients. *Pain, 67,* 253–258.

Csikszentmihalyi, M., & Larson, R. (1984). *Being adolescent: Conflict and growth in the teenage years.* New York: Basic Books.

Csikszentmihalyi, M., & Larson, R. (1987). Validity and reliability of the experience sampling method. *Journal of Nervous and Mental Disease, 175,* 526–537.

Csikszentmihalyi, M., Larson, R., & Prescott, S. (1977). The ecology of adolescent activity and experience. *Journal of Youth and Adolescence, 6*, 281–294.

Cutler, S. E., Larsen, R. J., & Bruce, S. C. (1996). Repressive coping style and the experience and recall of emotion: A naturalistic study of daily affect. *Journal of Personality, 64*, 379–405.

delle Fave, A., & Massimini, F. (1992). The ESM and the measurement of clinical change: A case of anxiety disorder. In M. W. deVries (Ed.), *The experience of psychopathology: investigating mental disorders in their natural settings* (pp. 280–289). New York: Cambridge University Press.

Diener, E., & Biswas-Diener, R. (2000). New directions in subjective well-being research: The cutting edge. *Indian Journal of Clinical Psychology, 27*, 21–23.

Diener, E., & Diener, C. (1996). Most people are happy. *Psychological Science, 7*, 181–185.

Diener, E., & Emmons, R. A. (1985). The independence of positive and negative affect. *Journal of Personality and Social Psychology, 47*, 1108–1117.

Diener, E., & Fujita, F. (1995). Resources, personal strivings, and subjective wellbeing: A nomthetic and idiographic approach. *Journal of Personality and Social Psychology, 68*, 926–935.

Diener, E., & Larsen, R. J. (1984). Temporal stability and cross-situational consistency of affective, behavioral, and cognitive responses. *Journal of Personality and Social Psychology, 47*, 871–883.

Diener, E., Larsen, R. J., & Emmons, R. A. (1984). Person × situation interactions: Choice of situations and congruence response models. *Journal of Personality and Social Psychology, 47*, 580–592.

Diener, E., Larsen, R. J., Levine, S., & Emmons, R. A. (1985). Intensity and frequency: Dimensions underlying positive and negative affect. *Journal of Personality and Social Psychology, 48*, 1253–1265.

Diener, E., Lucas, R. E., Oishi, S., & Suh, E. M. (2002). Looking up and looking down: Weighting good and bad information in life satisfaction judgments. *Personality and Social Psychology Bulletin, 28*, 437–445.

Diener, E., Smith, H., & Fujita, F. (1995). The personality structure of affect. *Journal of Personality and Social Psychology, 69*, 130–141.

Egloff, B., Tausch, A., Kohlmann, C.-W., & Krohne, H. W. (1995). Relationships between time of day, day of the week, and positive mood: Exploring the role of the mood measure. *Motivation and Emotion, 19*, 99–110.

Emmons, R. A. (1986). Personal strivings: An approach to personality and subjective well-being. *Journal of Personality and Social Psychology, 51*, 1058–1068.

Epstein, S. (1980). The stability of behavior: Implications for psychological research. *American Psychologist, 9*, 790–806.

Fahrenberg, J., & Myrtek, M. (Eds.). (2001). *Progress in ambulatory assessment: Computer-assisted psychological and psychophysiological methods in monitoring and field studies*. Kirkland, WA: Hogrefe and Huber Publishers.

Feldman Barrett, L. (1997). The relationships among momentary emotion experiences, personality descriptions, and retrospective ratings of emotion. *Personality and Social Psychology Bulletin, 23*, 1100–1110.

Fiske, D. (1971). *Measuring the concepts of personality*. Chicago: Aldine.

Flory, J. D., Raeikkoenen, K., Matthews, K. A., & Owens, J. F. (2000). Self-focused attention and mood during everyday social interactions. *Personality and Social Psychology Bulletin, 26*, 875–883.

Flügel, J. C. (1925). A quantitative study of feeling and emotion in every day life. *British Journal of Psychology, 15*, 318–355.

Funder, D. C. (2001). Personality. *Annual Review of Psychology, 52*, 197–221.

Han, J. J., Leichtman, M. D., & Wang, Q. (1998). Autobiographical memory in Korean, Chinese, and American children. *Developmental Psychology, 34*, 701–713.

Heiland, R. E., & Richardson, W. J. (1957). *Work sampling*. New York: McGraw-Hill.

Henry, B., Moffitt, T., Caspi, A., Langley, J., & Silva, P. A. (1994). On the "remembrance of things past": A longitudinal evaluation of the retrospective method. *Psychological Assessment, 6*, 92–101.

Hinricks, J. R. (1964). Communications activity of industrial research personnel. *Personnel Psychology, 17*, 193–204.

Hormuth, S. E. (1986). The sampling of experiences in situ. *Journal of Personality, 54*, 262–293.

Hurlburt, R. T. (1997). Randomly sampling thinking in the natural environment. *Journal of Consulting and Clinical Psychology, 65*, 941–949.

Isen, A. M. (1970). Success, failure, attention, and reaction to others: The warm glow of success. *Journal of Personality and Social Psychology, 15*, 294–301.

Isen, A. M., & Levin, P. F. (1972). Effect of feeling good on helping: Cookies and kindness. *Journal of Personality and Social Psychology, 21*, 384–388.

Ji, L.-J., Schwarz, N., & Nisbett, R. E. (2000). Culture, autobiographical memory, and behavioral frequency reports: Measurement issues in cross-cultural studies. *Personality and Social Psychology Bulletin, 26*, 585–593.

Kahneman, D. (1999). Objective happiness. In D. Kahneman, E. Diener, & N. Schwarz (Eds.), *Well-being: The foundations of hedonic psychology* (pp. 3–25). New York: Russell Sage Foundation.

Klinger, E. (1978–1979). Dimensions of thought an dimagery in normal waking states. *Journal of Altered States of Consciousness, 4*, 97–113.

Lamiell, J. T. (1997). Individuals and the differences between them. In R. Hogan, J. A. Johnson, & S. R. Briggs (Eds.), *Handbook of personality psychology* (pp. 117–141). San Diego, CA: Academic Press.

Larsen, R. J. (1987). The stability of mood variability: A spectral analytic approach to daily mood assessments. *Journal of Personality and Social Psychology, 52*, 1195–1204.

Larsen, R. J., & Diener, E. (1987). Affect intensity as an individual difference characteristic: A review. *Journal of Research in Personality, 21*, 1–39.

Larsen, R. J., & Kasimatis, M. (1990). Individual differences in entrainment of mood to the weekly calendar. *Journal of Personality and Social Psychology, 58*, 164–171.

Larson, R. W., Richards, M. H., & Perry-Jenkins, M. (1994). Divergent worlds: The daily emotional experience of mothers and fathers in the domestic and public spheres. *Journal of Personality and Social Psychology, 67*, 1034–1046.

Larson, R., & Delespaul, P. A. E. G. (1992). Analyzing experience sampling data: A guidebook for the perplexed. In M. W. deVries (Ed.), *The experience of psychopathology: Investigating mental disorders in their natural settings* (pp. 58–78). New York: Cambridge University Press.

Litt, M. D., Cooney, N. L., & Morse, P. (1998). Ecological momentary assessment (EMA) with treated alcoholics: Methodological problems and potential solutions. *Health Psychology, 17*, 48–52.

Lucas, R. E. (2000). *Pleasant affect and sociability: Towards a comprehensive model of extraverted feelings and behaviors.* Unpublished Doctoral Dissertation, University of Illinois, Urbana-Champaign.

Lynn, P. (2001). The impact of incentives on response rates to personal interview surveys: Role and perceptions of interviewers. *International Journal of Public Opinion Research, 13*, 326–336.

Mathews, A., & MacLeod, C. (1994). Cognitive approaches to emotion and emotional disorderes. *Annual Review of Psychology, 45*, 25–50.

McAdams, D. P. (1995). What do we know when we know a person? *Journal of Personality, 63*, 365–396.

McFarland, C., Ross, M., & DeCourville, N. (1989). Womens theories of menstruation and biases in recall of menstrual symptoms. *Journal of Personality and Social Psychology, 57*, 522–531.

Mehl, M. R., Pennebaker, J. W., Crow, M., Dabbs, J., & Price, J. (2001). The electronically activated recorder (EAR): A device for sampling naturalistic daily activities and conversations. *Behavioral Research Methods, Instruments, and Computers, 33*, 517–523.

Mischel, W. (1968). *Personality and assessment.* New York: Wiley.

Nolen-Hoeksema, S. (1993). Sex differences in control of depression. In P. D. M. Wegner & J. W. Pennebaker (Eds.), *Handbook of mental control* (pp. 306–324). New Jersey: Prentice-Hall.

Nowlis, D. P., & Cohen, A. Y. (1968). Mood-reports and the college natural setting: A day in the lives of three roommates under academic pressure. *Psychological Reports, 23,* 551–566.

Oishi, S. (2002). *The function of daily vs. retrospective judgments of satisfaction in relationship longevity.* Manuscript in preparation.

Oishi, S., Diener, E., Scollon, C. N., & Biswas-Diener, R. (2004). Cross-situational consistency of affective experiences across cultures. *Journal of Personality and Social Psychology, 86,* 460–472.

Pavot, W., Diener, E., & Fujita, F. (1990). Extraversion and happiness. *Personality and Individual Differences, 11,* 1299–1306.

Pelham, B. W. (1993). The idiographic nature of human personality: Examples of the idiographic self-concept. *Journal of Personality and Social Psychology, 64,* 665–677.

Ptacek, J. T., Smith, R. E., Espe, K., & Raffety, B. (1994). Limited correspondence between daily coping reports and retrospective coping recall. *Psychological Assessment, 6,* 41–49.

Redelmeier, D. A., & Kahneman, D. (1996). Patients memories of painful medical treatments: Real-time and retrospective evaluations of two minimally invasive procedures. *Pain, 66,* 3–8.

Reis, H. T., & Gable, S. L. (2000). Event-sampling and other methods for studying everyday experience. In H. T. Reis & C. M. Judd (Eds.), *Handbook of research methods in social and personality psychology* (pp. 190–222). New York: Cambridge University Press.

Robinson, D., & Clore, G. L. (2002). Episodic and semantic knowledge in emotional self-report: Evidence for two judgment processes. *Journal of Personality and Social Psychology, 83,* 198–215.

Ross, M. (1989). Relation of implicit theories to the construction of personal histories. *Psychological Review, 96,* 341–357.

Rusting, C. L., & Larsen, R. J. (1998). Diurnal patterns of unpleasant mood: Associations with neuroticism, depression, and anxiety. *Journal of Personality, 66,* 85–103.

Ruble, D. N. (1977). Premenstrual symptoms: A reinterpretation. *Science, 197,* 291–292.

Schimmack, U. (2003). Affect measurement in experience sampling research. *Journal of Happiness Studies, 4,* 79–106.

Schimmack, U. (2002). Frequency judgments of emotions: The cognitive basis of personality assessment. In P. Sedelmeier & T. Betsch (Eds.), *Frequency processing and cognition.* Oxford: Oxford University Press.

Schimmack, U., & Diener, E. (1997). Affect intensity. Separating intensity and frequency in repeatedly measured affect. *Journal of Personality and Social Psychology, 73,* 1313–1329.

Schimmack, U., Bockenholt, U., & Reisenzein, R. (2002). Response styles in affect ratings: Making a moutain out of a molehill. *Journal of Personality Assessment, 78,* 461–483.

Schwarz, N. (1994). Judgment in a social context: Biases, shortcomings, and the logic of conversation. In M. Zanna (Ed.), *Advances in experimental social psychology* (Vol. 26, pp. 123–162). San Diego, CA: Academic Press.

Schwarz, N. (1999). Self-reports: How the questions shape the answers. *American Psychologist, 54,* 93–105.

Shedler, J., Mayman, M., & Manis, M. (1993). The illusion of mental health. *American Psychologist, 48,* 1117–1131.

Scollon, C. N., Diener, E., Oishi, S., & Biswas-Diener, R. (2002). *Culture, selfconcept, and memory for emotions.* Manuscript under review.

Scollon, C. N., Diener, E., & Oishi, S. (2002). *An experience sampling and cross-cultural investigation of dialectical emotional experience.* Manuscript in preparation.

Snijders, T. A. B., & Bosker, R. J. (1999). *Multilevel analysis: An introduction to basic and advanced multilevel modeling.* Thousand Oaks, CA: Sage Publications.

Stone, A. A., Kessler, R. C., & Haythornwaite, J. A. (1991). Measuring daily events and experiences: Decisions for the researcher. *Journal of Personality, 59,* 575–607.

Stone, A. A., Schwartz, J. E., Neale, J. M., Shiffman, S., Marco, C. A., Hickcox, M., et al. (1998). A comparison of coping assessed by ecological momentary assessment and retrospective recall. *Journal of Personality and Social Psychology, 74*, 1670–1680.

Stone, A. A., Shiffman, S. S., & DeVries, M. W. (1999). Ecological momentary assessment. In D. Kahneman, E. Diener, & N. Schwarz (Eds.), *Well-being: Foundations of a hedonic psychology* (pp. 26–39). New York: Russell Sage Foundation.

Tennen, H., Suls, J., & Affleck, G. (1991). *Personality and daily experience: The promise and the challenge. Journal of Personality, 59*, 313–337.

Thomas, D. L., & Diener, E. (1990). Memory and accuracy in the recall of emotions. *Journal of Personality and Social Psychology, 59*, 291–297.

Tversky, A., & Kahneman, D. (1973). *Judgment under uncertainty: Heuristics and biases*. Eugene, OR: Oregon Research Institute.

Wang, Q. (2001). Culture effects on adults earliest childhood recollection and selfdescription: Implications for the relation between memory and the self. *Journal of Personality and Social Psychology, 81*, 220–233.

Wessman, A. E., & Ricks, D. F. (1966). Mood and personality. New York: Holt, Rinehart and Winston.

West, S. G., & Hepworth, J. T. (1991). Statistical issues in the study of temporal data: Daily experiences. *Journal of Personality, 59*, 609–662.

Wheeler, L., & Reis, H. T. (1991). Self-recordings of everyday life events: Origins, types, and uses. *Journal of Personality, 59*, 339–354.

Wilson, K. C. M., Hopkins, R., deVries, M. W., & Copeland, J. R. M. (1992). Research alliance and the limit of compliance: Experience sampling with the depressed elderly. In M. W. deVries (Ed.), *The experience of psychopathology: Investigating mental disorders in their natural settings*. New York: Cambridge University Press.

Winkielman, P., Knäuper, B., & Schwarz, N. (1998). Looking back at anger: Reference periods change the interpretation of (emotion) frequency questions. *Journal of Personality and Social Psychology, 75*, 719–728.

Wirtz, D., Kruger, J., Scollon, C. N., & Diener, E. (2003). What to do on spring break? The role of predicted, on-line, and remembered experience in future choice. *Psychological Science, 14*, 520–524.

Wong, M., & Csikszentmihalyi, M. (1991). Motivation and academic achievement: The effects of personality traits and the quality of experience. *Journal of Personality, 59*, 539–574.

Zelenski, M., & Larsen, R. J. (2000). The distribution of basic emotions in everyday life: A state and trait perspective from experience sampling data. *Journal of Research in Personality, 34*, 178–197.

Zirkel, S., & Cantor, N. (1990). Personal construal of life tasks: Those who struggle for independence. *Journal of Personality and Social Psychology, 58*, 172–185.

Life-Satisfaction Is a Momentary Judgment and a Stable Personality Characteristic: The Use of Chronically Accessible and Stable Sources

Ulrich Schimmack, Ed Diener, and Shigehiro Oishi

Abstract Social cognition research indicates that life-satisfaction judgments are based on a selected set of relevant information that is accessible at the time of the life-satisfaction judgment. Personality research indicates that life-satisfaction judgments are quite stable over extended periods of time and predicted by personality traits. The present article integrates these two research traditions. We propose that people rely on the same sources to form repeated life-satisfaction judgments over time. Some of these sources (e.g., memories of emotional experiences, academic performance) provide stable information that explains the stability in life-satisfaction judgments. Second, we propose that the influence of personality traits on life satisfaction is mediated by the use of chronically accessible sources because traits produce stability of these sources. Most important, the influence of extraversion and neuroticism is mediated by use of memories of past emotional experiences. To test this model, participants repeatedly judged life-satisfaction over the course of a semester. After each assessment, participants reported sources that they used for these judgements. Changes in reported sources were related to changes in life-satisfaction judgments. A path model demonstrated that chronically accessible and stable sources are related to stable individual differences in life-satisfaction. Furthermore, the model supported the hypothesis that personality effects were mediated by chronically accessible and stable sources. In sum, the results are consistent with our theory that life-satisfaction judgments are based on chronically accessible sources.

Over the past two decades research on the determinants of subjective well-being has increased dramatically (Argyle, 1987; Diener, Suh, Lucas, & Smith, 1999; Myers, 1992). Researchers typically distinguish an affective component and a cognitive component of subjective well-being. The present article focuses on the cognitive component of subjective well-being, that is, people's evaluations of their lives. This component of subjective well-being is typically assessed by life-satisfaction

U. Schimmack (✉)
Department of Psychology, University of Toronto at Mississauga, Erindale College,
Mississauga, Ontario, L5L 1C6, Canada
e-mail: uli.schimmack@utoronto.ca.

E. Diener (ed.), *Assessing Well-Being: The Collected Works of Ed Diener*,
Social Indicators Research Series 39, DOI 10.1007/978-90-481-2354-4_9,
© Springer Science+Business Media B.V. 2009

judgments, (e.g., "I am satisfied with my life"; cf., Diener, Emmons, Larsen, & Griffin, 1985). The use of judgments to assess life-satisfaction stimulated two research traditions. On the one hand, a social cognition tradition has studied the cognitive processes underlying judgments of life-satisfaction (see Schwarz and Strack, 1999, for a review). On the other hand, a personality tradition has studied predictors of individual differences in life-satisfaction (see Diener & Lucas, 1999, for a review). These traditions evolved relatively independent of each other. The present article presents an integrated model of life-satisfaction that incorporates the major findings of both traditions.

Integrating the Social Cognition and the Personality Tradition

The social-cognition tradition used experimental or quasi-experimental studies to study the processes underlying life-satisfaction judgments. For example, participants reported their life-satisfaction after a pleasant or unpleasant mood induction, before or after answering a question about dating, or in the presence or absence of a handicapped confederate (Schwarz and Strack, 1999). These studies demonstrate that life-satisfaction judgments are sometimes influenced by temporarily accessible information. Additional studies showed that people disregard accessible information that is considered irrelevant (Schwarz and Clore, 1983). To account for these findings, Schwarz and Strack (1999) developed a model of life-satisfaction judgments. The model assumes that life-satisfaction judgments are based on a few, easily accessible, and relevant sources. This model has been used to explain why life-satisfaction judgments often are unrelated to objective indicators of people's lives and why life-satisfaction judgments sometimes show low retest reliabilities. Based on this model, Schwarz and Strack (1999) suggested, "there is little to be learned from self-reports of global well-being. Although these reports do reflect subjectively meaningful assessments, what is being assessed, and how, seems to be too context-dependent to provide reliable information about a population's well-being, let alone information that can guide public policy" (p. 80).

The personality tradition usually relies on correlational studies in which individual differences in life-satisfaction are related to individual differences in predictor variables such as self-esteem (Diener & Diener, 1995) or the Big Five personality dimensions (Costa & McCrae, 1980; McCrae and Costa, 1991). These studies indicate that personality influences life-satisfaction, with extraversion and neuroticism being the most reliable predictors (cf. Diener & Lucas, 1999). Furthermore, research in this tradition demonstrated that life-satisfaction is quite stable over extended periods of time. For example, Pavot and Diener (1993) reported a retest-correlation of 0.82 over a 2-month period and a retest-correlation of 0.54 over a period of 4 years. These findings have been interpreted as evidence that "situational factors usually pale in comparison with long-term influences on well-being measures" (Diener, 2000, p. 35).

At first sight, the two traditions have produced conflicting results. However, we suggest that both traditions have provided valuable insights that can be integrated into a common model. Following Schwarz and Strack (1999), we propose that life-satisfaction judgments are based on accessible and relevant information. Sometimes people rely on *temporarily accessible* information. However, in addition, people are likely to use *chronically accessible* information (cf. Schwarz and Strack, 1999). For example, thoughts about the satisfaction with important life domains (e.g., work, social relationships) may automatically come to mind when asked about life-satisfaction. Furthermore, these chronically accessible sources may provide relatively stable information over time. For example, individual differences in income are relatively stable over time. If financial satisfaction were chronically accessible and people were drawing on this information in repeated life-satisfaction, then life-satisfaction judgments could be quite stable over time.

In short, we propose that participants draw on three types of sources to form life-satisfaction judgments, which have different implications for the stability and variability of life-satisfaction judgments. First, participants seem to use temporarily accessible sources that are salient in one assessment situation, but not in other situations (e.g., a handicapped confederate is present). The use of these sources produces variability in life-satisfaction judgments. Second, participants can use chronically accessible sources that provide variable information. For example, people may chronically use mood as information because it is a salient and relevant source (Schwarz and Clore, 1983). Use of mood should also produce variability in life-satisfaction judgments because mood fluctuates considerably over time (e.g., Schimmack, 1997; Schimmack & Grob, 2000). Finally, participants may use chronically accessible sources that provide stable information (e.g., satisfaction with income). The use of chronically accessible and stable sources could explain the stability of life-satisfaction judgments that has been demonstrated in the personality tradition (Pavot and Diener, 1993). Of course, stability and variability are extremes of a continuous dimension. Even chronically accessible and stable sources change over longer time intervals, which explains why life-satisfaction judgments are more stable over shorter time periods than over extended periods of time (Pavot and Diener, 1993).

Why Do People Use Certain Types of Information?

One key assumption in subjective well-being research is that people select sources because they are relevant and reflect important aspects of their lives (Diener & Lucas, 1999). Past research indicated that people use temporarily accessible information only when this information is relevant (Schwarz and Strack, 1999). For example, when the relevance of mood is drawn into question, people stop using mood as information (Schwarz and Clore, 1983). It seems plausible that chronically accessible sources are also relevant because relevant information is more accessible (Pelham, 1995; Pelham & Swann, 1989; Schwarz and Strack, 1999). For example, if somebody is married, marital satisfaction is salient and relevant for this individual. As a consequence, it is likely that the individual thinks about marital satisfaction to evaluate life-satisfaction. In contrast, this domain is less salient for singles or priests, and it is less likely that this domain comes to mind during a life-satisfaction judgment. Cross-cultural studies provide support for the hypothesis that people rely on chronically accessible sources because they are emphasized in a culture (Kwan, Bond, & Singelis, 1997; Oishi, Diener, Lucas, & Suh, 1999; Suh, Diener, Oishi, & Triandis, 1998). For example, people in collectivistic and poorer countries were more likely to rely on financial (dis)satisfaction (Oishi, Diener, Lucas, et al., 1999), social norms (Suh et al., 1998), and relationship harmony (Kwan et al., 1997), presumably because these sources are chronically accessible in these cultures. However, even within cultures, individuals are likely to use different sources to judge life-satisfaction because the relevance of sources is likely to differ across individuals. In short, we propose that chronically accessible sources reflect important aspects of people's lives. To the extent that a specific source is important to members of a particular group, it is likely to be used by most members of a group. For example, most students care about their academic performance. Hence, most students should consider this domain in their global life-satisfaction judgments. To the extent that sources vary in importance across individuals, we expect individual differences in the use of sources. For example, students may differ in the importance that they attach to the relationships with their family. In this case, we expect that students are more likely to use family satisfaction if this domain is important to them.

Integrating Top-Down and Bottom-Up Models of Life-Satisfaction

The hypothesis that people use chronically accessible and stable sources also integrates top-down and bottom-up theories of life-satisfaction (cf. Diener, 1984). Bottom-up theories assume that life-satisfaction is a summary evaluation of aspects of one's life. For example, one is satisfied with one's life because one has good social relations, enough money, and an interesting job. Top-down theories assume that life-satisfaction is due to personality influences. For example, a neurotic individual is more dissatisfied in general and with his or her job, social relations, and income in particular. Brief, Butcher, George, and Link (1993) presented an intriguing integration of these two seemingly contradictory models. Consistent with judgment theories of life-satisfaction (Schwarz and Strack, 1999), the authors proposed that life-satisfaction judgments are constructed bottom-up by considering chronically accessible sources. At the same time, personality traits produce stability in these sources. The authors presented strong support for this model for health satisfaction. The authors obtained measures of objective health (e.g., hospital visits), subjective health (participants' ratings of their health), neuroticism, and life-satisfaction. A path model indicated that health satisfaction was a joint function of objective health and neuroticism. This finding indicates a top-down influence of neuroticism on health satisfaction. The path model also indicated that life-satisfaction was based on health satisfaction. Hence, life-satisfaction was constructed in a bottom-up manner, using health as one source. The model also demonstrated that the influence of neuroticism on life-satisfaction was mediated by health satisfaction. Taken together, the model suggests that a chronically accessible and stable source (i.e., satisfaction with health) mediated the influence of neuroticism on global life-satisfaction.

Drawing on Brief et al.'s (1993) integrated model, we propose that other chronically accessible sources also mediate the influence of personality traits on life-satisfaction. As noted earlier, extraversion and neuroticism are the strongest predictors of life-satisfaction (Diener & Lucas, 1999). Furthermore, it is well known that extraversion is a disposition to experience more pleasure, whereas neuroticism is a disposition to experience more displeasure (Costa & McCrae, 1980; Diener & Lucas, 1999). Hence, these two personality traits are likely to produce stable individual differences in the actual amount of pleasure and displeasure in people's lives. Furthermore, previous research demonstrated that memories of past emotional experiences are an important chronically accessible source of life-satisfaction judgments, in particular in individualistic cultures (Ross, Eyman, & Kishchuck, 1986; Suh et al., 1998). Hence, it seems likely that memories of past emotional experiences are an important mediator of the relationship between extraversion and neuroticism and life-satisfaction. In short, we predict that personality traits are determinants of stability in chronically accessible sources of life-satisfaction judgments and that the influence of personality traits on life-satisfaction is mediated by chronically accessible sources. More specifically, we predict that the influence of extraversion and neuroticism on life-satisfaction judgments is mediated by memories of emotional experiences.

Studying Chronically Accessible Sources: The Validity of Source Reports

Previous research on life-satisfaction judgments has neglected chronically accessible sources. The reason might be the preference of social cognition researchers for experimental designs. Experimental studies have the advantage of high internal validity. However, they are not suitable to the investigation of chronically accessible information because these sources are by definition not subject to experimental manipulation. Correlational studies are also problematic because a significant correlation between life-satisfaction judgments and a source does not prove causality. For example, a significant correlation between life-satisfaction and marital status could be due to the fact that satisfied people are more likely to marry (cf. Myers, 2000). Hence, we needed a new empirical approach to study the influence of chronically accessible sources on life-satisfaction judgments. We decided to ask participants after they completed life-satisfaction judgments to report their thoughts during the judgment process. We refer to these reports as *source reports*.

After the decline of behaviorism, the assessment of people's thoughts has gained in acceptance in contemporary research, although this method is still controversial (cf. Crutcher, 1994). However, several findings over the past decades encouraged us to use this method to examine sources of life-satisfaction judgments. First, thought protocols are routinely and successfully used in persuasion research (cf. Eagly & Chaiken, 1993). For example, Osterhouse and Brock (1970) examined the influence of distraction on the effectiveness of a counter-attitudinal message with weak arguments. The authors demonstrated that higher levels of distraction produced larger attitude changes. Participants thought protocols revealed why this was the case. In the low distraction condition, participants were able to generate counterarguments to the weak messages, whereas high levels of distraction interfered with the generation of counterarguments. Further evidence for the usefulness of thought protocols stems from the cognitive literature (Ericsson & Simon, 1993). For example, Brown (1995) demonstrated that participants judge frequencies by enumerating exemplars when exemplars are easy to retrieve, but they use an intuitive estimation strategy when the retrieval of exemplars is difficult. This finding was first suggested by participants' reports of their judgment strategies and then confirmed by response latencies in a second study.

A few studies already examined sources of well-being judgments. Ross et al. (1986) asked participants to report the sources that they considered during life-satisfaction judgments. The authors found that participants often mentioned affective experiences as one source of their life-satisfaction judgments. Although the authors did not validate the reports, the reports are consistent with findings in other studies of life-satisfaction judgments (Schwarz and Clore, 1983; Suh et al., 1998). More direct evidence stems from a recent study of relationship satisfaction. Wilson and Kraft (1993) obtained thought-protocols of the reasons for romantic happiness and ratings of romantic happiness on four separate occasions from the same panel of participants. Independent raters determined the number of positive and negative statements in the thought-protocols. The scores were then related to participants' romantic happiness ratings. The correlations ranged from 0.25 to 0.81, with an average of 0.52. Schimmack (1998) obtained first evidence regarding the validity of source reports in the context of global happiness judgments. Participants rated whether they were happy or unhappy persons. Then they completed a check list with potential sources that they might have used to answer the well-being question. One question asked about mood because some participants were expected to use mood as information (Schwarz and Clore, 1983). After the source reports, participants reported their current mood. Roughly half of the participants reported using mood. Hence, it was possible to split the sample into participants who reported using mood (users, $N = 53$) and those who did not report mood (non-users, $N = 48$) and to compute the correlation between well-being judgments and current mood separately for users and for non-users. If users did indeed rely on their current mood when they answered the well-being question, then users' mood should be more highly correlated with the well-being judgment than non-users' mood. Consistent with this prediction, the correlation between mood and the well-being judgment was significantly higher for users ($r = 0.67$) than for non-users ($r = 0.25$), $z = 2.37$, $p < 0.05$ (one-tailed). We used one-tailed significance tests because we had a directed hypothesis that correlations are higher for users than for non-users. The present studies were designed to provide more definitive evidence regarding the validity of source reports. Based on the preliminary results in Schimmack's (1998) study and the usefulness of thought protocols in other research areas (cf. Ericsson & Simon, 1993), we predicted that source reports provide useful information about the determinants of life-satisfaction judgments.

Overview

The present article examines two related, yet distinct research questions. On the one hand, we examined the usefulness of source reports to study the cognitions that are underlying life-satisfaction judgments. On the other hand, we examined whether stability in chronically accessible sources that are used by a majority of participants is influenced by personality factors, and whether these sources mediate the relation between personality traits and life-satisfaction. In this part of the article we relied on findings from the first part of the article to identify chronically accessible sources that are repeatedly used by the majority of participants. We present the results in two parts. The first part examines the validity of source reports. The second part examines an integrated bottom-up, top-down model that specifies chronically accessible sources as mediators of the relation between personality traits and life-satisfaction.

Part I: The Validity of Source Reports

Pilot Study 1

Researchers have a variety of methods at their disposal to assess people's thoughts, namely (a) concurrent verbalization, (b) retrospective open-ended reports, and (c) retrospective questionnaires (e.g., Ericsson & Simon, 1993). One problem of concurrent verbalizations is that they can alter the judgment process. Retrospective questionnaires may invite participants to generate thoughts post hoc based on the questions. To avoid these potential problems, we used open-ended retrospective thought protocols in a preliminary study.

Method

Participants

Participants were 150 students at the University of Illinois, Urbana-Champaign. Students took part in the data collection as part of a semester-long course on subjective well-being (SWB).

Materials and Procedure

First participants completed the Satisfaction With Life Scale (SWLS; Diener et al., 1985) to measure life-satisfaction. The scale comprises five-items, namely (a) "In most ways my life is close to ideal," (b) "The conditions of my life are excellent," (c) "I am satisfied with my life," (d) "So far I have gotten the important things

I want in my life," and (e) "If I could live my life over, I would change almost nothing." Responses were made on a 7-point *agree-disagree* scale (Diener et al., 1985). Immediately afterwards, participants reported their thoughts during the life-satisfaction judgments on a blank page.

Results

The free responses were coded into several categories derived from the subjective well-being literature. Responses were coded as providing either clear or vague evidence that respondents had thought about a source. Respondents quite often thought about *family* (clear statements 33%, vague statements 16%), *romantic life* (22.5%, 21%), *relationships with friends* (26%, 12%), and *academic life* (20%, 16%), whereas *financial situation* (9%, 10%), *housing* (9%, 4%), and *health* (12%, 4%) were mentioned less frequently. Participants also frequently mentioned past emotional events (36%, 12%), whereas *social comparisons* (6%, 1%) and *using the past as a comparison standard* (1%, 0%) were mentioned infrequently. A classification into positive and negative statements revealed that participants thought more often about positive aspects (39%) than about negative aspects (30%).

Discussion

Study 1 provided encouraging evidence that people have access to some of their thoughts during life-satisfaction judgments. Furthermore, the results replicate Ross et al.'s (1986) finding that people often think about past emotional events when they form life-satisfaction judgments. In addition, Study 1 revealed that participants frequently mention important life domains such as relations with family, romantic partner, and friends as well as academic performance. In contrast, financial satisfaction was mentioned less frequently. This finding is consistent with evidence that financial satisfaction is a weak predictor of life-satisfaction in the United States. If people do not think about their financial situation when they form life-satisfaction judgments, then individual differences in income do not influence these judgments.

Although open-ended response formats decrease the likelihood of demand effects, they have other problems. It is most likely that participants omitted sources that they considered because they lacked the motivation to note all thoughts in writing and because they forgot some thoughts. A questionnaire overcomes these limitations because it requires the same effort to indicate that a source was used as it takes to indicate that a source was not used. Furthermore, a checklist can serve as a retrieval cue for thoughts that would have been forgotten in an open-ended report.

Pilot Study 2

Study 2 examined whether previous results from the open-ended study could be replicated with a closed-format assessment of sources. For this purpose, we focused on two life-domains that were mentioned with different frequencies in Study 1, namely satisfaction with family relationships (frequently mentioned) and satisfaction with housing (infrequently mentioned). Study 2 also tested the hypothesis that chronically accessible sources are more relevant. Hence, we also obtained ratings of the importance of the two domains. We predicted that (a) participants report using family satisfaction more frequently than housing satisfaction, (b) participants rate family satisfaction as more important than housing satisfaction, and (c) participants who report using family satisfaction or housing satisfaction rate these domains as more important than participants who report not using these domains.

Method

Participants

One-hundred and ninety students at the University of Illinois, Urbana-Champaign participated in the study. The data were collected at the beginning of a lecture in an introductory psychology class in return for extra course credit.

Materials and Procedure

Participants received a two-page questionnaire. On the first page was a five-item life-satisfaction questionnaire (cf. Schwarz and Clore, 1983). The internal consistency of the five-item scale was 0.86. At the beginning of the second page followed two dichotomous questions (yes/no) about the use of satisfaction with one's family relationships and satisfaction with one's housing situation. Next followed two items regarding the importance of the two life-domains ($0 = not\ at\ all\ important$ to $7 = of\ utmost\ importance$). The next two questions addressed how satisfied participants were with the two life-domains ($0 = totally\ dissatisfied$ to $10 = totally\ satisfied$).

Results

Consistent with the open-ended reports in Study 1, satisfaction with family relationships (83%) was reported significantly more often than satisfaction with housing (67%), sign-test $z = 3.78$, $p < 0.01$. As predicted, participants also rated family relationships as more important ($M = 6.29, SD = 1.09$) than housing ($M = 4.76, SD = 1.43$), $F(1, 189) = 151.69, p < 0.01$. Importance ratings were also related to individual differences in the report of the two domains in the source reports. Users of family relationships rated this domain as more important ($M = 6.56, SD = 0.67$) than non-users ($M = 5.03, SD = 1.67$), $F(1, 188) = 75.19, p < 0.01$, and users of housing satisfaction rated this domain as more important ($M = 5.23, SD = 1.08$) than non-users of housing satisfaction ($M = 3.79, SD = 1.59$), $F(1, 188,) = 54.36, p < 0.01$.

Next, we explored the validity of participants' source reports. The analyses follow the procedure outlined in the introduction (cf. Schimmack, 1998). We divided the sample into those participants who reported using family satisfaction (i.e., users) and those participants who reported not using family satisfaction (non-users). Then we computed the correlation between life-satisfaction and family satisfaction separately for users and for non-users. If source reports are valid, then the correlation between a source (i.e., family satisfaction) and life-satisfaction judgments should be stronger in the user-group than in the non-user group. Consistent with this prediction, the correlation between life-satisfaction and family satisfaction was higher among users ($N = 157, r = 0.44, p < 0.01$) than among non-users ($N = 33, r = 0.12, p = 0.51$), $z = 1.75, p < 0.05$ (one-tailed). The same analysis was performed for users and non-users of housing satisfaction. Again, the correlation among users ($N = 128, r = 0.35, p < 0.01$) was higher than the correlation among non-users ($N = 62, r = 0.03, p = 0.83$), $z = 2.15, p < 0.05$ (one-tailed).

Discussion

Study 2 revealed several findings. First, a closed-format questionnaire replicated the finding of Study 1 that participants report using family more often than housing. The convergent evidence with open-ended and closed-format assessments suggests that source reports reflect actual thoughts during life-satisfaction judgments. Study 2 also supported the hypothesis that relevance is related to the accessibility and use of sources. Overall, participants reported family satisfaction as more important than housing satisfaction, and they mentioned family satisfaction more often than housing information in the source report. In addition, individual differences in source reports were correlated with individual differences in importance ratings.

However, Study 2 suffers from several shortcomings. First, importance ratings were assessed after the source reports. Hence, participants may have relied on their responses on the source questionnaire to judge importance. Second, domain satisfaction was assessed shortly after the source reports. Participants may have biased their domain satisfaction judgments in order to be consistent with the life-satisfaction judgments and the source reports. To address these concerns, we conducted the main study.

Study 1: A Longitudinal Investigation

The study involved assessments of life-satisfaction in monthly intervals over the course of one semester. At each time, participants made life-satisfaction judgments, reported the use of various sources (e.g., use of current mood) and rated themselves on these dimensions (e.g., actual current mood). The study also used two types of life-satisfaction judgments. At the beginning and the end of the semester, participants made general life-satisfaction judgments without an explicit time frame. In the two assessments during the semester, participants made life-satisfaction judgments that were limited to the past month. We had two reasons for the use of monthly satisfaction judgments during the semester. First, general life-satisfaction judgments are highly stable over periods of a few months (Pavot and Diener, 1993). Hence, it would have been very difficult to observe changes are small. Assessments of satisfaction with the past month allow a better test of our hypothesis that changes in reported sources are related to changes in life-satisfaction judgments, because monthly satisfaction judgments are more variable. Second, we wanted to test whether people use different sources to evaluate longer or shorter time periods of their lives.

Method

Participants

One-hundred-and-thirty-six students at the University of Illinois, Urbana-Champaign, enrolled in a semester-long course on personality and life-satisfaction. Due to the longitudinal nature, some students missed one or more data collections. As a consequence, the final sample for the present data analyses consisted of 122 students (36 male, 86 female) who completed all data collections. On average, participants were 21 years old.

Materials

The materials are presented in the order as they appeared on the questionnaire.

Current mood. Current mood was assessed before the life-satisfaction judgments for several reasons. First, life-satisfaction judgments may influence people's moods. A participant who comes to the laboratory in a good mood, but then is made to think about his terrible family relationships, lack of a romantic partner, and bad grades might feel worse after the life-satisfaction judgments. In this case, mood ratings would be consistent with life-satisfaction judgments influenced mood. Second, mood assessments after source reports may introduce a demand to be consistent. If an individual just reported a high level of life-satisfaction and then reported using mood, he or she may feel compelled to report a positive mood to be consistent with the prior judgments. Mood assessments before the life-satisfaction judgments avoid these problems. Mood was assessed with the pleasure-displeasure subscale of the PAT questionnaire (Schimmack & Grob, 2000; see also Steyer, Schwenkmezger, Notz, & Eid, 1994). The questionnaire relies on three items to assess pleasure (pleasant, good, positive) and three items to assess displeasure (unpleasant, bad, negative). Ratings were made on 4-point intensity scale (*not at all, slightly, moderately, strongly*). We subtracted unpleasant items from pleasant items to create bipolar indicators. At all measurement occasions, the three indicators had good reliabilities (Cronbach's alpha > 0.80).

Satisfaction With Life Scale. After the mood ratings, we assessed life-satisfaction with the Satisfaction With Life Scale (Diener et al., 1985), a common five-item measure of life-satisfaction with good psychometric properties (cf. Pavot and Diener, 1993). At the beginning and the end of the semester, the SWLS was given with standard instructions. For the two assessments during the semester, the items were changed to assess satisfaction in the past month (e.g., "In the past month, I was satisfied with my life.") The internal consistency of the five-item scale was good at all four assessments (Cronbach's alpha > 0.80).

Most well-being researchers consider the use of mood as information as a source of error variance in the assessment of life-satisfaction because mood is variable and influenced by situational factors. To test whether the influence of this source can be reduced, we included explicit instructions not to use mood before the life-satisfaction judgments at Time 3 and Time 4. Incidentally, these instructions provide a conceptual replication of Schwarz and Clore's (1983) attribution manipulation. The authors found that participants do not use mood when moods are attributed to irrelevant factors like the weather. We reasoned that direct instructions might have the same effect as the indirect attribution manipulation.

Source reports. Immediately after the SWLS, participants completed source reports. The source report included 10 sources that could be used to judge life-satisfaction. Following the procedure of Pilot Study 2, participants reported the use of sources by means of dichotomous yes/no responses. The first question addressed whether participants used current mood because previous studies demonstrated that mood influences life-satisfaction judgments (Schwarz and Clore, 1983; Schimmack, 1998). The next question addressed the use of memories of past emotional experiences because previous studies found that this is another important source of life-satisfaction (Ross et al., 1986; Schimmack, 1998; Suh et al., 1998). The third question addressed use of progress towards goals because goal progress was an important determinant of life-satisfaction in a previous semester-long studies (Brunstein, 1993). Next we asked about several life-domains. We included family relations and housing to replicate the results of the pilot studies. We added academic performance, romantic relationships, and health, which were also mentioned in Pilot Study 1. Finally, we included two domains that were not mentioned in the open-ended pilot study. We included satisfaction with weather because previous studies demonstrated that people usually do not consider this source in life-satisfaction judgments (Schkade & Kahneman, 1998). The second irrelevant domain was the performance of the Illini men's basketball team. The inclusion of irrelevant sources has several advantages. They allow examining the influence of acquiescence response styles on dichotomous source reports, and they allow testing the hypothesis that people do not include irrelevant factors in life-satisfaction judgments. The second assessment of monthly satisfaction followed spring break. We speculated that students' satisfaction judgments would be influenced by their experiences during spring break. To examine whether participants report this source, we included spring break in the source questionnaire during this assessment only.

Hedonic balance. To assess the reliance on past emotions, we used a measure of hedonic balance. Participants estimated how much of the time on a typical day they experience pleasure versus displeasure. Consistent with the life-satisfaction judgment, we asked either about a typical day in general, or a typical day in the past month. The same six adjectives that were used for the mood assessment were used for the assessment of hedonic balance. However, the response format was an 8-point scale with the following response categories: 1 = *never* (0% of waking time), 2 = *slight amount* (1–5%), 3 = *some of the time* (5–25%), 4 = *less than half*

(25–50%), 5 = *more than half* (50–75%), 6 = *large amount* (75–95%), *almost always* (95–99%), *always* (100%). As for current mood, we computed a single pleasure-displeasure score (Cronbach's alphas > 0.78).

Goal progress. For global assessments, we asked about three major goals in life. For monthly assessments, we asked about three important goals in the past month. Participants first wrote a short description of the goals. Then they rated the progress that they had made toward the goal on a 4-point scale, ranging from 1 = *close to reaching this goal* to 4 = *not sure I will ever reach this goal.* We recoded the data so that high numbers reflect higher levels of goal progress. We averaged the three ratings to obtain a general index of goal progress. The internal consistency of progress toward the three different goals ranged from 0.22 to 0.38. The finding demonstrates that progress towards one goal is not strongly related to progress toward another goal. Nevertheless, the average of three goals might be a reasonable estimate of people's general sense of goal progress.

Domain satisfaction. Domain-satisfaction questions were either framed "in general" or "in the past month." Participants were asked about their satisfaction with the domains that were included in the source reports, namely academic performance, family relation-ships, romantic relationship (or the lack thereof), health, housing, weather, and the Illini men's basketball team. Each domain was rated on a 5-point scale, from 1 = *rock bottom cannot get worse* to 5 = *top cannot get better.* The second assessment of monthly satisfaction occurred after spring break. We used this opportunity to include satisfaction with spring break as a temporarily accessible source that might influence students' life-satisfaction.

Importance ratings. At the first assessment of life-satisfaction, participants also rated the importance of the seven life-domains. Importance ratings were made on a 6-point scale, ranging from 1 = *does not matter to me at all* to 6 = *is of vital importance to me.* Participants were also instructed to consider each domain separately to minimize the use of internal standards of comparison (cf. Schimmack, Oishi, Diener, & Suh, 2000).

Personality dimensions. The Big Five personality dimensions were assessed at the beginning of the semester in a session following the first assessment of life-satisfaction. We used Goldberg's 300-item questionnaire that assesses the Big Five with 60 items for each dimension (Goldberg, 1997). All scales had satisfactory reliabilities (alphas > 0.70).

Procedure

Participants completed the questionnaire with global instructions (i.e., all questions referred to life in general) at the beginning of the semester on the first measurement occasion. One month later, participants completed the questions with past-month instructions. After another month, participants repeated the questions with past-month instructions. At the end of the semester, another month later, participants repeated the life-satisfaction and source reports with global instructions. For the last two measurements, we also included special instructions before the life-satisfaction judgments. These instructions explained that mood is influenced by transient and irrelevant factors. For this reason participants were asked not to use mood in their life-satisfaction judgments.

Results

Effects described as significant met the conventional 5% level for type I errors. We present our empirical data in four sections. The first section explores the stability of life-satisfaction judgments and sources. These analyses test the claim that some sources provide rather stable information about one's life, whereas other sources provide more variable information. The analyses also address the question whether general judgments draw on more stable information than monthly judgments. The second section explores the use of sources. The results provide information about the consistency in the use of sources and about the influence of the time frame of the life-satisfaction judgments on source selection. In this section, we also explore the relation between source selection and importance of these sources. The third section explores the validity of source reports by comparing correlations between life-satisfaction judgments or changes in life-satisfaction judgments with sources.

Stability of Life-Satisfaction Judgments and Sources

First, we explored the stability of life-satisfaction judgments and sources (see Table 1). Consistent with previous studies, life-satisfaction judgments were highly stable (Pavot and Diener, 1993). The retest correlation of the two global life-satisfaction judgments at the beginning and the end of a three-month semester was high (0.73). The retest correlation of the monthly satisfaction judgments was lower (0.51), even though these were assessed only 1-month apart. This pattern of results indicates that people use more stable information to judge global life-satisfaction. Aggregating across all four assessments produced a highly reliable measure of life-satisfaction (see Table 1).

Consistent with previous findings, current mood shows low stability, whereas the moderate alpha indicates greater stability in average mood levels (e.g., Diener & Larsen, 1984; Schimmack, 1997; Steyer et al., 1994). Judgments of hedonic balance also confirm high stability in average levels of pleasure and displeasure (Costa & McCrae, 1980). The low stability of goal progress ratings might be due to the low reliability of our measures (see Method section). Most domain satisfaction judgments also revealed fairly high stability across measurements. The exceptions were satisfaction with weather and satisfaction with the Illini basketball team. The reason might be that weather and performance of the basketball team were objectively the same for all participants. Hence, variability can only be due to subjective evaluations. Interestingly, there seem to be very few stable differences in the subjective evaluation of these sources. This finding is inconsistent with the idea that generally satisfied people have a strong bias to evaluate all aspects—relevant and irrelevant—of their lives consistently more favorably than chronically dissatisfied individuals.

Table 1 Stability of life-satisfaction measures and sources

	Assessments			
	G1-G2	M1-M2	Mean *r*	Alpha
Life-Satisfaction	0.74	0.50	0.55	0.82
Sources				
Current Mood	0.30	0.29	0.29	0.62
Emotional Memories	0.65	0.59	0.58	0.85
Goal Progress	0.16	0.44	0.28	0.52
Family Relationships	0.56	0.65	0.60	0.85
Housing	0.44	0.59	0.54	0.83
Health	0.47	0.57	0.45	0.76
Academic Performance	0.51	0.57	0.52	0.81
Romantic Relationship	0.65	0.78	0.72	0.91
Weather	0.13	0.08	0.19	0.48
Illini	0.26	0.44	0.34	0.67

Note. G1-G2 = correlation between global assessments three months apart. M1-M2 = correlation between monthly assessments 1 month apart. Mean *r* = average correlation of all six pairwise combinations, alpha = reliability of the combined scale based on all four assessments.

Source Reports

Which Sources Do People Report?

Stability in source selection. Table 2 shows the percentages of source reports over the four assessments. Sources like emotional memories, goal progress, academic performance, and romantic relationships were reported by many participants, whereas very few participants reported weather and Illini basketball. To determine the stability of the source reports over time, we computed the rank order correlations of the percentages in Table 2. The correlation between the percentages of reported sources were 0.94 between the two global assessments at the beginning and the end of the semester, and 1.00 between the two monthly assessments during the semester. The average correlation among all four assessments was 0.94.

Importance ratings of life domains are consistent with previous findings that work (academic performance for students) and social life are more important than weather (Schkade & Kahneman, 1998). Next, we computed the rank order correlations between percentages of source reports and importance ratings of domains. These correlations were 0.67 or higher. This finding replicates the results of Study 2 that source reports are related to the relevance of a life domain. Romantic relationships are reported by most participants and rated as important; weather is reported by very few participants and rated as unimportant. This relationship persisted over time, in that importance ratings at the beginning of the semester predicted source reports three months later at the end of the semester. In sum, these findings indicate that source reports are not made in an ad-hoc random manner. Rather, they contain systematic information that is related to the importance of domains. This finding is consistent with our theory that relevant aspects of people's lives are chronically accessible and are easily accessible when people are asked to evaluate life-satisfaction.

Table 2 Percentages of reported sources in life-satisfaction judgments

		Assessments			
Source of Information	Importance	General 1	General 2	Monthly 1	Monthly 2
Current Mood	–	0.63	0.43	0.57	0.40
Hedonic Balance	–	0.70	0.76	0.90	0.85
Goal Progress	–	0.93	0.94	0.91	0.90
Satisfaction with...					
Family Relationships	5.26 (1)	0.78 (3)	0.81 (2)	0.53 (4)	0.69 (4)
Health	5.10 (2)	0.76 (4)	0.78 (3)	0.67 (3)	0.70 (3)
Academic Performance	4.99 (3)	0.90 (1)	0.88 (1)	0.86 (1)	0.87 (1)
Romantic Relationship	4.91 (4)	0.85 (2)	0.78 (3)	0.84 (2)	0.78 (2)
Housing (inc. Roommate)	4.02 (5)	0.57 (5)	0.50 (5)	0.48 (5)	0.55 (5)
Weather	2.38 (6)	0.09 (6)	0.07 (6)	0.12 (6)	0.07 (6)
Illini basketball team	1.22 (7)	0.01 (7)	0.03 (7)	0.01 (7)	0.03 (7)

Note. Numbers in parentheses are ranks for the domain satisfaction means in descending order.

Variability in source selection. The following analyses explored whether source reports varied significantly across the four assessments. We analyzed each source report in a *type of question* (general vs. monthly) × *time* (first vs. second assessment) repeated measurement ANOVA. Source reports of mood revealed a significant time effect, $F(1, 121) = 22.72$, $p < 0.01$. The main effect for type and the interaction were not significant. The time effect reveals that our instructions not to use mood significantly decreased reports of this information. The analyses of emotional memories revealed a main effect for type of question, $F(1, 121) = 19.30$, $p < 0.01$. Participants reported using emotional experiences more often in monthly satisfaction judgments than in global judgments. Furthermore, participants more often reported using family relationships in general satisfaction judgments than in monthly satisfaction judgements, $F(1, 121) = 29.36$, $p < 0.01$. A similar effect was observed for health satisfaction, $F(1, 121) = 6.76$, $p < 0.05$. We also analyzed the data with the non-parametric McNemar test because source reports are dichotomous variables. These analyses confirmed the results of the ANOVAs for mood, emotion memories, and family relationships, but the weaker effect for health did not reach significance. In sum, these analyses reveal that participants use slightly different sources to evaluate extended life-satisfaction and monthly life-satisfaction. This finding is inconsistent with the idea that source reports are based on implicit theories about the sources that people should use to evaluate life-satisfaction, unless one assumes that people hold different implicit theories for life-satisfaction judgments with varying time frames. Our results also provide additional evidence for the mood-as-information model. Although mood was as accessible during the last two assessments as it was during the first two assessments, fewer people reported this source because we told participants not to use this information.

Individual differences in source selection. Finally, we explored the stability of individual differences in the use of sources. These analyses were only meaningful for sources that revealed a sufficient amount of variability between individuals such as current mood, housing, and health. Regarding use of mood, we only could investigate source reports of the first two occasions because our intervention at times 3 and 4 influenced participants' natural selection of this source. Source reports of mood at time 1 and time 2 were significantly correlated (phi = 0.30). Regarding family relationships, source reports of the two monthly satisfaction judgments were significantly correlated (0.40), as were the source reports of the two general satisfaction judgments (0.45). The average correlation across all four assessments was 0.38. Regarding housing, source reports of the two monthly satisfaction judgments were significantly correlated (0.48), as were the source reports of the two general satisfaction judgments (0.30). The average correlation across all four assessments was 0.32. Finally, health-related source reports of the two monthly satisfaction judgments were significantly correlated (0.39), but the correlation for the two general satisfaction judgments did not approach significance (phi = 0.17). The average correlation across all four assessments was 0.32. Individual differences in source reports of life domains were also significantly related to importance ratings at the beginning of the semester. Importance ratings of family relationships predicted source reports of family satisfaction overall and at each of the four assessments over the semester (source reports at T1: $r = 0.36$, T2: $r = 0.34$, T3: $r = 0.23$, T4: $r = 0.25$, Average: $r = 0.41$, all $ps < 0.05$). Importance ratings of housing predicted source reports of housing satisfaction overall and at each of the four assessments over the semester (source reports at T1: $r = 0.43$, T2: $r = 0.27$, T3: $r = 0.26$, T4: $r = 0.25$, Average: $r = 0.43$, all $ps < 0.05$). The relation was weaker for health satisfaction, but the overall relationship was again significant (source reports at T1: $r = 0.18$, $p < 0.05$, T2: $r = 0.18$, $p < 0.05$, T3: $r = 0.12$, n.s., T4: $r = 0.08$, ns, Average: $r = 0.21$, all $ps < 0.05$). In sum, the results replicate the findings of Study 2 that individual differences in source reports are related to individual differences in the importance of life domains. Furthermore, for two out of three domains, the correlation remained significant for source reports three months after the importance ratings (although this relation was not significant for health satisfaction). This finding eliminates the concern that the relation is merely due to a pressure to provide consistent responses during a single assessment of both variables.

Concurrent Validation of Source Reports

Comparisons of users and non-users. The first validation relied on concurrent reports of sources, source reports, and life-satisfaction at one point in time. The analyses follow the procedure of Study 2. We first divided the sample into users and non-users on the basis of source reports. For example, participants were considered users of family satisfaction if they answered "yes" to family satisfaction in the source report questionnaire. Participants were considered non-users if they answered "no" to family relationships in the source report questionnaire. Then, we computed the correlations between a source (e.g., actual level of family satisfaction) and life-satisfaction among users and among non-users (Table 3). If users actually used family satisfaction in life-satisfaction judgments, then their family satisfaction and life-satisfaction should be more strongly correlated than the family satisfaction and life-satisfaction of non-users. Furthermore, the correlation between a source and life-satisfaction should be significant for users, but may not be significant for non-users. Table 3 confirms these predictions. First, nearly all correlations for users are significant with the notable exceptions of weather. For weather, the N is too small to obtain a reliable effect. Second, many of the correlations for non-users are non-significant. The findings for weather and Illini are particularly important because they are based on a large sample. Hence, the lack of a statistical association cannot be attributed to a lack of statistical power. Rather, these nonsignificant correlations indicate that participants' life-satisfaction judgments were indeed unrelated to satisfaction with the weather, just as one would expect on the basis of the source reports.

Table 3 Correlations between life-satisfaction and sources for users and non-users

	Assessments			
Source	General 1	General 2	Monthly 1	Monthly 2
Current Mood				
User	**0.47*** (77)	**0.64*** (53)	**0.56*** (70)	**0.42*** (49)
Non-User	0.15 (45)	0.23 (69)	0.32* (52)	0.27* (73)
Hedonic Balance				
User	**0.59*** (86)	**0.48*** (93)	**0.77*** (110)	**0.47*** (104)
Non-User	0.48* (36)	0.43 (29)	0.57 (12)	0.43 (18)
Goal Progress				
User	**0.33*** (113)	0.41* (115)	**0.52*** (111)	**0.50*** (110)
Non-User	−0.11 (9)	**0.64** (7)	−0.22 (11)	0.09 (12)
Satisfaction with...				
Family Relationships				
User	**0.34*** (95)	**0.46*** (99)	0.25 (64)	**0.23*** (84)
Non-User	0.12 (27)	0.24 (23)	−0.02 (57)	0.08 (38)
Housing				
User	**0.49*** (70)	**0.33*** (61)	**0.52*** (59)	**0.31*** (67)
Non-User	0.31* (52)	0.29* (61)	0.17 (63)	0.29* (55)
Health				
User	**0.35*** (93)	0.28* (95)	**0.43*** (82)	**0.48*** (86)
Non-User	0.06 (29)	**0.33** (27)	0.26 (40)	0.26 (36)
Academic Perform.				
User	**0.35*** (110)	**0.40*** (107)	**0.40*** (105)	**0.42*** (106)
Non-User	−0.51 (12)	0.25 (15)	−0.23 (17)	−0.23 (16)
Romantic Rel.				
User	**0.45*** (103)	**0.31*** (95)	**0.41*** (104)	**0.38*** (95)
Non-User	0.19 (19)	0.30 (27)	−0.01 (18)	0.25 (27)
Weather				
User	−0.20 (11)	**0.58** (9)	**0.20** (15)	**0.20** (9)
Non-User	**0.03** (111)	−0.07 (113)	0.16 (107)	−0.02 (113)
Illini				
User	−0.0 (1)	−0.0 (3)	−0.0 (1)	−0.0 (3)
Non-User	−0.11 (121)	−0.07 (119)	0.00 (121)	−0.01 (119)

Note. Higher correlations are printed in bold type. Number of participants in each group is printed in parentheses. Asterisks denote a correlation significantly different from zero at $p < .05$.

There are also a few significant correlations for non-users, most clearly for mood and monthly satisfaction judgments. This finding can indicate that source reports are not entirely accurate. However, it is also possible that these correlations are due to a third variable. For example, current mood may be correlated with hedonic balance in the past month. Hence, current mood can correlate with life-satisfaction when people use hedonic balance rather than mood as information.

Table 3 also allows a direct comparison of users and non-users. This comparison was not possible for the basketball team because too few participants reported using it. For the remaining nine sources, correlations for users nearly always exceeded the ones for non-users (33 of 36), $z = 4.83$, $p < 0.01$. Averaged across all 36 correlations in Table 2, the average correlation between a source and life-satisfaction was 0.41 when participants reported that they had used this source, whereas the same correlation was only 0.17 when participants reported that they had not used this information. The difference between these two correlations is significant, $t(35) = 6.03$, $p < 0.01$ (the t-test is based on z scores after Fisher r to z transformation). In sum, the results replicate the findings of Pilot Study 2 that sources are more strongly correlated with life-satisfaction judgments when participants reported using this source than when they reported not using this source. In addition, the present results generalize the results to a larger number of sources.

Weighted and unweighted domain satisfaction and life-satisfaction. The previous analyses examined one source at a time. In the following analyses, we examined the relation between life-satisfaction and multiple sources. If source reports reflect actual sources of life-satisfaction judgments, then weighing domain satisfaction by source reports should increase the relation between domain satisfaction and global life-satisfaction. To test this prediction, we created weighted and unweighted predictor variables based on the seven domains listed in Table 1. Unweighted domain satisfaction (UDS) was the average satisfaction in all seven domains. Weighted domain satisfaction (WDS) included only domains that were reported in the source reports. For example, if a participant reported using romantic satisfaction, academic satisfaction, and health satisfaction, then WDS was based on the average satisfaction in these three domains, whereas the other domains were not considered.

At each point in time, we computed hierarchical regression analyses with life-satisfaction as the criterion variable. In the first step, we entered UDS and in the second step we entered WDS into the regression equation. The incremental amount of explained variance reveals the ability of source reports to increase the fit between global life-satisfaction and domain satisfaction by taking individuals' use of domains into account. For the first assessment of life-satisfaction, UDS explained 24% of the variance. Entering WDS into the equation significantly increased the amount of explained variance in life-satisfaction by another 11% to a total of 35%. In the final equation, only WDS was significant (beta = 0.50), whereas UDS did not contribute unique variance to life-satisfaction (beta = 0.13, $p = 0.24$). Similar results were obtained at time 2 (incremental $R^2 = 10\%$, WDS beta = 0.49, UDS beta = 0.19, *ns*). At time 4, WDS still produced a significant increase in explained variance (incremental $R^2 = 4\%$), but the increase was smaller and the relation to

UDS remained significant (WDS beta $= 0.27$, UDS beta $= 0.30$). In sum, the results confirm that weighting domain satisfaction judgments by source reports improves the relationship between domain satisfaction judgments and global life-satisfaction judgments. This finding is consistent with the hypothesis that source reports reflect sources that people use to form global life-satisfaction judgments. The findings are also consistent with previous findings in the self-esteem literature that weighted esteem of self-aspects is more strongly related to global self-esteem than unweighted esteem of self-aspects (Pelham, 1995; Pelham & Swann, 1989).

Cross-Lagged Validation of Source Reports

The following analyses tested the hypothesis that source reports are related to actual changes in life-satisfaction judgments. To illustrate, consider mood as a source. Mood fluctuates considerable over time with very low stability from one life-satisfaction assessment to the next (see Table 1). The mood-as-information model assumes that people rely on their mood to judge life-satisfaction. In this case, mood should be related to changes in life-satisfaction judgments from one assessment to the next because they are influenced by a chronically accessible, yet variable, source. However, life-satisfaction judgments are also influenced by other factors that produce stability in life-satisfaction judgments over time (Pavot and Diener, 1993). In a longitudinal regression analysis, life-satisfaction at Time 2 should be influenced by life-satisfaction at Time 1 (stability) and by mood at time 2 (variability, mood-as-information effect). However, if some participants do not use mood as information, then mood should not be related to changes in life-satisfaction from Time 2 to Time 1. Hence, we predict that a source is only related to changes in life-satisfaction if participants reported using this source. That is, mood at Time 2 is a significant predictor of life-satisfaction at Time 2 above and beyond life-satisfaction at Time 1 for users, but not for non-users. Typically, researchers conduct a single regression analyses to test this prediction and interpret the beta coefficients. However, betas cannot be compared directly across samples. Hence, we conducted similar analyses that produced simple correlations instead. We first regressed life-satisfaction judgments onto previous life-satisfaction judgments. For example, life-satisfaction at Time 3 was regressed onto life-satisfaction at Time 1 and Time 2. We retained the standardized residuals of these analyses for further analyses. The standardized residuals represent changes in life-satisfaction judgments. Then, we computed separate correlations between sources at Time 3 and the standardized residuals for users and non-users. If source reports reflect actual sources, one would expect significant correlations for users, but not for non-users.

There is, however, one caveat. If a source is highly stable, using this source does not produce changes in life-satisfaction judgments. Hence, one can expect significant correlations for users only when there are valid changes in the source information. For example, we can expect stronger results for a variable source like mood than for a stable source like romantic satisfaction (see Table 1). The same reasoning also applies to the stability of life-satisfaction. As demonstrated earlier, monthly satisfaction judgments were more variable than general life-satisfaction judgments (see Table 1). Therefore, sources are more likely to predict changes in monthly satisfaction judgments than in global satisfaction judgments.

Table 4 shows the results. Overall, the results support the validity of source reports. Most comparisons (24 of 27) revealed higher correlations for users than for non-users, $z = 4.12$, $p < 0.01$. The average correlation between changes in life-satisfaction judgments and a source was 0.27 for users and 0.01 for non-users, $t(26) = 5.76$, $p < 0.01$. A closer inspection of Table 4 suggests an influence of the variability of sources and life-satisfaction judgments. Strong results were obtained for mood, a highly variable source. Table 4 also suggests that the more

Table 4 Correlations between changes in life-satisfaction and sources for users and non-users

Source	Assessments			
	General 1	General 2	Monthly 1	Monthly 2
Current Mood				
User	–	**0.40***	**0.52***	**0.38***
Non-User	–	0.06	0.29*	0.11
Emotional Memories				
User	–	**0.19**	**0.66***	**0.28***
Non-User	–	0.00	0.38	0.26
Goal Progress				
User	–	**0.19***	**0.43***	**0.41***
Non-User	–	0.03	−0.30	−0.04
Satisfaction with. . .				
Family Relationships				
User	–	**0.18**	**0.10**	**0.07**
Non-User	–	0.14	−0.26	0.01
Housing				
User	–	**0.08**	**0.40***	0.09
Non-User	–	−0.07	0.07	**0.13**
Health				
User	–	0.02	**0.35***	**0.32***
Non-User	–	0.02	0.24	0.24
Academic Perform.				
User	–	**0.16**	**0.24***	**0.32***
Non-User	–	−0.46	−0.34	−0.20
Romantic Rel.				
User	–	**0.10**	**0.29***	**0.25***
Non-User	–	−0.04	−0.16	0.18
Weather				
User	–	**0.34**	−0.03	**0.29**
Non-User	–	0.03	**0.19**	−0.02
Illini				
User	–	–	–	–
Non-User	–	0.16	0.08	−0.02

Note. Higher correlations are printed in bold type. The number of participants in each group is identical to the numbers in Table 2. Asterisks denote a correlation significantly different from zero at $p < .05$.

variable monthly satisfaction judgments produced stronger correlations than the more stable global judgments. In sum, the results indicate that source reports are related to the amount of change in life-satisfaction judgements when actual satisfaction with a source changed. For example, if family satisfaction changed over time, then life-satisfaction changed in the same direction when participants reported using this source, but not when participants did not report using this source. This finding is consistent with the hypothesis that source reports reflect actual sources of life-satisfaction judgments.

Spring Break: A Temporarily Accessible Source

The second monthly satisfaction assessment was given one week after spring break. We included questions about use and satisfaction with spring break to examine whether participants relied on this temporarily accessible source. Seventy-five percent of the participants reported using satisfaction with their spring break to judge monthly satisfaction. For users the correlation between life-satisfaction and spring-break satisfaction was significant (0.53). For non-users the correlation was significantly weaker ($r = -0.20$, difference $z = 3.60$, $p < 0.01$). Furthermore, users' satisfaction with spring break was not significantly correlated with previous life-satisfaction judgments at time 1 (0.12) and at time 2 (0.01). As a consequence, satisfaction with spring break was related to changes in life-satisfaction from before to after spring break for users ($r = 0.54$), but not for non-users ($r = -0.10$). This finding demonstrates that source reports of a temporarily accessible source reflect actual influences of temporarily accessible information on life-satisfaction.

Discussion

In the first part of this article, we presented evidence regarding source reports after completing a life-satisfaction questionnaire. The first question was whether participants have anything to report. If life-satisfaction judgements are made in an intuitive, unconscious manner, then participants would not be able to report the determinants of life-satisfaction judgments. However, our first pilot study with open-ended source reports demonstrated that participants have more to say then "I felt this way," "Six seemed to be the appropriate answer," or "I am just a happy guy." Rather, participants reported thinking about important life-domains such as their academic performance, romantic relationships, and family relationships.

Of course, these reports do not show that participants formed life-satisfaction judgments in a deliberate manner that is accessible to introspection. Alternatively, participants may have based their source reports on cultural theories of the factors that should influence life-satisfaction. For example, participants may recall the saying "Money doesn't buy happiness," and therefore report that they did not use financial satisfaction to evaluate life-satisfaction. Several findings challenge this account of source reports. First, participants reported some sources that are not salient in cultural theories of happiness, such as the use of mood as information (Schwarz and Clore, 1983). Nevertheless, participants reported this source, and mood was related to life-satisfaction judgments. On the other hand, cultural theories imply that weather is a determinant of life-satisfaction (Schkade & Kahneman, 1998). However, participants did not report this source, and it did not influence life-satisfaction judgments. Furthermore, cultural theories have problems to explain individual differences among individuals in the same culture. Although cultural theories may acknowledge variability within cultures, they do not explain these differences. However, our data show reliably individual differences in the use of sources, and these individual differences were related to the importance of life-domains. For example, participants who reported thinking about family relations also rated family relations as more important. In Study 4, this relationship was significant even when source reports and importance ratings were assessed three months apart. At the very least, our data show that source reports differed from individual to individual, and any theory of source reports has to account for this finding.

One possible explanation could be that participants spend a lot of time thinking about their lives (Diener et al., 1999). As a consequence, they have a pre-stored evaluation of their life and pre-stored theories about the determinants of their life that differ between individuals. At the time of the life-satisfaction judgment, participants may report a pre-stored evaluation. For the source reports, they may draw on pre-stored reflections about the determinants of life-satisfaction. One problem for this theory is to account for changes in life-satisfaction judgments, and for the countless examples of context effects on life-satisfaction judgments (cf. Schwarz and Strack, 1999). If life-satisfaction judgments were pre-stored in memory, why would they be influenced by a prior question about dating? In the present study, some participants reported using their mood at the time of the judgment, and life-satisfaction judgments actually changed in the direction of their current mood. Furthermore, ample evidence indicates that mood effects disappear, when participants believe that their mood is influenced by irrelevant factors (Schwarz and Clore, 1983). In the present study, fewer participants reported using mood as information when we told them that mood is an unreliable source. These findings are inconsistent with the idea that life-satisfaction judgments and source reports are based on pre-stored evaluations and personal theories of life-satisfaction.

The last alternative explanation assumes that our findings are an artifact. This theory assumes that participants have no insight into the determinants of life-satisfaction judgments based on introspection or based on prior personal theories. However, when they are confronted with source reports, they use a few simple heuristics to infer whether they used a source or not. For example, when they are asked to report whether they used family satisfaction to judge life-satisfaction, they compare the life-satisfaction judgment to their actual level of family satisfaction. If life-satisfaction and family satisfaction are consistent, they infer that they must have used family satisfaction to evaluate global life-satisfaction. If family satisfaction is inconsistent with life-satisfaction, they infer that they must not have used life-satisfaction. This explanation is inconsistent with several findings. First, participants report sources even when they are asked about sources in an open-ended format (Ross et al., 1986; Pilot Study 1). Second, this account cannot explain the infrequent endorsement of weather and Illini basketball in the source reports. The near zero correlations between satisfaction with these domains and life-satisfaction imply that satisfaction with these domains was consistent with life-satisfaction for several participants. Hence, more participants should have reported using this source, if source reports were inferred from the consistency between life-satisfaction judgments and domain satisfaction. In fact, if people rely on consistency and nobody reports using a domain in the source reports, then satisfaction with this domain should be strongly negatively correlated with life-satisfaction. Our data do not support this prediction. Rather, domains that participants reported not using were uncorrelated with life-satisfaction, which is consistent with the validity of source reports. If somebody is not thinking about a domain, then this domain should have no influence on life-satisfaction.

The final argument against this alternative explanation stems from our longitudinal data, which revealed that changes in variable life-domains are related to changes in global life-satisfaction. For example, satisfaction with spring break was related to life-satisfaction after spring break after controlling for life-satisfaction before spring break. This finding suggests that spring break influenced life-satisfaction judgments after spring break. Consistent with this conclusion, the majority of participants reported this source in their source reports. In this sense, source reports reflect actual sources of life-satisfaction that produced changes in life-satisfaction judgments over time. Any theory of source reports has to account for the relation between source reports and the relation between sources and life-satisfaction. An inference process that merely compares the consistencies between global life-satisfaction judgments and satisfaction with a particular domain is unable to do so because domains that were not used during a life-satisfaction judgment may be consistent with a global life-satisfaction judgment.

We realize that it is impossible to prove that source reports reflect actual thoughts during a life-satisfaction judgment. However, research in many other areas of psychology has benefited from examining participants' thoughts (Ericsson & Simon, 1993). Furthermore, we do not see any reason why participants should not form life-satisfaction judgments in a deliberate manner that is accessibly to introspection. One challenge to this view would be the behaviorists' notion that people do not have access to thoughts or feelings—a position that we find no longer defensible 40 years after the cognitive revolution (cf. Pashler, 1999). The second challenge seems to arise from Nisbett and Wilson's (1977) influential article, which revealed the limitation of introspection to explain behavior. However, even Nisbett and Wilson (1977) share our view that people have introspective access to thoughts and feelings: "It should be noted that *the individual's private access to content* [italics added] will sometimes allow him to be more accurate in his report about the causes of his behavior than an observer would be" (p. 256). It also has to be noted that source reports about thoughts during the formation of a judgment differ from inquires about causal explanations of behavior. "Did you think about the weather when you answered the previous question about life-satisfaction?" is different from asking "Did your parents' upbringing influence your level of life-satisfaction today?" The latter question goes beyond the evidence that could be accessible to introspection and forces people to rely on inferences. To avoid this problem, we deliberately limited our questions to the content of thoughts during the formation of a life-satisfaction judgement.

In sum, we believe that the present findings encourage the use of source reports in life-satisfaction research. We do not suggest that source reports are a magic bullet that can replace correlational and experimental research on actual determinants of life-satisfaction. However, we believe that they constitute an economical and useful tool for life-satisfaction researchers that can enrich future studies of life-satisfaction. Part II illustrates how source reports can be used to inform research on life-satisfaction with more traditional methods.

Part II: Chronically Accessible and Stable Sources Mediate the Influence of Personality Traits on Life-Satisfaction

One challenge for any theory of life-satisfaction judgments is to explain the high temporal stability of life-satisfaction judgments and the systematic relations between life-satisfaction and personality traits (Diener & Lucas, 1999; Pavot and Diener, 1993). We propose that the use of chronically accessible sources explains these findings. If people rely on chronically accessible sources, then their life-satisfaction judgments are based on the same sources in repeated life-satisfaction judgments. Furthermore, if satisfaction in these domains remains stable over time, then the global life-satisfaction judgment will remain stable as well. Personality traits may be related to global life-satisfaction because they predict stability of chronically accessible sources. We tested these hypotheses by means of a path model. The theoretical assumptions underlying this model were derived from (a) the source reports in the longitudinal study of source reports in Part I and (b) well-established findings in the subjective well-being literature.

We relied on the source reports to determine chronically accessible sources of life-satisfaction judgments. We focused on sources that were chronically accessible for the majority of participants. The major reason for this decision was the lack of appropriate statistical tools to test mediator models, in which a source is only a mediator for a subset of the full sample. For example, housing satisfaction should only mediate the relation between a personality predictor of housing satisfaction and global life-satisfaction for the one half of the sample that actually used housing satisfaction. In other words, the mediation of housing satisfaction should be moderated by the use of housing satisfaction. To avoid these difficulties, we focused on sources that were reported by a large majority of participants. These sources should mediate personality effects for (nearly) all participants, thus avoiding the problem of modeling moderator effects.

We derived a theoretical path model based on the source reports in the main study and previous findings in the well-being literature. The source reports suggested that hedonic balance, romantic satisfaction, academic satisfaction, family satisfaction, and health satisfaction were considered by a majority of the participants. Hence, we specified in the path model direct paths from these sources to global life-satisfaction.

Furthermore, we predicted that these sources fully mediate the relation between life-satisfaction and personality traits in the following manner.

The influence of personality traits on subjective well-being is best documented for the affective component of subjective well-being (Costa & McCrae, 1980). Extraversion is a predictor of pleasure, and neuroticism a predictor of displeasure. When the two affects are combined in a hedonic balance score, extraversion is a positive predictor and neuroticism a negative predictor. Furthermore, people rely on their hedonic balance as one source of information to judge life-satisfaction (Suh et al., 1998). We integrated these two findings by assuming that the influences of extraversion and neuroticism on life-satisfaction are mediated by hedonic balance. To test this mediation hypothesis, we specified that (a) neuroticism predicts hedonic balance (N–>HB), extraversion predicts hedonic balance (E–>HB), and hedonic balance predicts life-satisfaction (HB–>LS), but neuroticism and extraversion do not predict life-satisfaction directly (N–>LS = 0, E–>LS = 0).

McCrae and Costa (1991) proposed that love and work are predictors of subjective well-being beyond the influences of extraversion and neuroticism. Agreeableness is a predictor of love, whereas conscientiousness is a predictor of work. This idea is consistent with our findings that a majority of participants used satisfaction with academic performance (work) and with romantic relationships (love) in life-satisfaction judgments. To integrate these findings in a path model, we predicted that conscientiousness predicts academic satisfaction (C–>AS), and academic satisfaction predicts life-satisfaction (AS–>LS). Similarly we predicted that agreeableness predicts romantic satisfaction (A–>RS), and that romantic satisfaction predicts life-satisfaction (RS–>LS). Furthermore, the direct paths from conscientiousness and agreeableness to life-satisfaction should not be significant (A–>LS = 0; C–>LS = 0).

We also found that a majority of participants reported considering health satisfaction. Health satisfaction is influenced by neuroticism (Brief et al., 1993). Hence, we also predicted that N influences health satisfaction (N–>HS), and that health satisfaction predicts life-satisfaction (HS–>LS). Hence, influences of neuroticism on life-satisfaction can be mediated by two sources, namely hedonic balance and health satisfaction.

We were not aware of clear theoretical predictions about the relationship between personality dimensions and satisfaction with family relationships. Hence, we only predicted that family satisfaction predicts life-satisfaction (FS–>LS), but we did not assume that this domain is a mediator of personality traits.

Method

We used the data from the longitudinal study in Part I for our analyses (see Part I for methodological details. To simplify the analyses and to examine long-term life-satisfaction, we aggregated life-satisfaction judgments and sources across the four assessments (see Table 1 for reliabilities).

Results

After fitting the theoretically predicted model, we freed additional paths that were not theoretically predicted, but improved model fit. In addition, we removed agreeableness from the model because, contrary to our predictions, it was neither significantly related to romantic satisfaction nor to life-satisfaction. Figure 1 shows the final model. Not shown in the figure are the correlations between the personality traits, namely −0.55 between E and N, 0.28 between E and C, and −0.41 between N and C. Due to our modifications, the fit of the final model was acceptable, indicating that further modifications would not improve the fit of the model, $\chi^2(df = 14) = 21.76$, $p = 0.08$; AIC $= -0.6.24$, and RMSEA $= 0.069$ (see Bollen & Long, 1993, for tests of structural equation models). Figure 1 shows theoretically predicted paths as solid lines and added paths as dashed lines. Seven of the nine predicted paths showed statistically significant path coefficients. In addition, all paths predicted to be nonsignificant were nonsignificant. The most important result was that personality influences on life-satisfaction were mediated by sources that were used to judge life-satisfaction. The influence of extraversion and neuroticism was mediated primarily by hedonic balance. The influence of conscientiousness was mediated by academic satisfaction. Figure 1 also shows that hedonic balance, romantic satisfaction, and academic satisfaction were the strongest independent predictors of life-satisfaction. Together the five sources in Fig. 1 explained 68% of the variance in life-satisfaction. In sum, the path model confirms our prediction that chronically accessible sources mediate the influence of personality traits on life-satisfaction.

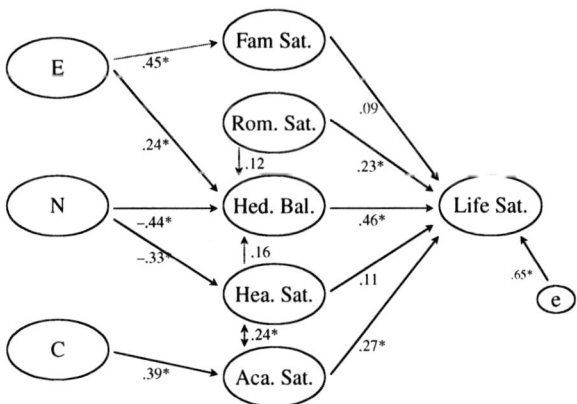

Fig. 1 Path model of the integrated top-down bottom-up model
Note. E = Extraversion, N = Neuroticism, C = Conscientiousness, Fam Sat. = Satisfaction with Family Relationships, Rom. Sat. = Satisfaction with Romantic Relationships, Hed. Bal. = Hedonic Balance, Hea. Sat. = Satisfaction with Health, Aca. Sat. = Satisfaction with Academic Performance, Life-Sat. = Life-Satisfaction, e = Error Variance, that is Variance not explained by predictor variables.

General Discussion

Our findings extend previous research on life-satisfaction in three ways. First, it was commonly assumed that individuals consider different types of information to judge life-satisfaction (e.g., Diener & Lucas, 1999; Oishi, Schimmack, & Diener, 2001). However, it was difficult to test this assumption in previous paradigms. We presented evidence that participants differ in the use of some sources, such as satisfaction with family relations, housing, and health. However, for other sources, we found that a majority of participants tended to use some sources (academic performance) and not to use others (weather). This consistency might be due to the homogeneity of the sample. We expect more variability in source reports in more diverse samples. Future research needs to test this prediction.

Our second contribution is the integration of personality theories and judgment theories of life-satisfaction. Consistent with judgment theories of life-satisfaction, we presented evidence that life-satisfaction judgments are constructed bottom-up from accessible and relevant sources of information. Consistent with the personality literature, we found that life-satisfaction judgments were quite stable over time. We demonstrated that this stability was due to the consistent use of chronically accessible sources that provided stable information.

Our third contribution was our support of Brief et al.'s (1993) integrated top-down and bottom-up model. Personality traits produced stability in sources such as hedonic balance, health satisfaction, and academic performance. At the same time, these sources were chronically accessible and consistently used in life-satisfaction judgments. As a consequence, personality traits predict stable individual differences in life-satisfaction.

The present findings pose several constraints on potential theories of life-satisfaction. Judgment theories that focus exclusively on temporarily accessible sources and highly variable sources like current mood fail to explain the temporal stability of life-satisfaction judgments and the relationship between life-satisfaction and personality traits. Life-satisfaction theories that regard life-satisfaction as a global trait cannot explain the changes in life-satisfaction judgments over time, nor can they account for the mood effects on life-satisfaction judgments. Exclusive top-down theories of life-satisfaction have difficulties explaining why global life-satisfaction should influence some domains (e.g., family satisfaction), but not other domains (e.g., weather). They also are inconsistent with the finding that participants reported the construction of life-satisfaction judgments in a bottom-up manner on the basis of important life domains. Although it may be possible to change these theories to accommodate inconsistent findings, we consider our integrated model as the most parsimonious account of all findings. People rely on multiple sources to form life-satisfaction judgments. Some sources, like mood and spring break, produce temporal changes in life-satisfaction, whereas other sources, like academic success, provide rather stable information. This explains the stability and variability of life-satisfaction judgments. Personality traits are responsible for some of the stability in chronically accessible sources. As a consequence, personality traits predict life-satisfaction, and this relation is mediated by chronically accessible sources. Finally, participants form life-satisfaction judgments partially in a consciously accessible, deliberate manner. As a consequence, source reports predict the strength of the relation between global life-satisfaction and life-domains. A conscious, deliberate process is also consistent with the evidence that life-satisfaction judgments are not influenced by accessible sources when these sources are considered uninformative (Schwarz and Strack, 1999). For example, when students are asked to judge dating prior to a life-satisfaction judgment, dating satisfaction heavily influences life-satisfaction judgments. However, when the instructions implied that dating should be excluded from the global judgment, a previous question about dating no longer influences global life-satisfaction. This finding is more in line with a deliberate judgment process that takes the context of the question into account. In sum, our integrative theory is a plausible and parsimonious account of the existing evidence. However, it is possible that other theories can explain the data as well or better. Furthermore, it is possible that the present results are limited to samples with predominantly female psychology students. Future research should test the integrated theory of life-satisfaction judgments with other methods and in other populations.

Acknowledgments This research was supported by a post-doctoral scholarship awarded to Ulrich Schimmack by the DFG.

References

Argyle, M. (1987). *The psychology of happiness*. London: Methuen.

Bollen, K. A., & Long, J. S. (Eds.). (1993). *Testing structural equation models*. Newbury Park, CA: Sage.

Brief, A. P., Butcher, A. H., George, J. M., & Link, K. E. (1993). Integrating bottom-up and top-down theories of subjective well-being: The case of health. *Journal of Personality and Social Psychology, 64,* 646-653.

Brown, N. R. (1995). Estimation strategies and the judgment of event frequencies. *Journal of Experimental Psychology: Learning, memory and cognition, 21,* 1539–1553.

Brunstein, J. C. (1993). Personal goals and subjective well-being: A longitudinal study. *Journal of Personality and Social Psychology, 65,* 1061–1070.

Costa, P. T., & McCrae, R. R. (1980). Influence of extraversion and neuroticism on subjective well-being: Happy and unhappy people. *Journal of Personality and Social Psychology, 38,* 668–678.

Crutcher, R. J. (1994). Telling what we know: The use of verbal report methodologies in psychological research. *Psychological Science, 5,* 241–244.

Diener, E. (1984). Subjective well-being. *Psychological Bulletin, 95,* 542–575.

Diener, E. (2000). Subjective well-being: The science of happiness and a proposal for a national index. *American Psychologist, 55,* 34–43.

Diener, E., & Diener, M. (1995). Cross-cultural correlates of life satisfaction and self-esteem. *Journal of Personality and Social Psychology, 68,* 653–663.

Diener, E., Emmons, R. A., Larsen, R. J., & Griffin, S. (1985). The Satisfaction With Life Scale. *Journal of Personality Assessment, 49,* 71–75.

Diener, E., & Larsen, R. J. (1984). Temporal stability and cross-situational consistency of affective, behavioral, and cognitive responses. *Journal of Personality and Social Psychology, 47,* 871–883.

Diener, E., & Lucas, R. E. (1999). Personality and subjective well-being. In D. Kahneman, E. Diener, & N. Schwarz (Eds.), *Well-being: The foundations of hedonic psychology* (pp. 213–229). New York: Russell Sage.

Diener, E., Suh, E. M., Lucas, R. E., & Smith, H. L. (1999). Subjective well-being: Three decades of progress. *Psychological Bulletin, 125*, 276–302.

Eagly, A. H., & Chaiken, S. (1993). *The psychology of attitudes.* Fort Worth, TX: HBJ.

Ericsson, K. A., & Simon, H. A. (1993). *Protocol analysis: Verbal reports as data* (rev. ed.). Cambridge, MA: MIT Press.

Goldberg, L. (1997). *A broad-bandwidth, public domain, personality inventory measuring the lower-level facets of several five-factor models.* [On line] Available: http://www.ipio.ori.org/ipip/.

Kwan, V. S. Y., Bond, M. H., & Singelis, T. M. (1997). Pancultural explanations for life-satisfaction: Adding relationship harmony to self-esteem. *Journal of Personality and Social Psychology, 73*, 1038–1051.

McCrae, R. R., & Costa, P. T. (1991). Adding Liebe and Arbeit: The full five-factor model of well-being. *Bulletin of Personality & Social Psychology, 17*, 227–232.

Myers, D. G. (1992). *The pursuit of happiness.* New York: Morrow.

Myers, D. G. (2000). The funds, friends, and faith of happy people. *American Psychologist, 55*, 56–67.

Nisbett, R. E., & Wilson, T. D. (1977). Telling more than we can know: Verbal reports on mental processes. *Psychological Review, 84*, 231–259.

Oishi, S., Diener, E. F., Lucas, R. E., & Suh, E. M. (1999). Cross-cultural variations in predictors of life satisfaction: Perspectives from needs and values. *Personality and Social Psychology Bulletin, 25*, 980–990.

Oishi, S., Diener, E., Suh, E., & Lucas, R. E. (1999). Value as a moderator in subjective well-being. *Journal of Personality, 67*, 157–184.

Oishi, S., Schimmack, U., & Diener, E. (2001). Pleasure and subjective well being. *European Journal of Personality, 15*, 153–167.

Osterhouse, R. A., & Brock, T. C. (1970). Distraction increases yielding to propaganda by inhibiting counterarguing. *Journal of Personality and Social Psychology, 15*, 344–358.

Pashler H. E. (1999). *The psychology of attention.* Cambridge, MA: MIT Press.

Pavot, W., & Diener, E. (1993). Review of the Satisfaction With Life Scale. *Psychological Assessment, 5*, 164–172.

Pelham, B. W. (1995). Self-investment and self-esteem: Evidence for a Jamesian model of self-worth. *Journal of Personality and Social Psychology, 69*, 1141–1150.

Pelham, B. W., & Swann, W. B. (1989). From self-conceptions to self-worth: On the sources and structure of global self-esteem. *Journal of Personality and Social Psychology, 57*, 672–680.

Ross, M., Eyman, A., & Kishchuck, N. (1986). Determinants of subjective well-being. In J. M. Olson, C. P. Herman, & M. Zanna (Eds.), *Relative deprivation and social comparison.* Hillsdale, NJ: Erlbaum.

Schimmack, U. (1997). Das Berliner-Alltagssprachliche-Stimmungsinventar (BASTI): Ein Vorschlag zur kontentvaliden Erfassung von Stimmungen [The Every-Day Language Mood Inventory (ELMI): Toward a content valid assessment of moods]. *Diagnostica, 43*, 150–173.

Schimmack, U. (1998, May). *Mood effects on life-satisfaction judgments: Conscious or unconscious?* Paper presented at the 70th annual convention of the Midwestern Psychological Association.

Schimmack, U., & Grob, A. (2000). Dimensional models of core affect: A quantitative comparison by means of structural equation modeling. *European Journal of Personality, 14*, 325–345.

Schimmack, U., Oishi, S., Diener, E., & Suh, E. (2000). Facets of affective experiences: A new look at the relation between pleasant and unpleasant affect. *Personality and Social Psychology Bulletin, 26*, 655–668.

Schkade, D. A., & Kahneman, D. (1998). Does living in California make people happy? A focusing illusion in judgments of life satisfaction. *Psychological Science, 9*, 340–346.

Schwarz, N., & Clore, G. L. (1983). Mood, misattribution, and judgments of well-being: Informative and directive functions of affective states. *Journal of Personality and Social Psychology, 45*, 513–523.

Schwarz, N., & Strack, F. (1999). Reports of subjective well-being: Judgmental processes and their methodological implications. In D. Kahneman, E. Diener, & N. Schwarz (Eds.), *Well-being: The foundations of hedonic psychology* (pp. 61–84). New York: Russell Sage.

Steyer, R., Schwenkmezger, P., Notz, P., & Eid, M. (1994). Testtheoretische Analysen des Mehrdimensionalen Befindlichkeitsfragebogens [Test theoretical analyses of the Multidimensional State Questionnaire]. *Diagnostica, 40*, 320–328.

Suh, M., Diener, E., Oishi, S., & Triandis, H. C. (1998). The shifting basis of life-satisfaction judgments across cultures: Emotions versus norms. *Journal of Personality and Social Psychology, 74*, 482–493.

Wilson, T. D., & Kraft, D. (1993). Why do I love thee? Effects of repeated introspection on attitudes. *Personality and Social Psychology Bulletin, 25*, 379–400.

Happiness is the Frequency, Not the Intensity, of Positive Versus Negative Affect

Ed Diener, Ed Sandvik, and William Pavot

Abstract In this chapter we suggest that "happiness," or high subjective well-being, is more strongly associated with the frequency and duration of people's positive feelings, not with the intensity of those feelings. People who rarely or never feel euphoria, for instance, can nonetheless report very high levels of well-being. We hypothesize that there are several reasons that subjective well-being is more strongly associated with the amount of time people feel positive versus negative feelings rather than with the intensity of their positive feelings. Intense positive feelings often have costs, including a tendency to more intense negative feelings in negative situations. Another hypothesis is that it is more difficult to accurately measure the intensity of feelings than their time-course, and this makes the amount of time people feel positive more amenable to study with self-report methods. The intensity of people's positive emotions should not be ignored, but should be studied in combination with the time-course (frequency and duration) of positive and negative feelings.

Introduction

When people seek happiness, some desire to be happy most of the time, even if only mildly so, whereas others appear to live and plan for rare but intense moments of ecstasy. The question addressed here is whether frequent positive affect, intense positive affect, or both are necessary and sufficient for happiness. One common sense view suggests that happiness is greatest when one has the maximum of both frequent positive affect *and* intense positive affect and only minimal amounts of non-intense, negative affect. But many people would suggest that either frequent (but mild) or intense (but infrequent) experiences of positive affect are necessary or sufficient to produce a happy life.

We will argue that happiness researchers should assess primarily the relative frequency of positive versus negative emotional experience. The first reason for this

E. Diener (✉)
Department of Psychology, University of Illinois, Champaign, IL 61820, USA
e-mail: ediener@uiuc.edu

E. Diener (ed.), *Assessing Well-Being: The Collected Works of Ed Diener,*
Social Indicators Research Series 39, DOI 10.1007/978-90-481-2354-4_10,
© Springer Science+Business Media B.V. 2009

contention is that the relative frequency of positive emotions can be more accurately and validly measured, a consideration that is fundamental to scientific work on the concept of happiness. A second reason that researchers should focus on the relative frequency of positive versus negative affect is that frequent positive affect is both necessary and sufficient to produce the state we call happiness, whereas intense positive experience is not. Thus, what we call happiness seems to actually be comprised of frequent positive affect and infrequent negative affect.

The final reason to emphasize the relative frequency of positive affect in the study of happiness is that intense positive experiences can, surprisingly, have undesirable features. These features tend to offset the benefit of intense positive emotions, making it questionable whether intense experiences in the long run are more valuable to the individual than less intense ones. Thus, although intense positive experiences are individually desirable at the time they are experienced, they may be less related to long-term well-being or happiness because of unattractive side effects, as well as because of their rarity.

In sum, there are several strong justifications for defining and studying happiness as the relative frequency of positive experiences rather than the intensity of positive affect. Although intense positive emotions are an interesting phenomenon in their own right, it is doubtful that they are closely related to the longer-term state we refer to as "happiness" or "subjective well-being."

In this paper we will refer to the "frequency of positive affect," which is a shorthand way of referring to the relative per cent of time individuals are happy versus unhappy. Although we call the percent of time experiencing predominantly positive affect the "relative frequency of positive affect" (Diener, 1984; Diener, Larsen, Levine, & Emmons, 1985), it should be noted that we mean frequency in terms of time sampling, and it is therefore the overall percentage of time the person is in a predominantly positive (as opposed to negative) emotional state. When the intensity of positive emotions is discussed, we mean the average intensity of affect when a person is experiencing positive emotions.

Measurement

One important reason for scientists to focus their attention on the frequency of positive affect in understanding happiness is that frequency of affect is more easily and accurately measured than affect intensity. Scientific research, in contrast to other approaches to knowledge, relies heavily on accurate measurement of the concepts which are studied. There are reasons to believe that frequency of positive affect measures are accurate, and perhaps approximate an interval or even ratio level of measurement. Frequency information can be encoded in memory, accurately recalled from memory, and can be reported in a way that is comparable across persons. Evidence has shown that people are more able to accurately estimate frequency of affect and are less biased in its recall than they assess the intensity of emotional experiences. This is perhaps one reason that most measures of happiness do in fact reflect the frequency of positive experiences to a much greater degree than they reflect intense positive emotions.

Brandstätter (1987) has argued that persons can clearly tell whether or not they are happy or unhappy at a particular time. In his terms, there is a natural "point of indifference" in emotion, above which people feel positive and below which they feel negative. The judgment of happiness versus unhappiness is facilitated by the fact that when one type of affect is dominant, the other type exists, if at all, at low levels (Diener & Iran-Nejad, 1986). Therefore, because individuals can tell when they are experiencing positive and/or negative affect and can usually judge which is stronger, it is possible for them to store frequency of affect information in memory.

In contrast to frequency information, the intensity of affect is likely to be more difficult to encode because there is no natural system by which to define or label emotional intensity. As one becomes more intensely joyful, it is difficult to calibrate this experience, and therefore, difficult to encode the intensity accurately. How can one clearly distinguish levels of emotional intensity and encode them in comparable ways from one occasion to the next? Frequency information can be encoded because people know whether they are happy or unhappy, joyful or fearful, whereas for intensity, there is no such discrete event. At best, individuals might be able to encode the intensity of their own emotional experiences in an ordinal way.

There is empirical evidence that frequency information can be more accurately recalled than intensity information. Hasher and Zacks (1979, 1984) have shown that people are particularly accurate at recalling frequency information in general. These researchers even hypothesize that humans may be biologically prepared to store such information, and review data which show that people can be accurate in retrieving the frequency of events and objects in their experience.

In the domain of internal experiences such as affect, people may also be much more accurate at recalling frequency information than intensity information. We have collected evidence which shows that people are less accurate in recalling intensity information, and that their intensity estimates are biased by the actual frequency of their emotions. In our laboratory Thomas (1987; Thomas & Diener, 1988) has examined the accuracy of memory for one's own moods. Across a series of studies he found that people are accurate at estimating the per cent of time they are happy. For example, in one study subjects estimated that they were happy 72% of the time on average and later mood recording indicated that they were happy 78% of the time. The estimates correlated substantially across subjects with their later experiences.

In contrast, subjects were much less accurate at recalling the intensity of their emotions. Their estimates were almost twice the actual daily values in an absolute sense and showed little correlation across subjects with the daily intensity figures. Because people's most emotional times are most salient in memory, they tend to greatly overestimate in an absolute sense their emotional intensity. Furthermore, subjects' intensity estimates correlated with how frequently they were actually happy more highly than they correlated with their emotional intensity as sampled over time. In other words, subjects seem to retrieve frequency information when they are trying to estimate intensity.

It is also likely that emotion reports are more comparable across people when they report frequency rather than intensity information. How can we ever know if mood intensity reports have similar meanings across respondents? A person can tell us if she is experiencing positive or negative affect and this appears to have very similar meaning across people because basic emotional experiences are largely universal. Reports of frequency are thus probably comparable across persons because they are the summation of positive and negative emotions which have cross-person meaning. But when a person tells us that she is *moderately* or *very* happy, what does this mean? There is simply no cross-person metric to make such judgments. Because the experiences are internal, it is hard to reach a consensual definition of response alternatives in the emotional intensity domain. Thus, it appears that frequency of positive affect should be easier to measure because it represents the summation over time of a discrete state variable, whereas intensity is very problematical to assess because it is a continuously distributed unobservable which can be scaled idiosyncratically by subjects. Furthermore, it should be noted that to some extent affect frequency reports are themselves unreliable because subjects label their emotions differently, the intensity of these emotions will thus be even more problematical to assess.

One other benefit in measuring the frequency of positive affect is that, in considering levels of measurement, frequency information has both interval and ratio properties. A person who is happy 40% of the time can legitimately be said to be happy 10% more of the time than a person who is happy only 30% of the time. Furthermore, it is meaningful to say that a person who is happy 80% of the time is twice as happy as a person who is happy only 40% of the time. In contrast, we cannot be sure that mood intensity information given by different subjects is even ordinal. For example, can one be sure that individuals who describe their positive moods as "quite strong" are really experiencing more intense affect than persons who describe their moods as "moderate"? Certainly we cannot be certain what response would be twice as strong as another because it is not even clear what this might mean. Thus, mood intensity measures are more likely to have nominal or perhaps ordinal properties rather than the more sophisticated measurement properties which characterize mood frequency measures.

Finally, response artifacts or biases appear to be a greater potential problem in measuring intensity than in assessing frequency of affect. For example, number-use response sets such as extremity bias (a subject's tendency to use very high or low numbers regardless of a question's content) are more likely to influence the reporting of intensity information. Frequency measures with concrete anchors such as the percentage of time the person is happy are less likely to be influenced by such response sets. When one uses time sampling methods of recording mood at particular moments, number use response sets are still a major potential problem for intensity reports, but seem to be unproblematical for reports of whether the person is happy or unhappy. When one "beeps" persons at random moments, their mood intensity report is still quite vulnerable to response artifacts such as extreme number use. But an indication of whether one was predominantly happy or unhappy when the pager sounded is much less susceptible to such artifacts. Social desirability is the tendency of some individuals to give responses which are desirable in that culture. In terms of social desirability, we (Diener, Sandvik, Gallagher, & Pavot, 1988) have found that the correlation between this variable and frequency of happiness reports reflects a substantive individual difference characteristic which actually enhances well-being. In other words, individuals who tend to respond in socially desirable ways are truly happier individuals (even when measured by nonself-report measures). Individual differences in social desirability are, therefore, not damaging response artifacts in the case of frequency of happiness reports.

In conclusion, there are both theoretical and empirical reasons for believing that frequency measures are more accurate, more comparable across subjects, and can be measured with scales which have more sophisticated properties. Therefore, it appears that the typical measurement of positive affect with a single self-report is much more likely to be veridical if it assesses frequency rather than intensity information because people can store and recall this information more accurately. In the next section evidence will be reviewed which shows that frequency of affect information is strongly reflected in subjects' questionnaire reports of happiness, again indicating that such frequency information must be stored in memory. The next question to be addressed relates to the validity of equating the frequency of positive affect with happiness. Although frequency of positive versus negative affect can be measured with some accuracy, is it really what we mean by happiness?

The Composition of Happiness

In this section it will be shown that frequent positive and infrequent negative affect correlate much more strongly with happiness measures than does the intensity of positive affect. Even more noteworthy, it will be demonstrated that relatively frequent positive affect is both *necessary and sufficient* to produce high scores on a variety of happiness measures. In contrast, those with intense positive emotions are sometimes happy, but are not always so. Thus, we maintain that happiness should be defined as relatively frequent positive affect and infrequent negative affect because this is the common ingredient reflected in widely varying measures of well-being. In other words, measures of subjective well-being all reflect an underlying unitary phenomenon (frequency of positive versus negative affect), and this state is separate from other phenomena such as intense positive affect. Subjective well-being measures all converge on the property of frequent positive affect, indicating that this experience is the essence of a phenomenon which can be labelled "happiness."

We have examined three major self-report measures of happiness as they relate to the frequency and intensity of positive affect in several samples. In the studies reported here we administered the Fordyce (1977) global happiness scale, along with two other widely used scales—Bradburn's (1969) Affect Balance Scale and the 7-point Delighted-Terrible scale of Andrews and Withey (1976). We then assessed the moods of our subjects over a period of six to eight weeks. During this time we measured both the frequency and intensity of positive affect (e.g. see Diener & Emmons, 1984; Diener et al., 1985). We have assessed these variables both at end of the day measurement times, as well as at random moments throughout each day, with parallel results. Frequency of positive affect was defined in our studies as the percentage of time individuals were experiencing positive affect at levels which exceeded their level of negative affect. Intensity of positive affect was the average

Table 1 Predicting happiness scale scores from frequency and intensity of positive affect

	Regression betas					
	Freq	N = 42 PI	Freq	N = 62 PI	Freq	N = 107 PI
Fordyce	0.58***	0.23	0.58***	0.22*	0.53***	0.29***
Bradburn	0.41**	0.22	0.39**	0.06	0.39***	0.21
Andrews and Withey[1]	0.42***	0.24	0.37***	0.23	0.49***	0.25**
	Partial correlations					
Freq with PI controlled	Partial r		Partial r		Partial r	
Fordyce	0.60***		0.57***		0.56***	
Bradburn	0.42**		0.38***		0.38***	
Andrews and Withey[1]	0.43**		0.38***		0.48***	
	PI with freq controlled					
Fordyce	0.28*		0.26*		0.34***	
Bradburn	0.24		0.07		0.20*	
Andrews and Withey[1]	0.27*		0.25*		0.25**	

[1] Reflected.
* $p < 0.05$.
** $p < 0.01$.
*** $p < 0.001$.

intensity of positive affect when the person was happy (experiencing more positive than negative affect). Table 1 shows how well the daily frequency and intensity of positive affect correlate with the happiness measures across the three groups. As can be seen, the results of the three studies are quite similar, as are the results across the three measures of happiness. The regression analyses shown in the top of the table reveal that frequency of positive affect is always a much stronger predictor of happiness reports than positive emotional intensity. The bottom half of Table 1 presents the partial correlations between the happiness reports and the frequency and intensity of positive affect. Because frequent and intense positive affect correlated in one of our samples, the partial correlations are given to show the amount of unique variance in the happiness reports associated with frequency and with intensity. Once again, it can be seen that traditional happiness measures are much more strongly related to the frequency of positive affect than to its intensity. These results are particularly striking when it is considered that these three happiness scales mention nothing about the frequency of positive or negative affect. Indeed, the wording in some of the measures reflects intensity content.

Further light can be shed on the question of the importance of frequency and intensity of positive affect for happiness by turning to the combined results of several of our studies. We were able to identify a number of individuals who were high in frequency (above 80%) and very low in intensity ("slightly" or "somewhat" intense positive affect). *All* seven of these individuals reported very happy scores on the Fordyce Scale ($M = 7.86$). In contrast, *none* of the three individuals who were very high in positive emotional intensity ("much" or "very" intense positive affect), but below 50% in frequency of positive affect, reported scores in the happy range on the Fordyce Scale ($M = 3.00$).

We have also examined affect balance scores derived from our daily mood recordings. Affect balance is computed by subtracting the average negative affect level for a day from the average positive affect level for a day. Subjects' frequency of positive affect scores correlated a very strong 0.86 with this affect balance score, whereas the positive intensity score correlated a more modest 0.28 with daily affect balance ($N = 62$). Thus, happiness measures sampled over time also reflect primarily the influence of frequency of positive versus negative affect rather than the intensity of positive affect.

What of the common sense idea that those who are happiest are actually those who have frequent and intense positive affect and infrequently experience only low intense negative affect? Certainly such a formula for happiness seems intuitively appealing, but we have thus far found little empirical support for it. For a sample of 107 subjects, we correlated happiness self-reports with the relative frequency of positive affect. We also correlated the happiness measures with the following formula: frequency of positive affect times positive affect intensity, minus frequency of negative affect times negative affect intensity. This formula score correlated $r = 0.95$ with the relative frequency of positive versus negative affect, suggesting that intensity information normally adds little to the prediction of happiness. Furthermore, this formula score correlated less well than the relative frequency of positive affect with the Fordyce Happiness score (r's of 0.67 versus 0.69), the Bradburn Affect Balance score (0.51 versus 0.53), and the Delighted-Terrible Scale (0.70 versus 0.72).

In addition to the above analysis, we correlated daily *average* positive affect and negative affect with the happiness scales. We also correlated the frequency that positive and negative emotions were each felt with the happiness scales. These frequencies correlated with the happiness scale scores as well as the daily affect averages. This is noteworthy because the averages reflect the intensity of one's emotions as well as the frequency. When average positive and average negative affect were used to predict the Fordyce happiness scale score, for example, a multiple correlation of 0.60 resulted. When the frequencies of positive and negative affect were used to predict the Fordyce score the multiple R was higher—0.63. Clearly, weighting the frequency of positive affect by its intensity seems to aid little in the prediction of happiness. Thus, the relative frequency of positive versus negative affect is the factor which appears to comprise affective well-being.

The above data indicate that self-reports of happiness reflect frequency of positive affect to a greater degree than the intensity of positive affect. Furthermore, these results generalize to nonself-report measures of well-being, suggesting that frequency of positive affect is not merely what subjects report on happiness scales. In one study we obtained several nonself-report measures of happiness: an expert rating of well-being based on a structured written interview; peer reports of happiness; and a memory based affect balance measure of well-being comprised of the number of happy versus unhappy life events subjects could recall in a timed period. Each of these well-being measures was predicted by the daily relative frequency and

Table 2 Multiple R's squared predicting nonself-report scales of happiness

	Memdiff[1]	Expert[2]	Peer[3]
Entering frequency first as predictor			
Frequency of positive affect	0.21***	0.30***	0.57***
Intensity of positive affect	0.23*	0.30	0.57
Entering positive affect intensity first as predictor			
Intensity of positive affect	0.14***	0.13***	0.22***
Frequency of positive affect	0.23***	0.30***	0.57***

[1] Memory difference measure of happiness.
[2] Expert rating of happiness based on structured interview.
[3] Peer-reported measure of happiness.
* $p < 0.05$.
** $p < 0.01$.
*** $p < 0.001$.

intensity of positive affect of subjects. As can be seen in Table 2, both predictors can predict significantly when entered first in the prediction equation. Only frequency, however, predicts when entered second, and it does so for all three measures. The results indicate that frequency and intensity share common variance in this sample which predicts the nonself-report happiness scales. In addition, frequency has unique variance which predicts the measures, but intensity does not. Self, peer, and expert ratings, as well as a memory based assessment of happiness, all seem to depend more heavily on the frequency of positive affect. This finding again suggests that the frequency of positive versus negative affect is at the core of a construct we can label happiness or affective well-being.

We turn now to the questions of whether frequency of positive affect is necessary and sufficient for happiness, and whether intense positive emotions are necessary or sufficient for happiness. Necessity and sufficiency are strong conditions which, if met, suggest that frequency or intensity are not merely influences on happiness, but may be the defining characteristics of happiness. Table 3 shows several happiness scores for individuals differing in their frequency of positive affect. In order to determine whether frequent positive affect is necessary or sufficient for happiness, individual data must be examined rather than group averages. This is because single individuals can invalidate the propositions that frequent positive affect or intense positive affect are necessary or sufficient for happiness by providing a single contradictory instance. The high frequency group is comprised of those thirteen individuals (out of 107 subjects) with complete data who showed predominantly positive affect on all forty-two days in which they were queried. The eight low frequency individuals were those who reported predominantly positive affect on fewer than one-half of these days. Because there were few individuals in this sample who were infrequently happy, a less stringent cutoff was mandated for the low group, a division which is not optimal for the present argument. Nonetheless, the results are quite revealing.

The Memdiff score shown in Table 3 refers to the number of positive events the subjects could recall and list from their life and last year in a five minute period, minus the number of negative events in his or her life and past year recalled in

Table 3 Happiness scores of individuals differing in frequency of positive affect

Subject number	Sex	High frequency Memdiff	Expert	Fordyce	PI
9	F	1	4	8	15.7
19	F	22	4	8	19.0
22	M	4	4	8	15.2
39	M	4	5	7	8.2
63	M	15	4	8	15.0
70	F	5	3	8	12.2
75	M	4	4	8	17.3
76	F	9	4	8	8.9
8	M	4	5	8	17.1
117	F	16	4	8	16.0
118	F	20	6	10	19.7
123	F	10	4	8	18.7
125	F	1	4	8	12.0
		Low frequency			
16	M	−4	2	6	6.5
69	M	−4	1	2	5.8
84	M	−13	1	2	5.3
86	M	7	2	5	8.4
96	F	−9	2	7	11.8
97	F	−1	2	4	9.1
132	M	−2	2	4	14.3
134	M	−7	1	2	10.2

a separate five minute period. As can be seen in Table 3, only one infrequently happy subject (number eighty-six) remembered more positive than negative events, whereas all of the frequent positive affect group did so. Similarly, the expert rating clearly discriminated between the two groups: in fact, virtually perfectly. The expert rating varied from zero (extremely unhappy) to six (extremely happy), with three being the neutral point. These ratings were made blind as to the subjects' identities, yet only one neutral rating (for subject number seventy) failed to perfectly place the individuals into happy versus unhappy groups. Finally, the subjects' Fordyce scores (varying from zero to ten, with five being the neutral point) properly classified individuals in almost every case. Peer reports were also collected but are not presented in Table 3. There was little overlap between the two frequency groups in the peer happiness ratings. Peers erred, however, in the direction of believing that the low frequency subjects were happier than the other happiness measures revealed them to be.

Given that some low frequency subjects were not that extreme in terms of frequency, and that some normally happy individuals may have been unhappy during the six week sampling period used to measure frequency, the discrimination among the groups is remarkable. Although a definitive case cannot be made for the idea that frequent positive affect is necessary and sufficient for happiness, these data indicate that this is a strong possibility. Every individual who experienced frequent positive affect was happy on virtually every measure. And every individual who experienced infrequent positive affect was unhappy on virtually all of the measures. From this pattern it appears that frequent positive affect is sufficient for happiness. Because no individual with infrequent positive affect scored in the happy range on more than one of the three scales reviewed above, it also seems likely that frequent positive affect is necessary for happiness. We suggest that if a more extreme infrequent positive affect group was examined (e.g. predominant positive affect 20% or less of the time), the case for the necessary and sufficient connection between happiness and frequency could be made without reservation.

In reference to intensity, there are several noteworthy findings in Table 3. Firstly, it can be seen that in this sample there is a tendency for the intensity and frequency of positive affect to be related, although we have not found this to be true in other samples. Secondly, it appears that intense positive affect is neither necessary nor sufficient for happiness. Low frequency subject number 132 experienced intense positive affect, yet was unhappy on every measure. In contrast, high frequency subject numbers thirty-nine and seventy-six had low intensity positive affect, yet were happy on every measure. It appears that frequent positive affect is sufficient for happiness regardless of its level of intensity, but that intense positive affect is neither necessary nor sufficient for happiness.

Intense Positive Affect

In this section it will be argued that intense positive experiences are less related to long-term well-being not simply because of measurement considerations. In other words, frequency of positive experiences are reflected to a greater degree in well-being measures not only because they can be accurately recalled or more validly measured across subjects. There are also even more substantive psychological reasons related to affective dynamics that intense positive emotions are only weakly related to the state of long-term happiness. In the first place, extremely positive experiences are quite rare and are therefore less likely to be important to global well-being. In the second place, there are both empirical and theoretical reasons to believe that intense positive experiences often carry emotional costs in terms of being accompanied by increased negative affect and lowered positivity of other good experiences. Thus, intense positive experiences may be counter-balanced by opposing forces in such a way that they do not greatly enhance long term well-being and are therefore not strongly reflected in happiness measures.

Rareness of Intense Positive Affect

It is unlikely that intense positive emotional experiences form the core of well-being because these experiences are so uncommon. In contrast, the frequent experience of mild levels of positive affect seems to occur quite often. Sigmund Freud recognized the difficulty in maintaining intense happiness when he wrote that the experience of intense positive affect is limited by our biological constitutions. Flugel (1925) found that the half life of extremely positive moods is very short—the more intense the mood, the shorter it lasted.

In our research based on time sampling, we have found that the extremely intense moods are quite unusual. For example, a sample of 133 subjects reported on their daily moods for forty-two days. Of the total 5,586 days assessed, extremely positive affect was reported on only 2.6% of the days. We also signalled the subjects at random moments at which time they completed mood reports. Of the 3,639 moment reports, 1.2% were marked as extremely intense on the positive mood adjectives. In another study of forty-two subjects, the respondents were asked to indicate their maximum mood for each day. Of the 1,756 reports, 266 or 15% showed a maximum mood sometime during the day of "extremely" happy. It is clear that extremely intense positive moods are quite rare. This is even more dramatic because the subjects were in general quite happy and in a youthful age group which more frequently experiences intense emotions than most adults (Diener, Sandvik, & Larsen, 1985). Because these subjects reached an extremely happy state about once a week and for about one per cent of their waking time, we would expect intensely happy moods very infrequently in older samples.

Finally, we have found that extremely positive events are relatively uncommon. In one study we asked subjects to write down the best thing which happened to them each day. We then had coders rate the events in terms of how good the events were on a 5-point scale ranging from neutral to extremely good. Only one of the 3,214 events was rated as extremely good and only thirty-seven or 1.2% were rated as very good. The vast majority of events were rated as slightly or moderately good. Again, we can see that intense positivity is a very scarce commodity. Indeed, if an event occurred frequently it would probably lose its intense character. It seems unlikely that subjective well-being is built on experiences which occur so seldom.

The Prevalence of Frequent Positive Affect

When we turn from intense positive emotions to positive affect in general, a very different picture emerges; positive moods at less intense levels occur most of the time for the majority of our subjects. This fact squares nicely with the finding in all large-scale surveys that the majority of respondents claim to be happy. In a sample of 210 subjects, our respondents reported a preponderance of positive over negative affect on 75% of their days. Only 8% of the subjects were happy less than half of the times. Figure 1 shows the distribution of the per cent of days these subjects were predominantly happy. As can be seen, the distribution is highly skewed, with a plurality of subjects reporting a high percentage of happy days. At the same time, the average intensity of the happy days was only 3.2 on a zero to six scale, a response anchored by "moderate" in reference to how intensely the positive mood adjectives were being felt. Thus, it appears that our subjects experience weak levels of positive affect most of the time.

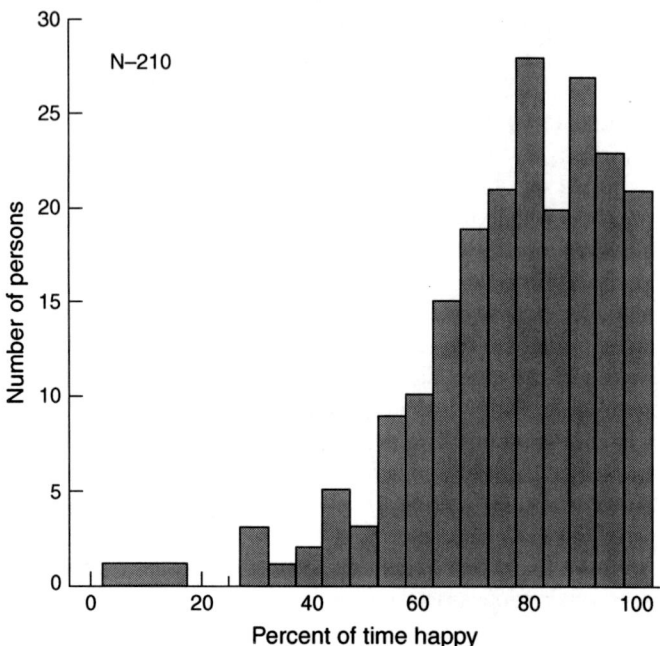

Fig. 1 Amount of time individuals experience positive versus negative affect

Costs of Positive Intensity

In addition to their rarity, there appear to be affective costs related to intense positive emotional experiences and these may counterbalance the good effects of these experiences in terms of long-term subjective well-being. Early thinkers recognized that intense positive emotions can involve a price. For example, the Epicureans counselled that happiness lies in quiet of the mind and not desiring things too strongly. Similarly, the Stoics believed that individuals should avoid extreme "highs." In *The Discourses*, Epictetus (1952) suggested that when we are delighted with a thing, we should temper this delight by thinking of its loss. Thus, if we lose the thing, we will be less disappointed. Epictetus recommends that we not allow our pleasures to go too far; we should check or curb them. Implicit in both Epicureanism and Stoicism is the idea that very intense positive affect can lead to more intense negative affect, a price that can be high. Similarly, Freud (1930) in *Civilization and Its Discontents* wrote that wild, untamed craving can lead to more intense satisfactions than curbed desires. On the other hand, he recognized that such unbridled desires also cause greater displeasure when they are not satisfied. Furthermore, he believed that we are so constituted that we can only intensely enjoy contrasts. It is impossible to attain uninterrupted intense positive affect. We will review theoretical and empirical works which indicate that one does indeed at times pay affectively for experiences of intense positive affect. Intense positive affect is not entirely a blessing and is therefore less related to long term emotional well-being.

In our studies on the temperament of emotional intensity, we have repeatedly found that those people who experience the most intense positive affect are likely to be those who will experience the most intense negative affect when unhappy (Larsen & Diener, 1987). For example, when we asked subjects to complete mood reports when they felt quite emotional, the relationship across persons between their intensity of positive feelings when they were happy and their intensity of negative feelings when feeling unhappy was strong $r = 0.80$. Thus, one reason that happiness reports do not correlate more strongly with positive emotions intensely is that the same individuals who are experiencing positive emotions intensely are also likely to be experiencing negative emotions more intensely.

If we examine factors which intuitively lead to intense positive affect, we find that most of these inputs can also heighten the intensity of negative affect. For instance, if a person works hard and long to gain some goal (high effort), intense positive affect will be experienced if the person is successful in reaching the goal. If the person fails to reach the goal, however, intense negative affect will ensue. One reason that subjects who experience positive events in an intense way are likely to experience negative events in an intense way also is that these individuals think of specific outcomes as quite important. For example, if a person thinks that the local team's winning of the next ball game is quite important because he identifies with the team, a win will produce more intense positive affect. But a loss will produce more intense negative affect. Similarly, if persons have their heart set on getting a particular job because it fulfils certain personal motives, receiving an employment call will make them quite happy. But they will also be more disappointed if they do not receive the offer. This phenomenon is what Freud meant by unbridled desires leading to more intense pleasure *or* to more intense displeasure. Thus, persons can achieve intense positive emotions by giving their goals a high subjective valence. If most of persons' goals are considered by them to be enormously important, they are likely to experience more intense positive emotions when the goals are reached. But in magnifying the importance of their goals, the persons will increase the intensity of their negative emotions whenever a goal is not attained.

Another related reason some people feel emotions intensely is because of certain cognitive styles. For example, the Freudian mechanism of repression would be likely to dampen the intensity of a person's negative affect. Interestingly, Davis and Schwartz (1987) found that repressors experienced both negative and positive affect less intensely. In other words, not only might repression lead to less intense negative affect, but the dynamics involved also seem to take the edge off positive emotions. Similarly, Gorman and Wessman (1974) found that repressive subjects reported less intense negative emotions, but were also less capable of hitting high peaks. The repressive subjects showed more shallow affect and less mood variability. Although repression has usually been studied in terms of negative affect, it may be that it blunts all types of emotions.

We have recently examined how cognitions can be used by individuals to blunt or dampen emotions. We asked subjects to list the best and worst event which happened to them each day for four days. We also requested that they write down each day their thoughts when these events occurred. Coders rated these thoughts for their emotional amplifying and emotional dampening qualities. It is noteworthy that those who showed the most amplifying thoughts for positive events also amplified their negative emotions the most, and a similar pattern occurred for dampening thoughts. What this and other laboratory studies (Colvin, Pavot, & Diener, 1988; Diener, Smith, Allman, & Pavot, 1988; Larsen, Diener, & Cropanzano, 1987) show is that when persons increase their use of either a dampening or an amplifying strategy in relation to positive stimuli, this is likely to carry over to negative stimuli as well. Thus, cognitions which allow high peaks or intense positive emotions will also lead to more extreme lows when one encounters a negative event.

Another reason that people are intense in their emotions is because of greater arousal or physiological reactivity. For example, Larsen and Scheffer (1987) showed that skin conductance was higher for emotionally intense subjects when they were exposed to either positive *or* emotional slides. Some individuals may have greater arousability and therefore experience intense positive affect in less extreme circumstances than others. These persons, however, are also likely to experience more intense negative emotions in unpleasant situations.

Our work and that of others suggests that a number of interrelated factors which influence the intensity of positive emotions also influence the intensity of negative emotions for the individual: high assessment of the importance of events; repression; cognitive amplifying and dampening strategies; and physiological reactivity. The end result of these mechanisms is the same: to amplify or dampen both positive and negative affective responses. Thus, it seems that in the long run in people's lives, many high peaks will be paid for to some extent by lower lows when the person becomes unhappy. There appear to be long-term individual differences in several of the factors which heighten emotional intensity. Therefore, some individuals will consistently show more intense positive reactions to the world, and also more intense negative reactions. In addition, an individual may show a more intense reaction to a particular event or situation. But factors such as being aroused or greatly wanting a particular outcome can heighten either the positive or negative response intensity in specific situations.

Opponent Process Theory

There are formal theories which maintain that there are costs related to intense positive emotions. Solomon's (1980) opponent process model predicts that intense emotional peaks often come at the cost of negative affect. According to this theory, novel positive events can produce high peaks. But these novel events are quickly habituated to and thereafter lead to only mild positive reactions. The other course to very positive emotional reactions is to have first suffered negative events. If a negative event occurs over time (e.g. being in prison) so that the person adapts to it, its withdrawal can then produce intense positive affect.

It can be predicted from the theory that extremely positive events will inevitably be quite rare. They must either be based on novelty (which is rare) or on habituation to a negative event which necessarily means that the person has suffered for a period of time in order to experience the intense positive event. Solomon also maintains that positive experiences can plant the seeds for unhappiness because the loss of the positive things will cause withdrawal or negative affect. The theory supports the current argument in suggesting that there are often emotional costs to intense positive experiences, especially those which are repeated.

Parducci's Range-Frequency Theory

Another theory which maintains that there are emotional costs to extremely good events is the range-frequency model of human judgments and happiness (Parducci, 1968, 1984; Smith, Wedell, & Diener, 1989). This theory is built on the presumption that all judgments are relative—events are judged in relation to other events. How good or bad an event is judged to be depends on the other events against which it is compared. For an event to produce happiness, it must be judged positively in the context of relevant events. What is noteworthy for the present argument is that extremely bad events create a context in which later good events can produce more intense happiness. Similarly, extremely good events can make future negative events even more negative. Parducci's theory predicts that the intensity of positive and negative experiences influence one another.

Richard Smith conducted a study in our laboratory to demonstrate how the relational property of judgements is affected by intensely good events. He showed subjects grade distributions they might receive in a difficult class. They were shown their scores on fifteen weekly quizzes on which the possible number of points was fifty per quiz. It was stressed that this was a very difficult class with a low grading distribution. The subjects were asked how happy they would feel when earning various grades. One group of subjects received a normal distribution of grades centering around twenty. Another group received the same distribution, but they had one score of fifty. The average happiness various scores would produce is shown in Fig. 2. Not surprisingly, the score of fifty would make people "extremely happy"—a 9.9 on the 11-point scale. But notice what happened to the other happiness values when an extremely high score was received. The lowest score (ten) is seen as more negative if the person had received a score of fifty. Even an otherwise high score (thirty) became less desirable if they had received a score of fifty. The extremely high score is very pleasing in itself, but it lowers the happiness one gains from other good events. Perhaps even worse, it makes the low scores even more painful. The above study is an empirical demonstration of the pleasure-pain connection about which Freud and the Stoics were concerned. The same effect was shown by Brickman, Coates, and Janoff-Bulman (1978) who found that those who won large lotteries were thereafter less happy when small positive everyday events occurred. To quote Parducci (1984):

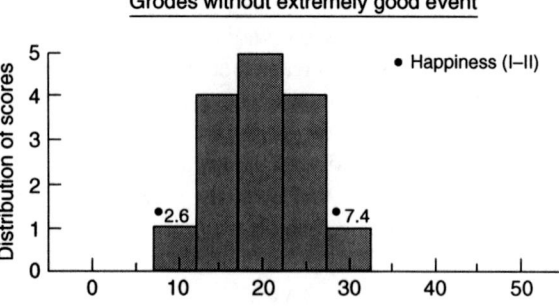

Fig. 2 Happiness judgments for various test scores

One type of "high" that can work against subsequent happiness comes from experiencing a new event better than any that had previously been experienced in the same domain. This new event extends the range upward so that lesser events become less satisfying. Although this makes an immediate positive contribution to the balance of happiness, its long-term effects are harmful unless the new upper endpoint can be experienced with high relative frequency ..." (p. 14)

Thus, it is clear that intense positive moments may lower the intensity of future positive moments, and that intense positive moments are often purchased at the price of past unhappy moments. It is unsurprising, therefore, that intense positive affect is not closely related to long-term happiness.

Conclusions

The basic tenet of this paper is that happiness or affective well-being can be equated with the relative amount of time a person experiences positive versus negative affect. Frequent positive affect is both necessary and sufficient for the experience of happiness and for high scores on happiness measures. Further study should certainly be devoted to examining the implications of this idea. This paper, however, advances a number of additional hypotheses which are researchable:

a. Intense positive affect is neither necessary nor sufficient for happiness, although intense positive experiences might sometimes heighten happiness among those who frequently experience positive affect.
b. The frequency of positive versus negative emotions can be measured across persons with accuracy and with a sophisticated level of measurement, whereas this is probably not true of the intensity of people's feelings.
c. Intense positive experiences often follow after a period of deprivation or suffering. In addition, intense positive experiences can cause later events and situations to be evaluated less positively. Thus, intense positive affect tends to be rare and to come with a price.

The above hypotheses are quite important to the field of subjective well-being because they are related to the most basic question of what comprises emotional well-being. Furthermore, these hypotheses are related to the fundamental issues about measuring well-being. Finally, the hypotheses raise interesting general questions about the causes of subjective well-being. The hypotheses we advance are of primary importance to the field, and yet are admittedly speculative. We have collected some data which support them but they have not yet received broad confirmation.

The above arguments raise a number of interesting researchable questions. When are the negative costs of positive emotional intensity exacted and when can they be avoided? That is, are there predictable times that a person will or will not suffer more negative emotions because of intense positive experiences? What factors increase positive emotional intensity and which of these generalize to negative emotional intensity? If seeking or obtaining intense positive experiences can have negative consequences for the individual, it seems imperative that we understand how this occurs because a large number of individuals in our culture are seeking such experiences. Theory should be developed which explains what personality and situational variables will effect the frequency of positive affect, its intensity, or both. A related set of questions has to do with the degree to which people seek and desire experiences which are intense versus those which produce mild happiness spread over time.

Another interesting question has to do with the independence of positive and negative affect (e.g. Bradburn, 1969; Diener & Emmons, 1984; Watson, Clark, & Tellegen, 1984). If these two types of emotions show some degree of independence across persons, it could be that looking separately at their frequencies would give even greater power in understanding happiness. In a sample of 100 college subjects, we found that the relative frequency of positive versus negative affect correlated with the Fordyce happiness scale, $r = 0.57$. When a regression was computed in which the Fordyce score was predicted by the frequency of positive affect and the frequency of negative affect, a multiple R of 0.59 was achieved. It appears that some small increment in knowledge can be gained by separately examining the frequencies of positive and negative affect, but further work on this issue is clearly required.

The arguments presented in this paper also have important applied implications. It appears that people who are successful at attaining frequent positive affect will be happy. Thus, interventions which aim at increasing happiness should centre on increasing the frequency and duration of happy experiences. The above arguments suggest that interventions or events which lead to intense but relatively infrequent positive experiences are unlikely to enhance long-term happiness to a substantial degree. It could be, however, that expectations about future intense events and the recall of past intense events may in some cases enhance long-term happiness. Therefore, the role of intense positive experiences to happiness needs to be explored in more depth.

References

Andrews, F. M., & Withey, S. B. (1976). *Social indicators of well-being: America's perception of life quality*, New York: Plenum Press.

Bradburn, N. M. (1969). *The structure of psychological well-being*. Chicago: Aldinc.

Brandstätter, H. (1987). Emotional responses to everyday life situations: An individual difference approach. *Paper delivered at the Colloquium on Subjective Well-Being*. Bad Homburg, Germany.

Brickman, P., Coates, D., & Janoff-Bulman, R. (1978). Lottery winners and accident victims: Is happiness relative? *Journal of Personality and Social Psychology, 36*, 917–927.

Colvin, C. R. Pavot, W., & Diener, E. (1988). *Emotional regulation: Affective amping and damping carryover*. In preparation, University of Illinois.

Davis, P. J., & Schwartz, G. E. (1987). Repression and the inaccessibility of affective memories. *Journal of Personality and Social Psychology, 52*, 155–162.

Diener, E. (1984). Subjective well-being. *Psychological Bulletin, 95*, 542–575.

Diener, E., & Emmons, R. A. (1984). The independence of positive and negative affect. *Journal of Personality and Social Psychology, 47*, 1105–1117.

Diener, E., & Iran-Nejad, A. (1986). The relationship in experience between various types of affect. *Journal of Personality and Social Psychology, 50*, 1031–1038.

Diener, E., Larsen, R. J., Levine, S., & Emmons, R. A. (1985). Intensity and frequency: Dimensions underlying positive and negative affect. *Journal of Personality and Social Psychology, 48*, 1253–1265.

Diener, E., Sandvik, E., & Larsen, R. J. (1985). Age and sex effects for emotional intensity. *Developmental Psychology, 21*, 542–546.

Diener, E., Sandvik, E., Gallagher, D., & Pavot, W. (1988). *The effects of response artifacts on measures of subjective well-being*. In preparation, University of Illinois.

Diener, E., Smith, R. H., Allman, A., & Pavot, W. (1988). *The costs of intense positive emotions*. In preparation, University of Illinois.

Epictetus. *The discourses*. Chicago: Encyclopaedia Brittanica, 1952.

Flugel, J. C. (1925). A quantitative study of feeling and emotion in everyday life. *British Journal of Psychology, 15*, 318–355.

Fordyce, M. W. (1977). *The happiness measures: A sixty-second index of emotional well-being and mental health*. Unpublished manuscript, Edison Community College, St. Meyers, Florida.

Freud, S. (1930). *Civilization and its discontents*. London: The Hogarth Press.

Gorman, B. S., & Wessman, A. E. (1974). The relationship of cognitive style and moods. *Journal of Clinical Psychology, 30*, 18–25.

Hasher, L., & Zacks, R. T. (1979). Automatic and effortful processes in memory. *Journal of Experimental Psychology: General, 108*, 356–388.

Hasher, L., & Zacks, R. T. (1984). Automatic processing of fundamental information: The case of frequency of occurrence. *American Psychologist, 39*, 1372–1388.

Larsen, R. J., & Diener, E. (1987). Emotional response intensity as an individual difference characteristic. *Journal of Research in Personality, 21*, 1–39.

Larsen, R. J., Diener, E., & Cropanzano, R. S. (1987). Cognitive operations associated with the characteristic of intense emotional responsiveness. *Journal of Personality and Social Psychology, 53*, 767–774.

Larsen, R. J., & Scheffer, S. (1987). *The influence of cognitive operations on physiological response to emotion-provoking stimuli.* Unpublished study, Purdue University.

Parducci, A. (1968). The relativism of absolute judgments. *Scientific American, 219*, 84–90.

Parducci, A. (1984). Value judgments: Toward a relational theory of happiness. In J. R. Eiser (Ed.), *Attitudinal judgment*. New York: Springer-Verlag.

Smith, R. H., Wedell, D., & Diener, E. (1989). Interpersonal and social comparison determinants of happiness. *Journal of Personality and Social Psychology, 56*, 317–325.

Solomon, R. L. (1980). The opponent-process theory of acquired motivation: The costs of pleasure and the benefits of pain. *American Psychologist, 35*, 691–712.

Thomas, D. (1987). *Memory bias in the recall of emotions.* Unpublished master's thesis, University of Illinois, 1987.

Thomas, D., & Diener, E. (1988). *Memory accuracy in the recall of emotions.* Paper submitted for publication.

Watson, D., Clark, L. A., & Tellegen, A. (1984). Cross-cultural convergence in the structure of mood: A Japanese replication and a comparison with US findings. *Journal of Personality and Social Psychology, 47*, 127–144.

Income's Differential Influence on Judgments of Life Versus Affective Well-Being

Ed Diener, Daniel Kahneman, Raksha Arora, James Harter, and William Tov

Abstract Findings are presented indicating that measures of subjective well-being can be ordered along a dimension varying from evaluative judgments of life at one end to experienced affect at the other. A debate in recent decades has focused on whether increasing income raises the experience of well-being. We found that judgment measures are more strongly associated with income and with the long-term changes of national income. Measures of affect showed lower correlations with income in cross-sectional analyses, as well as lower associations with long-term rising income. Measures of concepts such as "Happiness" and "Life Satisfaction" appear to be saturated with varying mixtures of judgment and affect, and this is reflected in the degree to which they correlate with income. The results indicate that measures of well-being fall along one dimension with different factors influencing scores at each end. Both types of well-being, judgment and affect, show very similar patterns of declining marginal utility with increasing income.

Introduction

Scholars have long pondered what leads to a happy life, and behavioral scientists have recently turned their attention to this question. However, in the past decade, attention has been drawn to the fact that "happiness" is not a single entity and can be divided into elements that differ from each other. Kahneman (1999) suggested that global judgments such as an evaluation of "life satisfaction" computed and reported at a single moment in time are quite different than the pleasantness of people's emotional lives, especially when it is sampled on-line over time rather than reported

E. Diener (✉)
Department of Psychology, University of Illinois, Champaign, IL 61820, USA
e-mail: ediener@uiuc.edu

This chapter is an alternative version of a paper that appears in: E. Diener, D. Kahneman,& J.F. Helliwell (Eds.). (2009). *International Differences in Well-Being*. Oxford, UK: Oxford University Press. The numbers in that paper differ slightly from the more preliminary analyses presented here, although the results here give a good account of the overall conclusions and pattern of findings.

globally. In support of this distinction, Lucas, Diener, and Suh (1996) found that various forms of well-being are empirically distinct and that their separability survives even when different measurement methods are employed. Thus, it is no longer satisfactory to inquire about "happiness." Rather, the various types of "happiness" should be individually analyzed and compared.

The major distinction that Kahneman drew was between global evaluative judgments and what he termed "objective happiness," the latter comprising people's feelings of pleasure and displeasure summated over time. One way to think of the distinction is to imagine that in global judgments, people step back and think of certain factors that they deem to be important and salient at the time of the judgment, whereas affect is determined in a less consciously controlled way as people react over time in their natural settings to ongoing events.

We suggest that the various self-report measures of subjective well-being are saturated to varying degrees with judgment and affect. Although no well-being measure is ever totally free of either of these components, it is plausible that a measure of "life satisfaction" might be more heavily weighted with judgment, whereas reports of "happiness" might be more saturated with affect. In the present study, we were fortunate to have two measures that seemed a priori to be close to the two opposite ends of the judgment–affect dimension: Cantril's Ladder (1965) and a report of daily affect. We analyzed two additional measures, life satisfaction and happiness, which we predicted would fall between the Ladder and affect measures on the judgment–affect dimension.

The goal of the study was to determine whether the judgment and affect measures performed differently and to identify the mix of the two processes reflected in specific measures. We pursued this goal by examining the intercorrelations among the measures at both the individual and national levels, as well as their correlations with external variables such as income. We also examined the distributions of the well-being measures and how the measures changed over time in response to changes in income. In this way, we sought to explore the characteristics of affect versus judgment measures of well-being.

In a classic 1974 article, Richard Easterlin asked whether economic growth makes people happier. The "Easterlin Paradox" consists of the puzzling fact that individual differences in income are usually correlated with differences in reports of well-being, but as national incomes have risen, there has often not been substantial growth in reported well-being. However, much debate has ensued in recent years about whether nations have, in fact, risen in average well-being over time in response to increasing income.

Hagerty and Veenhoven (2003), Stevenson and Wolfers (2008), and Inglehart, Foa, Peterson, and Welzel (2008) all claimed that, on the whole, the evidence suggests that there has been increasing happiness in many nations, and that it is associated with rising income. An examination of the data reported in these articles, however, indicates much variability in the pattern of findings. For example, in a response to Hagerty and Veenhoven, Easterlin (2005) pointed out that many nations, in fact, grew in income over time and did not increase in reported well-being. For instance, Easterlin presented reports of happiness over the decades in the United

States, which were essentially flat, and contrasted this trend with the substantial economic growth the country experienced during the same period of time. He concluded that across nations there are "quite disparate trends in happiness, suggesting that factors other than growth in income are responsible for the differential trends in happiness" (p. 429). In response, Veenhoven and Hagerty (2006) suggest that, on average, happiness increases occurred in nations where income rose the most. Stevenson and Wolfers (2008) argue that increasing income led to increases in happiness, but they also point to the substantial statistical uncertainty of some of their conclusions.

Inglehart et al. (2008) suggested that life satisfaction might be more influenced by economic conditions than is happiness, and this suggestion forms the starting point for our income analyses. We examine the possibility that various forms of well-being vary in their responsiveness to income change. Specifically, it could be that judgments and affective well-being vary with respect to how much they are influenced by economic growth. We analyze the association of four well-being variables that we propose vary along the judgment versus affect dimension with several economic variables—income, income change, and the ownership of modern conveniences such as television. Thus, we explore whether some of the past differences in conclusions about whether "happiness" has risen with income are due to the differential association of different types of well-being with income and which measures the researchers analyze.

We were fortunate to possess a representative sample of virtually the entire earth's adult population. Unlike many previous studies, the Gallup World Poll, on which we heavily relied, includes many less developed nations and a representative sample of rural residents outside of the major metropolitan areas. We were also fortunate that the survey included both a global judgment measure and an assessment of emotions experienced "yesterday." One issue with past research is that the wording of questions varies in different surveys conducted over the decades. Thus, we focused on surveys that used virtually identical wording and exactly the same response formats.

In our analyses, we relied heavily on the analyses of national data, not individual data, for several reasons. First, we have longitudinal data over time for nations and this forms a keystone in our analyses. Second, the Easterlin claim about income change is that in the aggregate at the societal level income increases do influence well-being because as the income of everyone rises, the standard for adequate income also rises at the same rate. Thus, our analyses focus on the nation-level, but we also examine individual data in the Gallup World Poll to determine whether the same dimensionality can be uncovered in the well-being measures, and whether the predictors are the same as at the nation-level.

In sum, we had several goals in the current study. First, we analyzed measures of well-being to determine whether they are separable, reflecting an underlying dimension related to global evaluative judgments versus the experience of affect. Second, we examined income and other predictors to determine whether they are most related to the judgment or affective ends of the well-being dimension, and whether income changes relate more to judgment or to affect. We also determined whether the distributions of the various measures of well-being were similar, and conformed to E. Diener and C. Diener's (1995) maxim that "most people are happy." Finally, we examined whether declining marginal utility of income shows the same pattern across all forms of well-being.

Methods

The Gallup Organization initiated its World Poll in 2005, and the first wave conducted from late 2005 to 2006 includes representative surveys of 132 societies representing over 95% of the world's population. The poll features a consistent set of standard questions in all surveys and uses nationwide samples (with the exception of Angola, Myanmar and Cuba where only urban populations were surveyed; and Afghanistan where there were only representative provinces).

Two sampling procedures were used in the World Poll: random-digit-dial (RDD) telephone surveys and face-to-face interviews. The RDD design was used in countries where the vast majority of the population had access to land line telephones. In all other countries, face-to-face surveys were conducted with clusters of households (obtained from census tract listings) serving as the basis for random sampling. The typical World Poll survey in a country consists of approximately 1,000 respondents. The total sample size for the present study was 141,741.

Wave 2 of the survey presented an additional well-being question on life satisfaction that was not included in the first wave. Thus, we analyzed the association of the well-being measures using also Wave 2, which included 84,225 respondents in 78 nations. Approximately 48,000 respondents were presented with the life satisfaction question.

From the survey, we employed several measures of well-being. Cantril asked respondents to evaluate their life (Ladder of Life) on a scale from 0 (*worst possible*) to 10 (*best possible*). Other measures assessed the recent experience of emotions, namely, positive feelings (enjoyment and smiling/laughter) and negative feelings (sadness, anger, worry, and depression). To reduce the extent of bias in recalling past experiences, respondents reported ("yes" or "no") whether they experienced these feelings during much of the previous day. At the individual level, we averaged Enjoyment and Smiling and subtracted the average of the four negative emotions to create an Affect Balance score. For each nation, we averaged the individual scores to create nation-level scores. The additional measure of well-being in Wave 2 on Life Satisfaction asked respondents how satisfied they were with their lives on a scale ranging from 0 (*Dissatisfied*) to 10 (*Satisfied*).

The Gallup World Poll queried respondents about their ownership of modern household conveniences, and we averaged five of these to create a composite Conveniences score: running water, electricity, telephone, television, and computer. In addition, we analyzed a question that asked how free subjects were in deciding how to spend their time. The question was answered by a dichotomous "yes" or "no" response, and asked: "Were you able to choose how you spent your time all day yesterday?"

In addition to the Gallup World Poll, we also obtained well-being measures for nations from Veenhoven's (2008) World Database on Happiness. We searched for those nations where the same 4-point happiness question was asked at two points in time separated by more than five years. When the scale had been administered more than two times, we used the first and last administrations. The question asked: "Taking all things together, would you say you are: 4—Very happy, 3—Quite happy, 2—Not very happy, or 1—Not at all happy," or small variants of these wordings. We also obtained Time 1 scores for nations where Cantril's Ladder had been administered previously and used the oldest date when the 0–10 response format was employed.

For life satisfaction at Time 1, we used the oldest existing survey in each nation where the same 0–10 format was used as in the Gallup World Poll. However, in order to increase our number of nations for life satisfaction, we also used instances where the response format was 1–10, as long as the earlier and later scales were available using the same response scale and were separated by more than five years. The Dominican Republic was dropped from the analyses of the Ladder scale because its score was an extreme outlier, far lower than any score ever reported, including very poor nations in the midst of turmoil. The score was so low that we suspect that it is an error, or a temporary response to some acute disaster.

Income scores were obtained from the Penn World Tables for years prior to 2005 (Heston, Summers, & Aten, 2006). Real GDP per capita in constant prices, chain series was used. For the years 2005–2007, we obtained income reports from the World Development Indicators database (World Bank, 2005–2007), and purchasing power parity in international dollars was used. Although the two methods yield some differences in estimated income, the differences are extremely small compared to the differences between nations, and the two types of income correlate almost perfectly.

Results

We hypothesized that measures that are more heavily weighted toward global life judgments will correlate more strongly with income and changes in income, whereas measures that more strongly reflect momentary affect will less strongly reflect income. In terms of widely used measures, we predicted that Cantril's Ladder will most heavily correlate with income, that affect will do so less strongly, and that measures that mix both elements such as global reports of "happiness" and "life satisfaction" will do so at intermediate levels. Most analyses were conducted at the level of nations, and not individuals, because it is at this level that the Easterlin debate focuses, and it is at this level that we obtain the most reliable measurements.

Our general plan is first to use the large Wave 1 of the Gallup World Poll to examine how well-being measures are related to one another in order to understand the nature of what each of them is assessing. We next determine how they relate to predictors such as income and satisfaction with standard of living. We also present the distributions of the various measures, as this too suggests a disjuncture between the judgment and affect measures. In addition, we analyze the patterns of declining marginal utility for the various measures to determine whether they are similar or different. Finally, we examine how changes in income over decades are associated with changes in the various well-being measures.

Cross-Sectional Analyses

Our analyses begin with cross-sectional correlations among the well-being measures themselves in order to explore their relationships with each other. We correlated the nation-level well-being averages for four measures of well-being at the most recent time of the surveys. As can be seen in Table 1, the correlations suggest a pattern of variables moving from the Ladder of Life Satisfaction, to Happiness, to Affect Balance. The Ladder and Affect Balance are least related, and the variables that are immediately adjacent to one another are most associated. The correlations suggest that the Ladder and Affect Balance are least related, and that the other two well-being variables are intermediate in their composition. The individual level correlations mirror this pattern.

We further explored the composition of Life Satisfaction and Happiness by predicting them simultaneously with both the Ladder and Affect Balance scores of nations. Life Satisfaction was predicted most strongly by the Ladder Score (Beta = 0.61, $p < 0.01$), although Affect Balance also significantly added to the prediction (Beta = 0.28, $p < 0.01$). In contrast, Happiness was most strongly predicted by Affect Balance (Beta 0.54, $p < 0.01$) with the Ladder predicting it positively, but not significantly so (Beta = 0.23). Thus, Life Satisfaction is more strongly saturated with judgment, but also includes an affective influence, whereas Happiness is more strongly reflective of affect.

We next analyzed the correlations of the four well-being measures with three predictors, and these associations are shown in Table 2. As can be seen, the Ladder correlated significantly more highly with income and conveniences, and lower with choosing how to spend one's time, than the other Subjective Well-Being (SWB)

Table 1 Intercorrelations of well-being measures

Well-being variables	Ladder	Life satisfaction	Happiness
Across Nations			
Life Satisfaction	0.74		
	N = 59		
Happiness	0.62	0.71	
	N = 48	N = 37	
Affect Balance	0.53	0.56	0.71
	N = 127	N = 58	N = 48
Across Individuals			
Life Satisfaction	0.54		
	N = 47,966		
Affect Balance	0.26	0.31	
	N = 78,238	N = 45,746	

Table 2 Nation-level correlates of measures of well-being

Well-being variables	Income per capita	Choose how to spend time	Possession of modern conveniences
Ladder Score			
Time 1	0.82 a		
	N = 18		
Time 2	0.83 c	0.33 a	0.80 a
	N = 119	N = 128	N = 128
Life Satisfaction			
Time 1	0.66 b		
	N = 38		
Time 2	0.58 d	0.51 b	0.46 b
	N = 62	N = 59	N = 59
Happiness			
Time 1	0.35 b		
	N = 48		
Time 2	0.34 de	0.54 b	0.16 bc
	N = 52	N = 48	N = 48
Affect Balance	0.31 e	0.57 b	0.16 c
(Time 1 only)	N = 118	N = 127	N = 127

Note. Correlations for the same time period in the same column which do not share a subscript letter in common differ by $p < 0.05$ or less.

variables. In some cases, the correlations for Life Satisfaction with the predictors differed from those for Happiness and Affect Balance, and in some cases not. Affect Balance and Happiness never differed significantly. The pattern of correlations clearly indicates that income and conveniences are more strongly associated with judgment forms of SWB, and that feelings tend to be more associated with the freedom to choose how to spend one's time.

Table 3 presents the correlations at the individual level between the well-being variables and the same three predictors as shown in Table 3. Because of the very large sample sizes, all with over 45,000 respondents, all correlations shown in the table differ significantly from one another by $p < 0.01$. The correlations with the material variables and well-being, as well as feelings of autonomy and well-being,

Table 3 Individual-level correlates of well-being

Well-being variables	Income per capita	Choose how to spend time	Possession of modern conveniences
Ladder Score	0.38	0.10	0.42
	N = 76,895	N = 81,534	N = 79,193
Life Satisfaction	0.34	0.16	0.27
	N = 36,898	N = 47,424	N = 47,962
Affect Balance	0.14	0.33	0.12
	N = 73,622	N = 78,191	N = 75,401

Note. All correlations are significantly different from zero at $p < 0.01$.

all closely mirror the pattern of associations found at the national level. The correlations are lower than those found with the nation-level variables, probably because there is random variation, and error of measurement and momentary mood effects tend to get averaged out when analyzing nation-level means. However, once again the two material variables were most strongly related to the Ladder, related least to Affect Balance, and at an intermediate level with Life Satisfaction.

A set of regression analyses in which Life Satisfaction was predicted by the other two variables at the individual level indicated that it was most closely associated with the Ladder, but that Affect Balance added significantly to its prediction as well (all p's < 0.01). When the Ladder was entered first as a predictor, it accounted for 29% of the variance, and Affect Balance added 3% more to the prediction when it was added. By contrast, when Affect Balance was entered first, it explained 10% of the variance in Life Satisfaction, but the Ladder added 22% additional variance. Thus, at the individual level, Life Satisfaction was both a judgment and affect variable, but much more strongly saturated with judgment.

The distributions of the well-being variables are also revealing. E. Diener and C. Diener (1995) hypothesized that most people are happy unless they are in dire circumstances, owing to the evolutionary advantages of being in a generally positive mood, and Cacioppo, Gardner, and Berntson (2002) similarly suggested that there is a "positivity offset" such that people tend to feel slightly pleasant in neutral situations. However, our findings indicate that this applies to affect, but not to judgments. Each of the four scales we employed has a neutral point above which is positive and below which is negative. For the Ladder and Life Satisfaction scales, above 5 indicates satisfaction or being closer to one's ideal life; and below 5 indicates dissatisfaction or being closer to the worst possible life one can imagine. For Affect Balance, above neutral means that there are more individuals who frequently experience pleasant than unpleasant emotions; and below 0 means the opposite. Finally, for "Happiness," the top two categories signify being happy and the bottom two signify being unhappy.

The distributions of scores for the four well-being measures are shown in Fig. 1. As can be seen, the distribution of the scores for the ladder is centered more closely around the midpoint, the neutral point, of the scale than the scores are for the other three measures. The percentage of nations below neutral for each measure at Time 2 was: Ladder—42%; Life Satisfaction—5%; Happiness—4%; Affect Balance—1%. Clearly, the distribution of scores around neutrality is dramatically different for the Ladder than for the other three scales.

People seem to be able to judge their lives to be closer to the worst possible than best possible lives they can imagine for themselves, and yet still feel generally positive in terms of their affect. Thus, conclusions about whether most nations are happy depend on whether we are discussing well-being judgments or affect. For judgments, many nations are not happy; but, for affect, almost all nations are above neutral in happiness. It appears that the affective influence on the happiness and life satisfaction scores tend to stabilize them in positive territory, at least at the level of nations, unless conditions have strongly deteriorated, whereas people are much more likely to step back from their lives and make a judgment that is more negative.

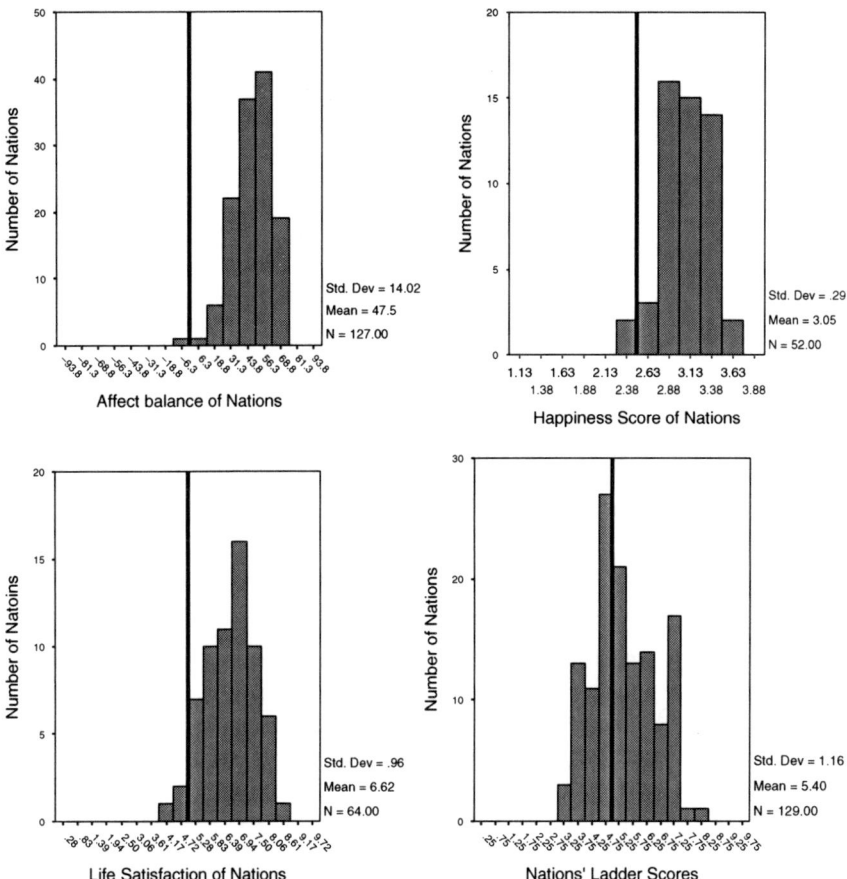

Fig. 1 Distributions of scores for four types of well-being measures

What of declining marginal utility, the tendency for money to have less and less impact as one obtains more and more of it? Is declining marginal utility similar for judgments and for affect balance? It might be, for example, that both types of well-being show declining marginal utility but have a different inflection point after which income makes less difference. In Fig. 2, we present the values of the two types of well-being for six levels of income. We standardized the measures of well-being in order to show them on the same scale. As can be seen, well-being increases rapidly as people rise out of poverty, but then improves more slowly after that. There is a very steep rise in well-being from dire poverty to about 20,000 dollars a year, and then a slow trend upwards, and then another slowing of the rise after about 50,000 dollars per year. Notably, the two lines are virtually identical, so close that they can barely be distinguished in the figure. Although affect is less influenced by income than are judgments of life, the association with income appears to decrease at the same rate for both.

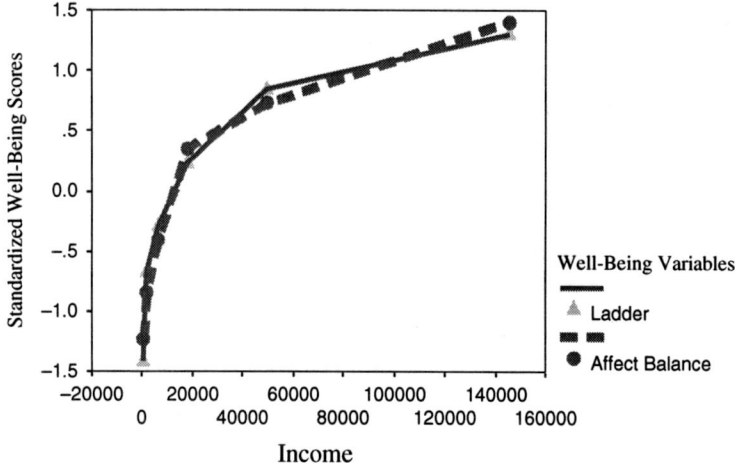

Fig. 2 Declining marginal utility

Longitudinal Analyses

We examined the correlations of each of the well-being measures with income and income change over longer periods of time greater than five years. In Table 4, we present the means for income and the well-being variables at the two points in time, as well as the average year of the surveys. As can be seen, on average the surveys were many years apart with intervals of 36, 21, and 19 years for three well-being measures. Furthermore, there were extremely large increases in income over those periods of time. Thus, if rising income has a long-term effect on well-being, it should be apparent during the periods of time we analyzed.

Table 4 Means and standard deviations of key variables for both waves

Wave & variables	Ladder	Life satisfaction	Happiness
Wave 1 Well-Being	5.58	6.68	3.01
	(1.04)	(1.15)	(.28)
Wave 2 Well-Being	6.31	6.91	3.08
	(1.01)	(.89)	(.28)
Wave 1 Year	1970	1983	1984
	(10.1)	(10.7)	(13.6)
Wave 2 Year	2006	2004	2003
	–	(4.4)	(2.9)
Wave 1 PPP/capita	8,148	10,702	11,187
	(6,475)	(5,478)	(7,385)
Wave 2 PPP/capita	19,938	22,114	20,332
	(13,756)	(14,039)	(12,498)
Number of Nations at Both Waves	18	32	48

We correlated the change in log per capita income with the change in well-being and found associations of: Ladder, $r = 0.56$, N = 18, $p < 0.05$; Life Satisfaction, $r = 0.33$, N = 32, $p < 0.10$; Happiness, $r = 0.24$, N = 0.48, $p < 0.10$. How large and consistent were the changes in well-being? Because income more than doubled, there ought to be a recognizable overall increase in well-being, not simply a correlation with changes in income if income influences well-being. For the Ladder and Happiness, there were significant national increases in well-being (p's < 0.01 and 0.05, respectively) during the periods we covered, whereas for Life Satisfaction, the difference was not significant. When the scale score changes are expressed in terms of the between-nation standard deviations in scores, well-being changed by the following amount: Ladder = 0.71 SD units; Life Satisfaction = 0.23 SD units; and Happiness = 0.25 SD units. As percentages of the total possible range of the scales, the differences between Times 1 and 2 were: Ladder = 7%; Life Satisfaction = 2%; and Happiness = 2%.

Discussion

Our findings indicate that measures of well-being vary along a dimension that is anchored by judgments about one's life at one end and by affect at the other. Selected measures can be placed on this continuum based on the relative amount they are influenced by the two types of subjective well-being. Cantril's Ladder of Life appears to reflect a judgment about one's life, whereas reports of emotions during the previous day stand at the other end of the dimension. Life Satisfaction is between the two anchors but appears to be closer to the Ladder, strongly reflecting a judgment but more heavily influenced by affect than is the Ladder. Reports of "Happiness" also fall toward the middle of the dimension but closer to the affective end than Life Satisfaction. Interestingly, on all of the measures that are influenced by affect most respondents score above the neutral point of the scale. By contrast, the Ladder is more evenly distributed around the neutral midpoint of the scale. Only for declining marginal utility do we see a very similar form for judgment and affect.

Not only do the measures differ in their relations with each other, but they also differ in their strength of associations with variables such as income and the ownership of modern conveniences. The Ladder was most strongly correlated with these material variables, and the Affect measure was least strongly associated with them. Life Satisfaction was significantly more strongly related to the material variables than Affect Balance, but significantly less strongly related to them than the Ladder. The strength of associations for Happiness and the material variables was significantly weaker than the Ladder correlations, but it did not differ significantly from either Life Satisfaction or Affect Balance. In contrast to income and the ownership of modern conveniences, feelings of autonomy in everyday life were more strongly associated with affect and less strongly associated with the Ladder. Thus, the pattern of correlations with the predictors confirms the dimensional ordering derived from the intercorrelations of the well-being variables with each other. The correlations suggest that material prosperity is strongly associated with judgments of life but much less correlated with affective well-being.

An examination of changes in well-being and income over time again supports the separability of the measures along the judgment–affect dimension. In terms of long-term changes in income, the Ladder showed a clear association, whereas the strength of this association for happiness and life satisfaction was more mixed across analyses and weaker. In terms of short-term changes in income, after controlling for income level, the Ladder showed the least association. By contrast, the more affective measures continued to show a significant inverse relation to short-term income change even after controlling for the level of income.

Is Easterlin correct, or his critics? The data on income and well-being are intricate, and like a Rorschach, one can see what one wants. On the one hand, life judgments are strongly related to income and have risen with income, and this is a pattern that is consistent across most nations. On the other hand, affect has benefited much less from long-term rising income. Similarly, one can point to the increases in well-being that have occurred in most nations, or one can point to the substantial number of nations that have declined in well-being even as their incomes have risen. Clearly, there is a more complex pattern than simply an input–output system in which income causes well-being in a one-to-one way. Other factors in societies must be considered, such as social trust and urbanization; psychological factors such as rising aspirations also play a role.

Easterlin was correct in his claim that rising incomes do not inevitably increase subjective well-being; and the critics are correct in their claim that rising incomes have often been associated with some increases in well-being. The challenge now is to understand when higher income leads to a higher well-being and when it does not.

In conclusion, we found that the judgment contained in Cantril's Ladder was much more associated with income and income changes than was the more purely affective measures. Thus, it is no longer productive simply to talk about income and general "happiness"; well-being must be parsed into the judgmental versus affective components. Whether income causes an increase in well-being appears to depend heavily on what type of well-being is being discussed. In future research, judgments of life and affect ought to be distinguished in all research on well-being, even though in some instances they will produce similar conclusions.

References

Cacioppo, J. T., Gardner, W. L., & Berntson, G. G. (2002). The affect system has parallel and integrative processing components: Form follows function. In J. T. Cacioppo, G. G. Berntson, et al. (Eds.), *Foundations in social neuroscience* (pp. 493–522). Cambridge, MA: MIT Press.
Cantril, H. (1965). *The pattern of human concerns*. New Brunswick, NJ: Rutgers University Press.
Diener, E., & Diener, C. (1995). Most people are happy. *Psychological Science, 7,* 181–185.
Easterlin, R. A. (1974). Does economic growth improve the human lot? Some empirical evidence. In P. A. David & M. W. Reder (Eds.), *Nations and households in economic growth*. New York: Academic Press.

Easterlin, R. A. (2005). Feeding the illusion of growth and happiness: A reply to Hagerty and Veenhoven. *Social Indicators Research, 74*, 429–443.

Hagerty, M., & Veenhoven, R. (2003). Wealth and happiness revisited – Growing national income does go with greater happiness. *Social Indicators Research, 64*, 1–27.

Heston, A., Summers, R., & Aten, B. (2006). *Penn World Table Version 6.2.* Center for International Comparisons of Production, Income, and Prices, Philadelphia, PA.

Inglehart, R., Foa, R., Peterson, C., & Welzel, C. (2008). Development, freedom, and rising happiness: A global perspective (1981–2007). *Perspectives on Psychological Science, 3*, 264–285.

Kahneman, D. (1999). Objective happiness. In D. Kahneman, E. Diener, & N. Schwarz (Eds.), *Well-being: The foundations of hedonic psychology.* New York: Russell Sage Foundation.

Lucas, R. E., Diener, E., & Suh, E. (1996). Discriminant validity of well-being measures. *Journal of Personality and Social Psychology, 71*, 616–628.

Stevenson, B., & Wolfers. J. (2008, April 15). *Economic growth and subjective well-being: Reassessing the Easterlin Paradox.* Working Paper Series. Available at SSRN: http://ssrn.com/abstract=1121237

Veenhoven, R. (2008). *World database of happiness, Trends in nations.* Roterdam: Erasmus University, September 10, 2008. http://worlddatabaseofhappiness.eur.nl/

Veenhoven, R., & Hagerty, M. (2006). Rising happiness in nations 1946–2004. *Social Indicators Research, 79*, 421–436.

World Bank. (2005–2007). *World development indicators.* http://web.worldbank.org/WBSITE/EXTERNAL/DATASTATISTICS/0,,contentMDK:21725423~pagePK:64133150~piPK:64133175~theSitePK:239419,00.html

New Measures of Well-Being

Ed Diener, Derrick Wirtz, Robert Biswas-Diener, William Tov,
Chu Kim-Prieto, Dong-won Choi, and Shigehiro Oishi

Abstract We present new measures of well-being to assess the following concepts: 1. Psychological Well-Being (PWB); 2. Positive Feelings, Negative Feelings, and the balance between the two (SPANE-P, N, B); and 3. Positive Thinking. The PWB scale is a short 8-item summary survey of the person's self-perceived functioning in important areas such as relationships, self-esteem, purpose and meaning, and optimism. The scale is substantially correlated with other psychological well-being scales, but is briefer. The scale provides a single overall psychological well-being score and does not yield scores for various components of well-being. The Scale of Positive and Negative Experience (SPANE) yields a score for positive experience and feelings (6 items), a score for negative experience and feelings (6 items), and the two can be combined to create an experience balance score. This 12-item brief scale has a number of desirable features compared to earlier measures of positive and negative feelings. In particular, the scale assesses with a few items a broad range of negative and positive experiences and feelings, not just those of a certain type, and is based on the frequency of feelings during the past month. A scale to measure Positive Thinking is also presented. Basic psychometric statistics are presented for the scales based on 573 college students at five universities.

New Measures of Well-Being

When examining the standard scales for assessing well-being, we were impressed with the need for measurement scales in several domains—positive and negative feelings, positive thinking, and a brief scale of psychological well-being (PWB).

E. Diener (✉)
Department of Psychology, University of Illinois, Urbana-Champaign, Champaign, IL 61820, USA
e-mail: ediener@uiuc.edu

The scale in this article entitled Psychological Well-Being has since been renamed as the Flourishing Scale. Further psychometrics and other data concerning the scale can be found in the article:

Diener, E., Wirtz, D., Tov, W., Kim-Prieto, C., Choi, D., Oishi, S., & Biswas-Diener, R. (2009). New measures of well-being: Flourishing and Positive and Negative Feelings.

E. Diener (ed.), *Assessing Well-Being: The Collected Works of Ed Diener*,
Social Indicators Research Series 39, DOI 10.1007/978-90-481-2354-4_12,
© Springer Science+Business Media B.V. 2009

These concepts are related to one another and to life satisfaction, although the types of well-being are separable (Lucas, Diener, & Suh, 1996; Ryff, 1989) and must, therefore, be assessed separately. Although scales exist to measure several of these constructs, the instruments have limitations that make additional measures desirable. We present a short measure of psychological well-being (PWB) designed to complement the longer scales that are available and a measure of negative and positive feelings that is designed to better assess ongoing feelings of well-being. An initial scale to assess positive thinking contains both positive and negative items. We present the psychometric properties of the scales, such as reliabilities and convergent correlations with other relevant measures.

The scales in this chapter are similar to measures that were first presented in Diener and Biswas-Diener's *Happiness: Unlocking the Mysteries of Psychological Wealth* (2008). Several items were altered or dropped, and we report here psychometric analyses that examined features of the revised scales such as internal and temporal reliability, factor structure, discriminant validity of the scales from one another, and convergent validity with other similar scales. The measures in this chapter, and their shortened names, are:

> Positive Experience (SPANE-P)
> Negative Experience (SPANE-N)
> The Balance of Positive and Negative Experience (SPANE-B)
> Positive Thinking (PTS)
> Psychological Well-being (PWB)

Why New Scales?

Positive and Negative Feelings

Scales exist to assess pleasant and unpleasant emotions, and probably the most widely used is Watson, Clark, and Tellegen's (1988) Positive and Negative Affect Schedule, called the PANAS. There are several limitations of this measure that motivated us to develop an alternative scale to assess pleasant versus unpleasant feelings. The PANAS was designed to measure a specific conception of emotional well-being and ill-being, and thus assesses some states that are usually not considered to be feelings. In addition, the scale fails to measure a number of important positive and negative feelings that are considered to be important to well-being. For example, the Positive Affect items of the PANAS include "strong," "alert," "active," and "determined," which many would not consider to be feelings. One can feel "active" and "alert" if one is scared, and "strong" when one does not feel emotional. "Determined" can be seen as a motivational state, but is not necessarily a pleasant or desirable one in all instances. For example, respondents might be "determined" because they are angry and vengeful. In addition, some feelings on the PANAS, such as "inspired," are rare and very specific. Thus, the scale does not with certainty reflect feelings that will enhance well-being.

The Negative Affect items include many adjectives that are more widely agreed to be emotional experiences, but some feelings are notable by their absence. For example, the scale does not include "sad" or "depressed," which are core negative feelings. Indeed, the "depression" facet of neuroticism predicts life satisfaction better than all facets of neuroticism (e.g., anxiety, anger, vulnerability) combined (Schimmack, Oishi, Furr, & Funder, 2004), suggesting the centrality of "sad" and "depressed" in understanding people's well-being. Furthermore, some feelings are represented by a number of similar adjectives, such as "jittery," "nervous," "scared," and "afraid." The inclusion of four synonyms for anxiety means that the scale is heavily weighted with one specific type of feeling. Thus, fully forty percent of the items represent various forms of fear, whereas sadness is not represented at all. This derives from the fact that Watson and colleagues consider negative feelings to be both negative and aroused, and, therefore, unaroused, unpleasant feelings were omitted from their scale. Thus, the PANAS represents a narrow definition of positive and negative feelings based on highly aroused forms of these feelings. However, well-being and ill-being include many feelings that are not of the highly aroused type.

As reviewed above, there are a number of important feelings that are omitted from the PANAS. For example, love and other terms referring to affectionate feelings are usually considered to be important emotions but are omitted from the PANAS. Feelings such as pride, envy and jealousy, contentment, joy, and happiness are not assessed. Although the expanded PANAS-X (Watson & Clark, 1994) includes many of these feelings, this scale is not used frequently in the well-being field, in part because of its length, and in part because it measures attentiveness, joviality, and self-assurance that are not precisely the types of feelings that well-being researchers want to assess.

Another important shortcoming of the PANAS and other existing scales is the problem that they omit feelings that might be important in some cultures or to certain individuals. For example, *schadenfreude* is an emotion that is often mentioned as a German emotion-word for which there is no word in English. Scollon, Diener, Oishi, and Biswas-Diener (2004) mention words such as "sukhi" and "aviman" in India and "shitashima" and "fureai" in Japan, which do not exist in English or in many other cultures. Furthermore, East Asians deem low-arousal positive emotions such as "calm" and "relaxed" to be more desirable than North Americans do (Tsai, Knutson, & Fund, 2006), suggesting that low arousal positive emotions that are missing from the PANAS might be important correlates of well-being in other cultures. Finally, high arousal positive emotions are stronger predictors of life satisfaction among sensation seekers than among non-sensation seekers, on weekends than on weekdays, and when the concept "excitement" is experimentally primed than when the concept "peace" is primed (Oishi, Schimmack, & Colcombe, 2003). In sum, the PANAS is limited in that it includes descriptors that are not feelings and omits other feelings that are widely believed to be core emotional feelings, as well as emotions that are important in some cultures, to some individuals, and in certain situations. The scale does not reflect the difference in the desirability of feelings in different contexts and cultures.

An example of why the adequate sampling of feelings is essential for an adequate measure of well-being can be offered based on a hypothetical comparison of young and old adults. On the PANAS positive emotions scale, young adults might score higher than the elderly simply because they are more energetic and lead lives that are more active and arousing. Young people are likely to score higher on terms such as "active" and "strong," even if they feel no more positive than old people. In contrast, the elderly might score higher on pleasant terms such as "contented" and "happy," although these feelings are not assessed by the PANAS. Thus, the PANAS might yield conclusions that would be completely reversed if a different set of adjectives were employed. The PANAS assesses highly activated or aroused states rather than the full range of pleasant/desirable and unpleasant/undesirable feelings.

What of other scales designed to measure positive and negative feelings? Lucas, Diener, and Larsen (2003) review measures of positive emotions, including the PANAS and other scales. Several of the scales they review are very long, and each of them suffers from certain deficiencies. For example, some of the scales are based on a checklist format that yields less reliable results, and several of the scales measure concepts such as surprise, joviality, and vigor that do not adequately sample the positive feelings composing well-being.

In conclusion, we created a scale called the Scale of Positive and Negative Experience, or SPANE for short. The SPANE brief name is followed by a P, N, or B to indicate the scales for Positive Experience, Negative Experience, and the Balance between the two. The SPANE includes broad descriptors for positive and negative feelings, as well as a number of positive and negative emotions that are central to the experience of well-being.

How can we avoid the omission of feelings, which is a major shortcoming of the PANAS, and include all positive and negative feelings without making an exhaustive list that would create a scale that is prohibitively long? Our solution was to include broad desirable and undesirable words that describe in general terms the feelings people approach and avoid. For the desirable feelings we included three descriptors: "Good," "Positive," and "Pleasant." These three adjectives all describe the feelings people seek and value, and should apply to a wide range of more specific feelings. Thus, our scale can reflect the indefinite number of positive feelings because it uses broad words that apply to all of these experiences. The three adjectives are each alternative ways of describing the feelings that people desire and enjoy, regardless of arousal and other qualities.

Similarly, for negative feelings, we used three general descriptors that apply to all feelings that people avoid: "Bad," "Negative," and "Unpleasant." Again, these items should allow us to reflect specific feelings that a scale with narrower items might miss. If people were to mean something different by "bad" and "unpleasant," this will be revealed in our empirical findings. In other words, if there are still concerns because the three good and three bad words are not identical in meaning and refer to different qualities of feelings, this should become evident when we analyze the associations of the items.

Another problem in measuring affective well-being is that some feelings might be experienced as positive in some cultures and as negative in other cultures, for example "pride" and "gratitude" (Kitayama, Markus, & Kurosawa, 2000; Scollon et al., 2004; Oishi, 2007). By inclusion of general desirable feelings (good, positive, and pleasant) and undesirable feelings (bad, negative, and unpleasant), we largely avoid this problem because we allow the respondents themselves to determine whether their experience is pleasant/desirable or unpleasant/undesirable. If people think of certain pleasant feelings as being undesirable, this will be uncovered in our findings.

By using the general labels for feelings, we also side-step the knotty debate about which feelings are truly emotional. Regardless of whether an experience is an emotion, a mood, or neither, it is captured in our measure if it is perceived to be a desirable or undesirable feeling. For example, our scale should reflect states that are pleasant and desirable but might not be emotions, for example "interested" and "engaged." In addition, if people are interested, but unpleasantly so, this will be reflected in our three general negative terms. Thus, the use of general feelings allows us to assess a full range of positive and negative feelings regardless of their source, and this approach seems to be the most sensible one when it is people's subjective well-being that is of interest. Our scale reflects pleasures and pains as well as emotions. We need not constrain ourselves to emotion scales, which were created by researchers whose goal was to study emotions.

Besides the six items used to measure general feelings, our positive and negative feelings scales also included a number of important emotions. For positive feelings beyond the general three, we included: "Contented," "Happy," and "Joyful." These were all considered to be so important and widely desirable that they were deemed worthy of assessment beyond the general adjectives. Schimmack (2003) found that "happy" predicts life satisfaction beyond specific positive emotions such as pride, being affectionate, or excited, but that these emotions did not predict life satisfaction after "happy" was controlled. For negative feelings we included: "Sad," "Afraid," and "Depressed." Thus, beyond the general descriptors of negative and positive feelings, we included feelings that are often considered to be the most important forms of these experiences related to feelings of well-being and ill-being. Furthermore, these terms reflect a range of activation from low to high arousal, and, therefore, capture feelings from around the emotion circumplex (see Larsen & Diener, 1992, for a description of this structure).

Psychological Well-Being

In recent years, a form of well-being in addition to subjective well-being has emerged from theorists such as Deci and Ryan (e.g., Ryan & Deci, 2000, 2001) and Ryff (1989) based on the idea of universal human needs and effective functioning. These approaches are labeled "psychological well-being" and are based in part on humanistic theories of positive functioning. The authors argue that they are distinct from subjective feelings of well-being even if they overlap empirically. Whereas subjective well-being is defined as people's evaluations of their lives, psychological well-being is thought to represent optimal human functioning. The aspects of psychological well-being we assess in the Psychological Well-Being Scale (PWB), and names of some of those who have been advocates for the desirability of these states are:

> Meaning and purpose (Ryff; Seligman)
> Supportive and rewarding relationships (Ryff; Deci and Ryan)
> Engaged and interested (Csikszentmihalyi; Ryff; Seligman)
> Contribute to the well-being of others (Maslow; Ryff; Deci and Ryan)
> Competency (Ryff; Deci and Ryan)
> Self-acceptance (Maslow; Ryff)
> Optimism (Seligman)
> Being respected (Maslow; Ryff)

Our goal was to be very brief, and yet reasonably comprehensive. Importantly, we do not claim to fully measure each of the separate components of PWB because our goal of brevity precluded this. Our aim was to create a broad overview of a person's PWB, and researchers who need valid measures of the specific components must employ longer scales.

Why not simply use the existing scales by Ryff or Deci and Ryan? First, we wanted a very brief scale because many surveys cannot include measures with more than a short number of items. Second, we hoped to include several aspects of well-being that are not included in the existing scales, for example "engagement and interest," and "optimism." Csikszentmihalyi (1990) has made the case that engagement and flow are core components of well-being and psychological capital, and, therefore, we included one item measuring this domain. Seligman (2002) suggested that well-being is made up of feelings of engagement and interest, pleasure, and meaning and purpose. Peterson and Seligman (2004) made the case that optimism is important to healthy functioning, and, therefore, we assessed this concept. We employed an item on feeling respected, a human need listed by Maslow (1958). Finally, we included an item on contributing to the well-being and happiness of others, in part because this has been related to health (Brown, Nesse, Vinokur, & Smith, 2003). In addition, some models of effective functioning have been criticized for being too individualistic and not weighting a person's contributions to others. From the Ryff and Deci and Ryan theories, we created items to assess: meaning, positive social relationships (including helping others and one's community), self-esteem, and competence and mastery. Thus, our scale is a broad measure of a number of aspects of psychological well-being using a very brief format.

Positive and Negative Thinking

A major recommendation for people seeking happiness has been that they need to develop positive thinking and decrease their propensity for negative thinking. Norman Vincent Peale (1956) popularized this notion with his bestseller *The Power of Positive Thinking*. Although his advice was seen as naïve in some academic circles, the idea that people's habits of thoughts could influence their subjective well-being became respectable with the proven effectiveness of cognitive behavioral therapy (Meichenbaum, 1977). Aaron Beck, Rush, Shaw, and Emery (1979) and Albert Ellis (2001) advanced the idea that the way people think about the world can influence their emotions and feelings of well-being. Richard Lazarus (1982) demonstrated in laboratory experiments that the way people thought about perceived stimuli has a large influence on their responses to them. Thus, Peale's ideas became more respectable among psychologists. At the same time, Buddhist and other Eastern approaches to contentment began to receive attention and study in the west (Tsai, Miao, & Seppala, 2007).

People's habits of positive thinking are not the sole determinant of happiness because circumstances can influence well-being as well. Some circumstances and societies are so overwhelmingly negative as to overpower positive thinkers. However, the propensity to positive or negative thinking can influence a person's feelings of well-being, controlling for environmental circumstances. Thus, we developed and assessed a measure of the propensity to view things in positive versus negative terms. This tendency was measured earlier by Judge and Bretz (1993), who assessed people's responses to neutral objects such as standard paper, and to things that are common within a culture and therefore constant across people, such as speed limits.

Our approach to measuring a propensity to positive thinking was to assess people's positive versus negative thinking about important aspects of their lives—themselves, one's past and future, other people, and the world in general. Our Positive Thinking Scale (PTS) focused primarily on people's view of themselves and other people. Rather than examine people's positivity about neutral objects, we chose to examine people's thought propensities about important aspects of life, of oneself, and of others. Which approach leads to an assessment that best reflects one's general thought tendencies will be a question for future research, as will be the incremental validity beyond other types of measures.

Satisfaction with Life

In our study, we included an existing measure, the Satisfaction with Life Scale (Diener, Emmons, Larsen, & Griffin, 1985) that has received extensive psychometric testing. Several thorough reviews of the scale exist (Pavot & Diener, 1993; Pavot & Diener, 2008). The primary reason for inclusion of the life satisfaction scale in the current study was to examine the associations of our new scales with it, and to determine whether they can predict life satisfaction.

The Current Study

Measures

The Scale of Positive and Negative Experience (SPANE)

This measure is a brief 12-item scale with six items devoted to positive experience and six items designed to assess negative experience. Because the scale includes very general positive and negative experience and feelings, it assesses the full range of positive and negative experience, including specific feelings that may be defined by one's culture. Because of the general items included in the scale, it can assess not only the pleasant and unpleasant emotional feelings that are the focus of most scales, but also reflects other states such as interest, flow and engagement, and physical pleasure.

The SPANE has several other desirable features. It asks people to recall their activities and experiences during the past four weeks and to report these feelings. The period of one month was selected in order to give an adequate sample of feelings, rather than focusing on a short time that might not have been representative. At the same time, events occurring during the previous month can be easily recalled, and are, therefore, more likely to be based on experience, not just on a person's general self-concept. Thus, one month was selected in order to provide a balance between sampling adequacy and memory accuracy. The scale items, however, can be used with other time frames, such as "Yesterday," "Past week," or "In general."

Another desirable feature of the SPANE is that the responses are in terms of the amount of time during which the respondent has experienced each feeling. Responses linked to time, such as "Very rarely or never" and "Very often or always," might possibly vary in interpretation across respondents but are much more likely than many types of descriptors to be used in a similar way across people. After all, "Always" and "Never" are absolute terms that should have the same meaning to all respondents. In contrast, measures that inquire how much a person had particular experiences, but without indicating either time or intensity, are open to greater ambiguity. Intensity is harder to calibrate across respondents because they can mean different things by "a lot" or "slightly." Furthermore, when scales inquire as to how much a person experiences a particular feeling, and they do not indicate time or intensity, the response is ambiguous in terms of whether the person felt the feeling rarely but very intensely, frequently but very mildly, or some other combination of time and intensity. Thus, our scale makes explicit the time duration frame of reference and uses response categories that are tied to objective time.

Another advantage of using the time response format is that it is more closely related to global well-being than is emotional intensity. Diener, Sandvik, and Pavot (1991) argued that global reports of well-being are more closely linked to the duration of positive versus negative experiences than to the intensity of the experiences. For one thing, it is possible that people who experience positive emotions in a generally intense way are also more likely to experience negative emotions in an intense way as well, thus negating the enhanced value of intense positive experiences. Diener, Colvin, Pavot, and Allman (1991) demonstrated that some of the factors that lead to intense positive feelings when a person succeeds will create more intense negative feelings when the person fails, for example. Diener et al. showed that the duration of positive versus negative experiences is empirically a stronger predictor of general well-being than is the intensity of these feelings. Thus, our use of the time response format should enhance the validity of our feelings scale.

The SPANE consists of 12 items, six of which are positive and six of which are negative. Each item is scored on a scale ranging from 1 to 5, where 1 represents "very rarely or never" and 5 represents "very often or always." The positive and negative scales are scored separately because of the partial independence or separability of the two types of feelings. The summed positive score can range from 6 to 30, and the negative scale has the same range. The two scores can be combined by subtracting the negative score from the positive score, and the resulting SPANE-B scores can range from −24 to 24. The SPANE is shown in the Appendix.

Psychological Well-Being (PWB)

The Psychological Well-Being scale (PWB) consists of eight items describing important aspects of human functioning ranging from positive relationships, to feelings of competence, to having meaning and purpose in life. Each item is answered on a 1–7 scale that ranges from Strong Disagreement to Strong Agreement. All items are phrased in a positive direction. Scores can range from 8 (Strong Disagreement with all items) to 56 (Strong Agreement with all items). High scores signify that respondents view themselves in very positive terms in diverse areas of functioning. Although the scale does not individually measure facets of psychological well-being, it does yield an overview of positive functioning across the domains that are widely believed to be important. The PWB is shown in the Appendix.

Positive Thinking Scale (PTS)

The Positive Thinking Scale (PTS) is composed of 22 items, 11 of which represent positive thoughts and perceptions and 11 of which represent low negative thinking. The 22 items are answered on a yes–no format. The negative items are reverse scored with a "no" response counting as a "1"; and for the positive items a "yes" response counts as a "1." After reversing the negative items, the 22 items are added, thus yielding scores that range from 0 to 22. The scale is presented in the Appendix.

Participants

Data collection occurred for all samples in the fall of 2008. The N's for different analyses vary in size because a few participants had missing data, and because the ancillary scales were given at some locations but not at others.

> *Sample 1.* Respondents from the Introductory Psychology participant pool at the University of Illinois volunteered to participate in order to earn course bonus points during the fall semester of 2008. The sample included 61 women and 13 men. Participants answered the survey twice, approximately one month apart. Besides the core new scales, respondents at this and some other locations completed additional surveys for the purpose of examining convergent validity.

Sample 2. College of New Jersey had 75 women and 11 men who responded to the survey at one particular time only.

Sample 3. Singapore Management University had 115 female and 66 male respondents.

Sample 4. California State University East Bay had 64 respondents, with 10 males, 41 females, and 13 who did not indicate their sex.

Sample 5. Students at East Carolina University responded twice to the core survey scales, with 31 male and 104 female participants, and 33 who did not indicate their sex.

Convergent Validity Scales

We used a number of well-being measures in order to determine the convergence of the new scales with established measures. For traditional subjective well-being, we included the Satisfaction with Life Scale (Diener, Emmons, Larsen, & Griffin, 1985), and, at some locations, Fordyce's (1988) single item measure of happiness, which is answered on a 11-point scale ranging from "Extremely happy (feeling ecstatic, joyous, fantastic!" down to "Extremely unhappy (utterly depressed, completely down)". Lyubomirsky and Lepper's (1999) 4-item scale of happiness was also used at some universities. The Lyubomirsky scale (SHS) asks how happy the respondent is in four different ways. We also included the Watson and colleagues' PANAS (1988), which is currently the most widespread measure of positive and negative feelings. We also included at some locations Scheier, Carver, and Bridges' LOT-R (1994), which assesses optimism, and the UCLA Loneliness Scale (Russell, 1996), which is a marker of poor social relationships. We also included Deci and Ryan's Basic Need Satisfaction Scale (BSN; 2000), which has 21 items to assess competence, supportive relationships, and autonomy. Finally, we administered the 54-item version of Ryff's (2008) scale with 9 items to measure each of the following concepts: Autonomy, Growth, Mastery, Relationships, Self-esteem, and Purpose and Meaning. Thus, we can determine the associations of our new scales with a wide variety of other well-being measures.

Results

Table 1 shows the means and standard deviations for each of the new scales, as well as the internal reliabilities, temporal reliabilities, and scale ranges. As can be seen, the mean score for each of the scales is in the positive range above the neutral point of the scales. The internal reliabilities are adequate, and the temporal stabilities show that some changes occurred over the period of one month, but that there was nonetheless substantial stability over time in the scores.

Table 2 presents the scores for the scales that correspond to approximate percentiles, in order to provide norms for the scales. It must be remembered, however,

Table 1 Psychometric statistics on the new scales

	Mean (SD)[1]	Cronbach's alpha	Temporal stability[2]	Scale range
Psychological Well-Being				
PWB	45.4	0.86	0.71	8–56
	(6.2)	N=568	N=261	
SPANE (Feelings)				
P (Positive)	22.1	0.84	0.62	6–30
	(3.7)	N=572	N=261	
N (Negative)	15.6	0.80	0.62	6–30
	(3.9)	N=567	N=261	
B (Balance)	6.5	0.88	0.68	−24 to 24
	(6.7)	N=566	N=261	
Positive Attitudes (PTS)				
Positive	9.2	0.70	0.73	0–11
	(2.0)	N=564	N= 261	
Negative[3]	6.4	0.75	0.76	0–11
	(2.8)	N=563	N=261	
Total	15.5	0.81	0.79	0–22
	(4.2)	N=555	N=261	

[1]N was 573 for the means.
[2]All values $p < 0.001$.
[3]High score signifies low negative attitudes.

that these norms are based only on college students. Norms for broader groups will need to be generated in future research.

Table 3 shows the correlations of the new scales with each other, and with the Satisfaction with Life Scale. As can be seen, the scales correlate at a moderate level with each other and with life satisfaction. This suggests that there are some common influences that affect feelings, attitudes, life satisfaction, and psychological well-being. It is possible that response styles, self-perceptions, and general well-being affect all of the scales, and these different influences will need to be explored in future studies.

Table 4 presents the correlations of the new feeling-scales with other scales that measure similar concepts in order to examine the convergent validity of the scales. As can be seen, the SPANE scales are substantially associated with the PANAS scales and the more global measures of happiness as well. The convergence of the SPANE scales and the corresponding PANAS scales was 0.59, 0.70, and 0.77. The SPANE positive and negative experience scales correlate more strongly with the SHS and Fordyce scales than do the corresponding PANAS scales; but the PANAS does as well when it comes to the balance score, perhaps because the balance score reflects the positive–negative dimension more strongly, with less influence from arousal than occurs in the individual positive and negative scales of the PANAS. Whereas the individual PANAS scales are highly saturated with high arousal emotions, the difference between the positive and negative scales may better capture the

Table 2 Norms for new scales approximate percentile rankings

Scale	Approximate percentile	Score
PWB	10	36
(Range 8–56)	20	40
	50	46
	80	50
	90	52
SPANE-P	10	17
(Range 6–30)	20	18
	50	22
	80	25
	90	26
SPANE-N	10	10
(Range 6–30)	20	12
	50	15
	80	18
	90	20
SPANE-B	10	−3
(Range −24 to 24)	20	0
	50	6
	80	11
	90	14
PTS	10	9
(Range 0–22)	20	12
	50	16
	80	19
	90	20

Table 3 Intercorrelations of scales

	PWB	SPANE-P	SPANE-N	SPANE-B	PTS-P	PTS-N	PTS-Tot
PWB							
SPANE-P	0.62						
SPANE-N	0.51	0.58					
SPANE-B	0.64	0.88	0.90				
PTS-P	0.60	0.45	0.40	0.48			
PTS-N	0.53	0.46	0.50	0.54	0.48		
PTS-Tot	0.64	0.53	0.53	0.59	0.81	0.91	
SWLS	0.62	0.55	0.42	0.54	0.50	0.52	0.59

$N = 563$; all p's < 0.001.

Table 4 Correlations of feelings scales

	SPANE-P	SPANE-N	SPANE-B	PANAS-PA	PANAS-NA	PANAS-BAL
PANAS-PA	0.59	−0.41	0.57			
PANAS-NA	−0.41	0.70	−0.63	−0.24		
PANAS-BAL	0.65	−0.71	0.77	0.77	−0.80	
SHS	0.66	−0.52	0.67	0.60	−0.45	0.68
Fordyce	0.65	−0.51	0.66	0.56	−0.46	0.65

$N = 563$, all p's < 0.001.

Table 5 Correlations of psychological well-being scales

	PWB	BSN total
BSN-Total	0.69	
Ryff Scales		
Autonomy	0.39	0.41
Mastery	0.73	0.76
Growth	0.67	0.65
Relationships	0.65	0.81
Purpose	0.63	0.66
Self-Acceptance	0.70	0.76
Total	0.80	0.86

$N = 74$; all p's $< .001$.

pleasantness dimension of emotions, and, therefore, reflect well-being more than the individual PANAS scales.

Table 5 represents the correlations of the Psychological Well-Being scale with two other related scales, Ryff's (2008) and Ryan and Deci's (2000). These scales provide yardsticks against which to assess the convergent validity of the shorter PWB. As can be seen, PWB correlated with the other scales moderately to strongly, except for the two Autonomy scales, which were more modestly associated with PWB.

Factor Structure of the Scales

Each of the scales was subjected to a principal axis factor analysis. For the SPANE-P of positive feelings, there was one eigenvalue above 1.0 (3.6), which explained 60% of the variance in the scale items. The factor scores ranged from 0.57 for Contented to 0.82 for Happy. For the SPANE-N scale of negative feelings, there was one eigenvalue above 1.0 (3.1), which explained 52% of the variance in the items. The factor scores varied from 0.49 for Afraid to 0.77 for Bad. For the SPANE-B score reflecting the balance of positive and negative feelings, the first factor was strong, accounting for 45% of the variance in responses.

However, for SPANE-B, a second factor emerged with an eigenvalue above 1.0 (1.4) and accounted for 12% additional variance in responses. An examination of the scree plot of eigenvalues also suggested a two-factor solution. The two rotated factors were correlated −0.54, with an oblimin rotation that did not restrict the factors to being orthogonal. The six positive items loaded 0.65 (Contented) to 0.84 (Happy) on the first factor, and −0.36 (Joyful) to −0.51 (Positive) on the second factor. The negative items loaded 0.61 (Afraid) to 0.80 (Bad) on the first factor, and −0.28 (Angry) to −0.53 (Negative) on the second factor. Thus, there were two separate factors for the valence of experience, although the two factors were inversely related. The greater independence of the PANAS positive and negative scales is due in part to their placement in the emotion circumplex in the high arousal quadrants. Furthermore, the time format of the SPANE is likely to lead to stronger inverse correlations between the two types of feelings (Diener & Emmons, 1985).

For the PWB, there was a single factor with an eigenvalue above 1.0 (4.0), which explained 50% of the variance in responses. The factor scores varied from 0.58 for feeling respected to 0.76 for leading a purposeful and meaningful life. Thus, a single and clear single factor described the PWB. The factor structure of the Positive Thinking Scale was less clear, possibly because of the single yes–no response format, or possibly there are many different facets of positive and negative thinking. It may be that the tendency to positive thinking is domain-specific rather than being universal across various areas of content.

Discussion

Psychological Well-Being Scale (PWB)

The brief PWB performed well, with high internal and temporal reliabilities and high convergence with other similar scales. Because of the brevity of the scale, its psychometric strength is slightly lower than the two other scales that assess PWB, but still quite good. The PWB correlated very strongly with the total scores for the other psychological well-being scales, at 0.80 and 0.69. Thus, the PWB provides a good assessment of overall self-reported psychological well-being, although it does not assess the individual components of psychological well-being that are described in some theories. It should be noted, however, that Ryff's (2008) scale has been criticized because the subscales do not clearly form six separate factors, but overlap with each other and produce fewer than six separate factors. The PWB seems to reflect the common elements of the other scales. If an overall psychological well-being score is needed, and a brief scale is desirable, the PWB should be adequate. If separate subscale scores are needed, one of the other two scales should be used.

The PWB scale predicts the total Ryff score even when the Deci/Ryan score is entered first. In terms of predicting measures of SWB, the scale picks up about 70–80% of the predictable variance compared to the longer Ryff scale. That is, the Ryff scale performs better in prediction, but the PWB scale does substantially as well. In conclusion, the PWB scale assesses a strong first factor that converges with the other scales.

Feelings Scale (SPANE)

The SPANE measure of feelings performed well in terms of reliability and convergent validity with other measures of emotion, well-being, happiness, and life satisfaction. The scale has several advantages over previous measures of feelings. For one thing, because of the general descriptors such as "positive" and "negative," it can assess all positive and negative feelings, not just those specific feelings that are listed on the scale. For another, it can reflect the fact that some feelings are considered desirable by some and less desirable by others because it reflects the respondent's own categorization of the pleasantness and desirability of the feelings. The scale should perform well across cultures because it is focused on the respondent's evaluations of their feelings, which can vary to some degree across cultures. Furthermore, the scale can reflect feelings such as physical pleasure, engagement, interest, pain, and boredom that are omitted from most measures of emotions. The scale also can reflect the full range of feelings, whether they are low or high in arousal. The SPANE is based on the duration during which people experience the feelings, with the advantage that this aspect of feelings predicts long-term well-being, and can also be better calibrated across respondents. Furthermore, the SPANE is based on feelings that occurred during the previous four weeks, and thus reflects a balance between memory accuracy and experience sampling. Thus, for measuring experiences that are related to well-being, the SPANE has a number of advantages over other measures. Although more research is needed on the scale, it should perform well in many contexts.

Positive Thinking Scale

Although this scale performed in an adequate way, with decent reliabilities and correlations with other measures of well-being, it is the scale in most need of further testing and development. Several questions are important. Might the measure perform better if responses were on a graded scale rather than simply being yes–no? Greater sampling of memories is needed, including both rumination and savoring, for example, and not just attention and interpretation. Another desirable future extension of the scale would be to include thoughts about nonsocial aspects of the world. An important question is whether the scale provides additional valid information beyond personality characteristics, such as neuroticism. Thus, the positive thinking scale shows initial promise but requires more psychometric work.

Future Research

The initial psychometric data we collected here are encouraging, but obviously more work is needed. All of the scales can use more validation in terms of correlations with other relevant scales, with non-self-report measures such as informant reports, and in various populations and cultural groups. We included only college student samples, and, therefore, broader participant samples are a high priority for future research. Another priority for future research is to examine how the new scales and existing scales differ and converge when comparing groups and cultures. Finally, an important question for this entire area of research is to determine the sources of unique and common variance in the scales. Across types of well-being there is substantial convergence of the scales, and the source of this overlap, as well as the unique contributions of the scales, is an important avenue for future research.

Permission for Using the Scales

Although copyrighted, the measures in this chapter may be used as long as proper credit is given. Permission is not needed to employ the scales and requests to use the scales cannot be answered because permission is granted here. This chapter can be used as the citation for the scales.

Appendix: The Scales

Scale of Positive and Negative Experience (SPANE)

© Copyright by Ed Diener and Robert Biswas-Diener, January 2009.

Please think about what you have been doing and experiencing during the past four weeks. Then report how much you experienced each of the following feelings, using the scale below. For each item, select a number from 1 to 5, and indicate that number on your response sheet.

1. Very Rarely or Never
2. Rarely
3. Sometimes
4. Often
5. Very Often or Always

> Positive
> Negative
> Good
> Bad
> Pleasant
> Unpleasant
> Happy
> Sad
> Afraid
> Joyful
> Angry
> Contented

Scoring: The measure can be used to derive an overall affect balance score, but can also be divided into positive and negative feelings scales, and can be divided even further into general and specific feelings.

Positive Feelings (SPANE-P): Add the scores, varying from 1 to 5, for the six items: positive, good, pleasant, happy, joyful, and contented. The score can vary from 6 (lowest possible) to 30 (highest positive feelings score).

Negative Feelings (SPANE-N): Add the scores, varying from 1 to 5, for the six items: negative, bad, unpleasant, sad, afraid, and angry. The score can vary from 6 (lowest possible) to 30 (highest negative feelings score).

Affect Balance (SPANE-B): The negative feelings score is subtracted from the positive feelings score, and the resultant difference can vary from -24 (unhappiest possible) to 24 (highest affect balance possible). A respondent with a very high score of 24 reports that she or he rarely or never has any of the negative feelings, and very often or always has all of the positive feelings.

Psychological Well-Being Scale (PWB)

© Copyright by Ed Diener and Robert Biswas-Diener, January 2009.

Below are 8 statements with which you may agree or disagree. Using the 1–7 scale below, indicate your agreement with each item by indicating that response for each statement.

7 Strongly agree
6 Agree
5 Slightly agree
4 Mixed or neither agree nor disagree
3 Slightly disagree
2 Disagree
1 Strongly disagree

    I lead a purposeful and meaningful life.
    My social relationships are supportive and rewarding.
    I am engaged and interested in my daily activities
    I actively contribute to the happiness and well-being of others
    I am competent and capable in the activities that are important to me
    I am a good person and live a good life
    I am optimistic about my future
    People respect me

Scoring: Add the responses, varying from 1 to 7, for all eight items. The possible range of scores is from 8 (lowest possible) to 56 (highest PWB possible). A high score represents a person with many psychological resources and strengths.

Positive Thinking Scale (PTS)

The following items are to be answered "Yes" or "No." Write an answer next to each item to indicate your response.

    I see my community as a place full of problems. (N)
    I see much beauty around me. (P)
    I see the good in most people. (P)
    When I think of myself, I think of many shortcomings. (N)
    I think of myself as a person with many strengths. (P)

I am optimistic about my future. (P)

When somebody does something for me, I usually wonder if they have an ulterior motive. (N)

When something bad happens, I often see a "silver lining," something good in the bad event. (P)

I sometimes think about how fortunate I have been in life. (P)

When good things happen, I wonder if they might have been even better. (N)

I frequently compare myself to others. (N)

I think frequently about opportunities that I missed. (N)

When I think of the past, the happy times are most salient to me. (P)

I savor memories of pleasant past times. (P)

I regret many things from my past. (N)

When I see others prosper, even strangers, I am happy for them. (P)

When I think of the past, for some reason the bad things stand out. (N)

I know the word has problems, but it seems like a wonderful place anyway. (P)

When something bad happens, I ruminate on it for a long time. (N)

When good things happen, I wonder if they will soon turn sour. (N)

When I see others prosper, it makes me feel bad about myself. (N)

I believe in the good qualities of other people. (P)

Scoring: Add a "1" for each of the "yes" responses to the 11 positive items, indicated by a (P). Add a "1" for each of the "no" responses to each of the negative responses (N). The (N) and (P) designations appear here for scoring purposes only, but should not be presented in the scales given to respondents.

The possible range of scores is 0 (most negative thinking) to 22 (most positive thinking). A high score indicates that the respondent sees much that is positive in the world and himself or herself, and in other people. A high score thus represents a tendency to think in positive ways and to not think in negative ways.

References

Beck, A. T., Rush, A. J., Shaw, B. F., & Emery, G. (1979). *Cognitive therapy of depression.* New York: Guilford Press.

Brown, S. L., Nesse, R. M., Vinokur, A. D., & Smith, D. M. (2003). Providing support may be more beneficial than receiving it: Results from a prospective study of mortality. *Psychological Science, 14,* 320–327.

Csikszentmihalyi, M. (1990). *Flow: The psychology of optimal experience.* New York: Harper & Row.

Diener, E., & Biswas-Diener, R. (2008). *Happiness: Unlocking the mysteries of psychological wealth.* Malden, MA: Blackwell Publishing.

Diener, E., Colvin, C. R., Pavot, W. G., & Allman, A. (1991). The psychic costs of intense positive affect. *Journal of Personality & Social Psychology, 61,* 492–503.

Diener, E., & Emmons, R. A. (1985). The independence of positive and negative affect. *Journal of Personality and Social Psychology, 47,* 1105–1117.

Diener, E., Emmons, R. A., Larsen, R. J., & Griffin, S. (1985). The satisfaction with life scale. *Journal of Personality Assessment, 49,* 71–75.

Diener, E., Sandvik, E., & Pavot, W. (1991). Happiness is the frequency, not the intensity, of positive versus negative affect. In F. Strack, M. Argyle, & N. Schwarz (Eds.), *Subjective well-being: An interdisciplinary perspective* (pp. 119–139). New York: Pergamon.

Ellis, A. (2001). *Overcoming destructive beliefs, feelings, and behaviors: New directions for rational emotive behavior therapy.* New York: Prometheus Books.

Fordyce, M. W. (1988). A review of research on happiness measures: a sixty second index of happiness and mental health. *Social Indicators Research, 20,* 355–381.

Judge, T. A., & Bretz, R. D. (1993). Report on an alternative measure of affective disposition. *Educational and Psychological Measurement, 53,* 1095–1104.

Kitayama, S., Markus, H. R., & Kurosawa, M. (2000). Culture, emotion, and well-being: Good feelings in Japan and the United States. *Cognition & Emotion, 14,* 93–124.

Larsen, R. J., & Diener, E. (1992). Promises and problems with the circumplex model of emotion. In M. S. Clark (Ed.), *Emotion: Review of personality and social psychology* (pp. 25–59). Newbury Park, CA: Sage.

Lazarus, R. S. (1982). Thoughts on the relations between emotion and cognition. *American Psychologist, 37,* 1019–1024.

Lucas, R. E., Diener, E., & Larsen, R. J. (2003). Measuring positive emotions. In S. J. Lopez & C. R. Snyder (Eds.), *Positive psychological assessment: A handbook of models and measures* (pp. 201–218). Washington, DC: American Psychological Association.

Lucas, R. E., Diener, E., & Suh, E. (1996). Discriminant validity of well-being measures. *Journal of Personality and Social Psychology, 71,* 616–628.

Lyubomirsky, S., & Lepper, H. S. (1999). A measure of subjective happiness: Preliminary reliability and construct validation. *Social Indicators Research, 46,* 137–155.

Maslow, A. H. (1958). *Motivation and personality.* New York: Harper & Brothers.

Meichenbaum, D. (1977). *Cognitive behavior modification: An integrative approach.* New York: Plenum Press.

Oishi, S. (2007). The application of structural equation modeling and item response theory to cross-cultural positive psychology research. In A. Ong, & M. van Dulmen (Eds.), *Oxford handbook of methods in positive psychology* (pp. 126–138). New York: Oxford University Press.

Oishi, S., Schimmack, U., & Colcombe, S. (2003). The contextual and systematic nature of life satisfaction judgments. *Journal of Experimental Social Psychology, 39,* 232–247.

Pavot, W., & Diener, E. (1993). Review of the satisfaction with life scale. *Psychological Assessment, 5,* 164–172.

Pavot, W., & Diener, E. (2008). The satisfaction with life scale and the emerging construct of life satisfaction. *Journal of Positive Psychology, 3,* 137–152.

Peale, N. V. (1956). *The power of positive thinking.* New York: Prentice Hall.

Peterson, C., & Seligman, M. E. P. (2004). *Character strengths and virtues.* Oxford: Oxford University Press.

Russell, D. W. (1996). UCLA loneliness scale (version 3): Reliability, validity, and factor structure. *Journal of Personality Assessment, 66,* 20–40.

Ryan, R. M., & Deci, E. L. (2000). Self-determination theory and the facilitation of intrinsic motivation, social development, and well-being. *American Psychologist, 55,* 68–78.

Ryan, R. M., & Deci, E. L. (2001). On happiness and human potentials: A review of research on hedonic and eudaimonic well-being. *Annual Review of Psychology, 52,* 141–166.

Ryff, C. D. (1989). Happiness is everything, or is it? Explorations on the meaning of psychological well-being. *Journal of Personality and Social Psychology, 57,* 1069–1081.

Ryff, C. D. (2008). *Scales of psychological well-being.* Obtained from Carol Ryff, University of Wisconsin, Institute on Aging.

Scollon, C. N., Diener, E., Oishi, S., & Biswas-Diener, R. (2004). Emotions across cultures and methods. *Journal of Cross-Cultural Psychology, 35,* 304–326.

Scheier, M. F., Carver, C. S., & Bridges, M. W. (1994). Distinguishing optimism from neuroticism (and trait anxiety, self-mastery, and self-esteem): A reevaluation of the Life Orientation Test. *Journal of Personality and Social Psychology, 67,* 1063–1078.

Schimmack, U. (2003). Affect measurement in experience sampling research.*Journal of Happiness Studies, 4,* 79–106.

Schimmack, U., Oishi, S., Furr, F. M., & Funder, D. C. (2004). Personality and life satisfaction: A facet level analysis. *Personality and Social Psychology Bulletin, 30,* 1062–1075.

Seligman, M. E. P. (2002). *Authentic happiness: Using the new positive psychology to realize your potential for lasting fulfillment.* New York: Free Press.

Tsai, J. L., Knutson, B., & Fund, H. H. (2006). Cultural variation in affect valuation. *Journal of Personality and Social Psychology, 90,* 288–307.

Tsai, J. L., Miao, F., & Seppala, E. (2007). Good feelings in Christianity and Buddhism: Religious differences in ideal affect. *Personality and Social Psychology Bulletin, 33,* 409–421.

Watson, D., & Clark, L. A. (1994). *PANAS-X. Manual for the positive and negative affect schedule-expanded form.* Iowa City, IA: The University of Iowa.

Watson, D., Clark, L. A., & Tellegen, A. (1988). Development and validation of brief measures of positive and negative affect: The PANAS scales. *Journal of Personality and Social Psychology, 54,* 1063–1070.

Conclusion: Future Directions in Measuring Well-Being

Ed Diener

What We Have Learned So Far

The studies in the present volume point to several facts that we have learned about defining and measuring well-being. First, we know with a degree of certainty that there are separable components of well-being, such as life judgments versus positive emotions, and we know some of the factors that are more likely to be more associated with certain components versus others. Lucas, Diener, and Suh (1996) showed clearly in a multi-trait multi-method study that several types of well-being are discriminable, and the Diener, Kahneman, et al. chapter in this volume shows that these types of well-being are sometimes predicted by very different factors.

Second, we know that the self-report measures of well-being have a degree of validity—they converge in expected ways with each other and with non-self-report measures, and they are associated in understandable ways with predictors. At the same time, there are certain artifacts or biases in the measures, although these appear in many instances to have small effects. Nonetheless, these effects are sufficiently large to produce significant differences between groups in some instances. A problem is that unless we assess or control the artifacts, we often cannot be certain whether the differences we find in well-being are substantive or due in part to the artifacts. Conversely, we must be careful in controlling "artifacts" that might have substantive implications for well-being. We know that the measures are valid across nations, although there are effects reviewed in Volume 38 that influence the interpretations we make of cultural differences.

Besides the survey self-report measures of well-being, we have gained knowledge of some alternative measures that ought more frequently to be used in conjunction with the self-report scales. For example, the Experience Sampling Method (ESM) and its relatives, such as the Daily Reconstruction Method (DRM; Kahneman, Krueger, Schkade, Schwarz, & Stone, 2004), should be used in many more studies to obtain more accurate assessments of people's feelings, and to gain measures of their feelings within specific situations and activities. Informant reports of well-being from a participant's family and friends (see Schneider & Schimmack, 2008) should also be used more frequently.

When the other types of measures besides one-tone self-report measures yield conclusions that converge with the self-report survey measures, we will have greater confidence in the findings. When the conclusions from different measures diverge, we will have learned something perhaps even more important and will gain deeper insight into the nature of well-being and its causes. A major goal for the decade ahead is to understand why different factors are differentially associated with the various forms of well-being. There are other possible measurement methods (see Sandvik, Diener, & Seidlitz, 1993; Lucas, Diener, & Larsen, 2003) for assessing well-being that have been created, but so far have not been thoroughly tested and developed. These methods hold promise, but they need more exploration, and this is an important area of future study for aspiring researchers. For example, we created measures of happiness based on the good and bad events people can recall from their lives in a timed period and (Robinson & Kirkeby,2005; Robinson & Compton, 2007) have invented reaction time measures to assess well-being.

Kim (Kim, 2004; Jang & Kim, in press) created an implicit Association Test (IAT) approach to assessing life satisfaction. The implicit approach seeks through a reaction-time task to map positive and negative associations in people's minds. For life satisfaction, the method assesses the degree to which negative versus positive things are associated with a person's life. Each of these alternative methods shows promise, but they need much more development and testing. We will have a much stronger basis for scientific understanding when we have conclusions from different types of measures examining different theoretical questions.

Another domain where we have made progress but need much more work is on the cognitive processes related to our measures. For example, we know from the work of Ulrich Schimmack the types of information that people seem to call on when they make life satisfaction judgments. We know some things about how people misremember their moods and how this affects their future behavior (Thomas & Diener, 1990; Wirtz, Kruger, Scollon, & Diener, 2003; Oishi et al., 2007). From the creative work of Michael Robinson (Robinson & Kirkeby, 2005; Robinson & Compton, 2007) and his colleagues we understand that cognitive structures in the memory networks of happy and unhappy people differ. Robinson explores these structures through reaction-time studies and other laboratory approaches and finds that happy and unhappy people respond differently to positive and negative stimuli, helping to explain some of the underlying psychological processes that are related to people's responses to the measures. From the work of Norbert Schwarz and Fritz Strack (1999), we understand how situational factors can sometimes influence self-reports of well-being. Thus, we have initial knowledge of the psychological processes affecting some of the measures, but we do not yet have a complete and thorough theoretical model of these factors.

In sum, we have made much progress, but have much farther to go. We know that many of the measures have a degree of validity, even the simplest self-report surveys, and we understand some of the underlying psychological processes involved in the measures. What we need now is a concerted effort to further understand the measures and when they perform well and poorly.

Methodological Issues Beyond Measurement

In this volume I focused on measurement, but there are additional critical methodological issues. After all, even if we measure well-being well, we may not understand the processes leading to it. A major issue is causality. The majority of the
studies in this field, virtually all, are conducted using cross-sectional correlational
designs. Because of this tendency, we usually do not know whether the correlates
we discover of well-being are causes of well-being, results of well-being, or that
they both result from some common third variable such as personality. Until we
begin understanding more about causality, we will not understand the true structures
underlying what we study.

Several methodologies can help us discern the causal structures associated with
well-being. First, we can use experiments and quasi-experiments. Experimental
interventions to change happiness or positive thinking, for example with control
groups, are a way to help explore the causes of well-being. In laboratory studies, people's moods or thoughts can be manipulated to determine the short-range
influence of the manipulated variable. Quasi-experiments can examine the effects
of natural events, such as a devastating earthquake, on people's well-being in an
affected area and a similar area elsewhere. If there were measures of well-being
collected before the earthquake, the before–after design is a quasi-experiment that
gives clues about causality. Similarly, longitudinal designs can help to discern
the direction of influence and to rule out certain causal paths. When experience-
sampling is used over time in people's lives, the time-course of daily events and
daily well-being can be studied and help estimate the direction of causal influence.
No design, even experimentation, is ever definitive in a single study. However, all
of these designs should be used much more often to help describe the structures
leading to well-being, and also to explore how feelings of well-being affect other
behaviors.

One issue that has not been stressed enough thus far is the same-source overlap in the measures between predictors and the well-being outcome measures.
Often a person reports her or his well-being and then reports her or his feelings about other variables, such as work or health. Such designs allow for the
exploration of interesting issues, but the interpretation of the findings is often
clouded by the fact that some third variable such as personality could influence
both measured variables with no direct connection between them. Furthermore,
there could be a "top–down" influence of general well-being on feelings in the
more specific area, rather than vice-versa, or both directions of influence might
hold. Even worse, method variance, such as the person's propensity to avoid the
extremes of scales, could influence both measured variables. In other words, when
two variables are measured by the same method, higher correlations are often the
result, but the interpretation of the association is difficult. Thus, when variables
can be measured by different methods, and when one is more objective and the
well-being variable is more subjective, the interpretation of findings is usually
clearer.

What We Do Not Need

The discussion above should make clear the types of studies that we need fewer of, and the types which are currently under-represented in our literature. We will not profit that much from most cross-sectional studies on samples of convenience such as college students when all of the measured variables are based on self-report, especially when the variables primarily represent subjective assessments and feelings. Even when a "new" variable is measured, it is often "old wine in new bottles" in the sense that the new variable correlates highly with others that have been assessed in the past. Much effort is expended conducting cross-sectional studies where well-being is correlated with other variables that represent the way the person sees himself or herself. Early in the history of research in this area, these studies provided new insights; they are now largely redundant in most instances. These types of studies are conducted in part because they are much easier than longitudinal, experience sampling, and other methods that require more time but can produce more definitive conclusions. It is time to move to more demanding methods, however, which can more rigorously explore the phenomena that are central to quality of life. There are so many very important questions that are still unanswered that we cannot afford to continue studies that add little to what we already know and are merely "science fair" projects that demonstrate what is already known.

One type of study that has nearly reached its maximum payoff is the analysis of the association of well-being with demographic characteristics such as age, income, sex, and education. A few excellent studies are still being conducted in these areas, for example Deaton's (2008) study of age and well-being around the globe. The findings are informative in that the trends vary systematically across nations, with well-being decreasing with age in the former Soviet bloc nations, and showing a curvilinear pattern in many European countries. Similarly, the data on income and well-being in the chapters presented in Diener, Kahneman, and Helliwell (2009) reveal that progress is being made in our understanding of the effects of money, primarily because many of the studies presented there rely on longitudinal data from around the globe. That is, the studies are able to add to what has gone before because they use much better samples and designs. In many cases, however, the added knowledge gained from simple cross-sectional correlational studies of the association of demographic factors and well-being add little to what is already known. When multi-method measurement and longitudinal designs are used, these studies can sometimes prove worthwhile. One factor that can give this research added-value is the inclusion of mediational variables in the design that help explain why the predictor is related to the well-being outcome.

What We Need Now

As mentioned above, we need more studies designed to explore causality, and we need more studies in which different types of well-being are measured, and with different methods. When we begin to understand which findings replicate across types of well-being and different measurement methods, and which show divergent patterns across methods or types, we will begin to much more fully understand what well-being is in a scientific way, as well as its boundaries and causes. For example, when Oishi et al. (2007) found that Asians and European-Americans had similar emotions when monitored on-line, but different emotions when they were asked to recall their week, this was extremely informative in terms of understanding the well-being experienced by the two groups. If this finding replicates, it can explain a lot about why Europeans often report higher well-being than Asians. The divergence between the on-line and memory measures need not be viewed simply as a disappointing failure of convergent validity. It was an important finding that could help advance theory, and probably more important in this regard than if the measures had converged.

Another example is when informant and self-reports diverge and converge. Schneider and Schimmack (2008) found that in general the two methods of measuring well-being correlated 0.42 across 81 studies they reviewed. The correlations across studies varied, however, from 0.06 to 0.66. Schneider and Schimmack found that studies with multiple informants, and those using multi-item well-being scales, produced higher correlations than research using single-item measures and single informants. In addition, the agreement between self- and informant-reports was greater for older participants. For older participants in studies where multiple informants and multi-item scales were used, agreement was 0.49. What will be interesting is to understand why different levels of convergence are reached, and thus to better understand the psychological processes underlying each type of measure.

We also need more studies in which both objective and subjective measures of the same predictors are obtained. Take income as an example—we can measure people's objective income as reported by their employer or tax return, their self-report of income, their perceived income relative to others, and their income satisfaction—and relate all of these to well-being. When we examine the differences between objective income, perceived income, and income satisfaction, and how they relate to well-being, we can build a model of the psychological processes leading to well-being. If we include personality and other moderator variables, we have the potential to gain an even deeper theoretical understanding. We should not be in the business of having subjective and objective indicators compete with one another to see which is larger—the subjective predictor will usually be larger because it is closer in the causal chain to well-being. Instead, we need to determine how the objective world is filtered by the person's perceptions, for this type of modeling of both objective and subjective predictors can be quite helpful.

Another interesting issue is the relation between psychological well-being and subjective well-being. Ryff and Keyes (1995) and Ryan and Deci (2000) both proposed theories of psychological well-being or effective functioning, which differ from people's feelings of well-being even though the two are related. The two types of well-being can be distinguished conceptually, although Kashdan, Biswas-Diener, and King (2008) suggest that some of the distinction has been overdrawn. Certainly, some processes that affect responding, such as positivity, will influence people's scores on measures of both PWB and SWB. What is sorely needed is a careful examination of the ways in which the two types of well-being converge and diverge, and measurement is an essential feature of examining this. Methods such as multi-method multi-trait are important in this endeavor because they can help delineate which of the differences between PWB and SWB are superficial, due to self-labeling tendencies for example, and which are deeper and refer to core psychological characteristics. Again, measurement is not merely a technical nicety here; a deep theoretical understanding of measures is needed in order to understand the differences between the concepts.

A final important area for measurement studies is the examination of the influence of artifacts or measurement biases. However, the idea that measurement is merely a technical exercise will interfere with true advances in this area because researchers will not understand that many, or most, "artifacts" are not simply measurement mistakes, but are related to true underlying phenomena that are relevant to well-being. For instance, "social desirability" was once thought to be merely responding to scales in such a way as to make oneself look better, but it is now widely appreciated that it is a deeper personality factor (e.g., Carstensen & Cone, 1983; McCrae & Costa, 1983) that is related to psychological processes and outcomes, including well-being. People who score high on social desirability scales might be, for example, more eager to please others, and this could be related to well-being.

Another example of how an "artifact" might actually be a substantive response tendency comes from the way people use number scales. For instance, Asians might avoid the extremes of scales more than Europeans, not wanting to appear unusual or extreme, and use the midpoints of the scales more. This tendency, however, might be related to how Asians view and approach the world and could conceivably influence the way they experience well-being. Thus, the issue of artifacts is deeper than the notion of response errors that need to be corrected. What we do need are analyses of the way response tendencies, including those called "artifacts," are related to actual psychological phenomena.

A final example of research needed in this area comes from norms for emotions. People in different cultures differ in terms of what emotions they believe are most desirable and least desirable (Diener & Tov, 2007; Eid & Diener, 2001). People report experiencing more of the emotions they value and less of the emotions they devalue. However, the reason for this association is unclear. It could merely be an "artifact" of people reporting their experiences in a socially desirable way that reflects the values of their culture. In contrast, it could be because the emotions that are valued are socialized in people in that culture (Tsai, Louie, Chen, & Uchida, 2007), and they do actually experience the valued emotions more. Just because reporting could be due to an "artifact" does not mean that it is, or that the "artifact" has no actual psychological consequences. If multiple types of measures of well-being are collected, there is a greater probability of understanding the structure, causes, and consequences of well-being.

Conclusions

Despite the low esteem often accorded in scientific articles to measurement, it is, in fact, a core element of understanding, and involves not only technical skills such as knowledge of measurement statistics, but also a deep theoretical understanding of the psychological processes involved in the phenomenon being measured. Measuring well-being well is ultimately equivalent to understanding well-being, although many do not seem to understand this connection. Much more research is needed on the development and validation of measures, including non-self-report measures. However, the use of the alternative measures in addition to self-report can often be very helpful in current studies. As our measurement gains in sophistication, so will our scientific understanding.

References

Carstensen, L. L., & Cone, J. D. (1983). Social desirability and the measurement of psychological well-being in elderly persons. *Journal of Gerontology, 38*, 713–715.

Deaton, A. (2008). Income, health, and well-being around the world: Evidence from the Gallup World Poll. *Journal of Economic Perspectives, 22*, 53–72.

Diener, E., Kahneman, D., & Helliwell, J. (Eds.). (2009). *International comparisons of well-being.* Oxford, UK: Oxford University Press.

Diener, E., & Tov, W. (2007). Culture and subjective well-being. In S. Kitayama & D. Cohen (Eds.), *Handbook of cultural psychology* (pp. 691–713). New York: Guilford.

Eid, M., & Diener, E. (2001). Norms for experiencing emotions in different cultures: Inter- and intra-national differences. *Journal of Personality and Social Psychology, 81*, 869–885.

Jang, D., & Kim, D.-Y. (in press). Two faces of human happiness: Explicit and implicit life satisfaction. *Asian Journal of Social Psychology.*

Kahneman, D., Krueger, A. B., Schkade, D. A., Schwarz, N., & Stone, A. A. (2004). A survey method for characterizing daily life experience: The day reconstruction method. *Science, 306*, 1776–1780.

Kashdan, T. B., Biswas-Diener, R., & King, L. A. (2008). Reconsidering happiness: The costs of distinguishing between hedonics and eudaimonia. *Journal of Positive Psychology, 3*, 219–233.

Kim, D. (2004). The implicit life satisfaction measure. *Asian Journal of Social Psychology, 7*, 236–262.

Lucas, R. E., Diener, E., & Larsen, R. J. (2003). Measuring positive emotions. In S. J. Lopez & C. R. Snyder (Eds.), *Positive psychological assessment: A handbook of models and measures* (pp. 201–218). Washington, DC: American Psychological Association.

Lucas, R. E., Diener, E., & Suh, E. (1996). Discriminant validity of well-being measures. *Journal of Personality and Social Psychology, 71*, 616–628.

McCrae, R. R., & Costa, P. T. (1983). Social desirability scales: More substance than style. *Journal of Consulting and Clinical Psychology, 51*, 882–888.

Oishi, S., Schimmack, U., Diener, E., Kim-Prieto, C., Scollon, C. N., & Choi, D. (2007). The value-congruence model of memory for emotional experiences: An explanation for cultural and individual differences in emotional self-reports. *Journal of Personality and Social Psychology, 93*, 897–905.

Robinson, M. D., & Compton, R. J. (2007). The happy mind in action: The cognitive basis of subjective well-being. In M. Eid & R. J. Larsen (Eds.), *The science of subjective well-being* (pp. 220–238). New York: Guilford Press.

Robinson, M. D., & Kirkeby, B. S. (2005). Happiness as a belief system: Individual differences and priming in emotion judgments. *Personality and Social Psychology Bulletin, 31*, 1134–1144.

Ryan, R. M., & Deci, E. L. (2000). Self-determination theory and the facilitation of intrinsic motivation, social development, and well-being. *American Psychologist, 55*, 68–78.

Ryff, C., & Keyes, C. (1995). The structure of psychological well-being revisited. *Journal of Personality and Social Psychology, 69*, 719–727.

Sandvik, E., Diener, E., & Seidlitz, L. (1993). Subjective well-being: The convergence and stability of self-report and non-self-report measures. *Journal of Personality, 61*, 317–342.

Schneider, L., & Schimmack, U. (2008). *Self-informant agreement in well-being ratings: A meta-analysis.* Study submitted for publication, University of Toronto, Mississauga.

Schwarz, N., & Strack, F. (1999). Reports of subjective well-being: Judgmental processes and their methodological implications. In D. Kahneman, E. Diener, & N. Schwarz (Eds.), *Well-being: The foundations of hedonic psychology* (pp. 61–84). New York: Russell Sage Foundation.

Thomas, D. L., & Diener, E. (1990). Memory accuracy in the recall of emotions. *Journal of Personality and Social Psychology, 59*, 291–297.

Tsai, J. L., Louie, J. Y., Chen, E. E., & Uchida, Y. (2007). Learning what feelings to desire: Socialization of ideal affect through children's storybooks. *Personality and Social Psychology Bulletin, 33*, 17–30.

Wirtz, D., Kruger, J., Scollon, C. N., & Diener, E. (2003). What to do on spring break? The role of predicted, on-line, and remembered experience in future choice. *Psychological Science, 14*, 520–524.

CPSIA information can be obtained at www.ICGtesting.com
Printed in the USA
LVOW070058030713

341301LV00002B/51/P